MENTAL HEALTH
Psycho-Social Perspectives

VOLUME FOUR: Therapeutic Applications

The details of the volumes: Mental Health

Volume 1: Issues and Interventions

Volume 2: Multigroup Analysis

Volume 3: Strength of Human Resources

Volume 4: Therapeutic Applications

About the Editors

Anubhuti Dubey is Associate Professor of Psychology in Department of Psychology, DDU Gorakhpur University, Gorakhpur. Her research interest includes Health Psychology, Applied Social Psychology, Gender and Health and Counselling. She had published a book entitled "Psychological Perspectives on Chronic Illness". She had also completed a research project sponsored by ICSSR on "Psychological Dynamics of Health and Illness in Women of Eastern Uttar Pradesh." She had published 25 research papers in journals of national and international repute and also contributed 11 chapters in different edited volumes. Four students had been awarded their Ph.D. thesis under her supervision. She had received university gold medals at under-graduate and post-graduate levels. She is also a Master Trainer and Supportive Supervisor for Training HIV/AIDS counsellors under GFATM-Round 7 programmes.

Aradhana Shukla is Professor and former Head, Department of Psychology, Kumaun University Campus, Almora, Uttarakhand. Currently, she is Campus Dean (Arts) at Kumaun University Campus, Almora. She has served in Department of Pediatrics of Banaras Hindu University, Post Doctoral fellow (U.G.C.) at University of Gorakhpur and has been serving here for last 27 years. She has published 100 research papers of national and international repute, ten books in which nine are published by national agencies and one from Germany (LAP). She has carried out 4 major projects from ICSSR and UGC and co-worked in UNICEF and GFATM-round 7 projects. She has guided 45 Ph.D. students and prepared 26 psychological tests. Moreover, she has attended 40 seminars of national and international repute and organized 4 seminars in her department. Her major thrust areas are: developmental psychology, personality psychology, cultural psychology, environmental psychology and mental health care system.

MENTAL HEALTH
Psycho-Social Perspectives

Volume Four
Therapeutic Applications

Edited by
Anubhuti Dubey
Aradhana Shukla

CONCEPT PUBLISHING COMPANY PVT. LTD.
NEW DELHI-110059

ISBN-13: 978-93-5125-173-6 (Series)
ISBN-13: 978-93-5125-172-9 (Vol. IV)

First Published 2017

Published and Printed by

Concept
Since 1974

Concept Publishing Company Pvt. Ltd.
Regd. Office:
A/15-16, Commercial Block, Mohan Garden,
New Delhi-110059 (INDIA)
Phones : 25351460, 25351794, *Fax* : 091-11-25357109
E-mail : publishing@conceptpub.com
Website: www.conceptpub.com

Editorial Office: H-13, Bali Nagar, New Delhi-110 015, India.

Cataloging in Publication Data—DK Courtesy: D.K. Agencies (P) Ltd. <docinfo@dkagencies.com>

Mental health : psycho-social perspectives / edited by Aradhana Shukla, Anubhuti Dubey.
pages cm
Contributed articles.
Includes bibliographical references and index.
Contents: volume three. Strength of human resources — volume four. Therapeutic applications
ISBN 9789351251712 (vol. III)
ISBN 9789351251729 (vol. IV)
ISBN 9789351251736 (series)

1. Mental health—Social aspects—India. 2. Mental health—India. I. Shukla, Aradhana, editor. II. Dubey, Anubhuti, editor.

RA790.7.I5M46 2017 DDC 362.20954 23

Preface

We desire to live a healthy and happy life. It is a common and well accepted fact that everyone desires to live a healthy life. The mind and bodily functions are closely embedded hence, the relative significance of mental health along with physical wellness cannot be denied. As mind and bodily functions are closely embedded we cannot deny the relative significances of mental health along with physical wellness. Mental health is an integral part of health, mental health is more than the absence of mental illness, and mental health is intimately connected with physical health and behaviour. Mental health is the foundation for well-being and effective functioning for an individual and for a community. Good mental health is a sense of well-being, confidence and self-esteem. It enables us to fully enjoy and appreciate other people, day-to-day life and our environment.

Mental health is the sheer responsibility of a person himself. The mental health field aims to deal with (1) mentally ill people, (2) people at risk, and (3) promoting mental health of normal people so that their normality can be sustained.

If we go back into the history of mental health we can see that it was treated either as "boon of God" (good or positive mental health) or "curse of God" bad or negative mental health). Both the eastern and western evidences support the notion. Not only in abroad but our ancient evidences also support this notion. The Western literatures on mental health were seen hallucinations as communication of humans with bad souls, ghosts and witches. Moreover, in the ancient Indian literature of Ayurveda, Mental disorders are represented as various forms. The aetio-genesis of these disorders was thought to be endogenous because of provoked humours like *Vata*, *Pitta* and *Kapha*. Exogenously the causes were attributed to sudden fear or association with ill influence of certain mythological gods or demon. *Charaka Samhita* listed Psychiatry as *'Bhuta Vidya'*. Psychotherapy was known as *Ilaj-I-Nafsani* in Unani Medicine. But time never remains stable. Years and years were passed and the outlook of people towards mentally ill people become more and more aversive and they were treated like an undesirable social being for whom only such behaviour was required that was only meant for animals or criminals. Even with the advent of modern scientific methods and practical thoughts, the stigma and discrimination against mentally illnesses prevail the society. However, the advocates of Psychology started a touch and healing approach for the mentally ill people. Again it took decades to develop behaviour and psycho-therapies against tying mentally ill people with iron chain, and treat them like prisoners. A complete soft and medico-human environment under single roof was constructed for them and it was termed as asylum or mental hospital. Psychologists attempted such patients to get out from the boundaries and from the trap of *ojhas, neem-haquims* and other such traditional healers and placed them at asylum. The patients were properly medicated along with different psychotherapies and many of them got complete recovery. At first, the asylums were established in abroad but in India the first asylum was established in 1787 by Surgeon Kenderline in Calcutta and thereafter many asylums were made. This period was relatively longer but it opened the doors of a new era for the support and care of mental ill-health. They not only paid attention to treat the mentally ill people but also concentrated on maintaining and nurturing public health, and trying to eradicate the stigma and discrimination faced by people with mental disorders. Psychologists and mental health care professionals are still trying to launch innovative programmes for the same. The focal theme of these developmental programmes are the utilization of community resources for mental health care. These programmes have given new vision to the mental health care professionals to prevent mental disorders and promote mental health. This also needs a greater role for the non-medical mental health care professionals and better utilization of cultural resources in terms of belief, practice and important social institutions like family and community groups. The contemporary world's realization about mental health and mental illness has come to a point where we find passionate discussions and caring mental health professionals to deal with mental disorder and promote well-being.

Keeping these views into consideration, the innovative thought of this series appeared in our mind and we decided to pool the thoughts of psychologists and healthcare professionals regarding various concerns of mental health. The basic aim of this series was: (i) to bring concepts, issues, strengths and treatment in a single jacket; (ii) bring a sense of mental health awareness in people so that they can make their health safe with additional attention on social health; (iii) to carve the research competence in young researchers; and (iv) to put forth the mental health policies before the readers, so that a better understanding of mental health can be developed.

About the series Mental Health: Psycho-Social Perspectives

It is a series on the psychology of mental health and we have tried to cover as many areas as possible and we could justify its name, i.e. rethinking. Many traditional notions of mental health have been reconceptualised and many concepts in a new framework have been introduced. Initially we planned to bring out only four volumes in this series, as detailed below:

1. ***Mental Health: Psychological Issues and Interventions:*** In this volume we have covered various issues that foster or hamper mental health. Also, strategies to minimize negative mental health and improve positive mental health are discussed.
2. ***Mental Health: Multigroup Analysis:*** This volume covers the conceptual background and psycho-social perspective of mental health in various social settings.
3. ***Mental Health: Strength of Human Resources:*** In this volume we have tried to throw light on the promotional strategies of mental health following which a person can be relieved from negative mental health.
4. ***Mental Health: Therapeutic Applications:*** This volume covers a range of behavioural therapies which were found effective to minimize or overcome mental ill health.

The first two volumes, after publication, were well received among the scholars and students. Just afterwards we started receiving encouraging responses from the intellectuals and the research scholars to continue this series. Now, we have decided to make this project "an ongoing series" and we invite the academic world to contribute their words of knowledge to share with the next generation.

We have exercised our best attempt to seek out as many experiences as possible and we also anticipate that this will open new foresight for the researchers. However, we will be highly blessed to obtain the healthy and critical comments from our colleagues, seniors and friends and we will appreciate them from the bottom of our hearts.

Anubhuti Dubey
Aradhana Shukla

Acknowledgements

We, the editors, feel immense pleasure to present our series on mental health before the august readers. We hope that it will be admired by you all and the comments will be highly appreciated.

We feel our deep sense of gratitude and thankfulness to our respected contributors. It was only their support that the volumes came in the shape. We are thankful to Mr. Abhishek and Mr. Pankaj Tewari for computer task.

Last but not least, we are thankful to Mr. Ashok Mittal, M/s. Concept Publishing Company Pvt. Ltd., New Delhi to shape our dreams in concrete form.

15 January, 2016
Makar Sankranti

Anubhuti Dubey
Aradhana Shukla

Acknowledgments

Contents

Introduction

Anubhuti Dubey and *Aradhana Shukla*

Mental health problems in India are more rampant than collectively the cancer and heart diseases. And, the robust markers suggest that mental healthcare in the country is not good. Regardless of the excessive prevalence of mental disorders, more than 80 per cent of people enduring any form mental disorders are not receiving appropriate treatment in the existing healthcare system. The key explanations for this massive treatment gap—the disparity between the number of persons have need of treatment and number of persons who actually be given treatment—are the scarcity of mental health professionals including clinical psychologists and psychological counsellors, stigma associated with seeking treatment from mental health professionals, limited mental- health facilities and the high cost of treatment. These untreated cases are not only a great liability on the family and society, but also these untreated mental disorders lead to many other complications too. The penalty of untreated mental disorders incorporates homelessness, incarceration and exploitation.

Indian Lunacy Act, 1912 was the governing mental health in India till the Independence. It was revoked with the Mental Health Act (MHA) in 1987 so as to walk along with the advances in psychopathology and psychopharmacology. A number of constructive modifications in the MHA, 1987 integrated a more humane approach to problems of the mentally ill by substituting the terminology like, lunatics and criminal lunatics by the term mentally ill person and mentally ill prisoner. The new provisions on management of their property and protection of human rights were included, as well as, the Central and State Mental Health Authorities were formed for protection the interests of the mentally ill person under one authority and the procedure for admission and discharge of voluntary patients was make simpler and straightforward.

However, over the period of time, the voices from different corners started coming out that India again need clear mental health policy to cater the needs of those affected and their caregivers as well as the demands of mental health professionals. Moreover, in order to comply with United Nations Conventions on Rights of Persons with Disability (UNCRPD), the Government of India, in 2013, decided to make amendments in the MHA. During the process of amendments, the government become conscious that the existing act have need of leading revision and decided to make new legislation rather than amending the existing one.

The new act is labelled as Mental Health Care Bill (MHCB), 2013. The experts believe that the proposed legislation MHCB, 2013 has major shortcomings. The major problems are that the Bill marginalises the families, who, in India endure the foremost burden of care of the mentally ill. In reality, as compared to the west, where family support has broken down, joint and extended family system is still a substantial Indian cultural feature. The MHCB entirely disregards the parents and families and, for the first time put forward that the patient can nominate any person as his/her nominated representative who will take all the major decisions regarding his/her care and property.

The biggest challenge in the treatment of mental illness is the rehabilitation and now-a-days, psychologists are increasingly challenged in delivering mental health services to clients who do not share their cultural background. The therapy requires the counsellor to relate to individuals who feel unable to relate to other people in their lives at home, at work, or elsewhere. Sometimes these injured persons have withdrawn from human beings into a private world of their own. Stress is the antecedent to a considerable number of mental health issues. A large number of persons suffering from mental disorders lack proper treatment which results in facing discrimination and human rights violations.

The introductory chapter by *Anubhuti Dubey* and *Aradhana Shukla* appear in this volume have presented a brief overview of the different widely used psychotherapies with their theoretical background. The role of psychotherapy in stress management is examined by *Mohammad Ali Khalid.* Based on the ideology of *Buddhism, Tien Liang, Narendra Singh Thagunna* and *Gurjeet Sindhu* has coined the term "Mansik Psychotherapy" and discussed its theoretical orientation and treatment approach. The next chapter of this volume written by *Arun Pratap Singh* has dealt with the effectiveness of Yogic lifestyle in promoting mental health and well being. *Aradhana Shukla* has reviewed the therapeutic application of both Indian and western music. Another chapter of the volume by *Anubhuti Dubey* and *Radha Maddhesia* has evaluated the status of psychotherapy in India from past to present. *Piyali Chakrabarti* and *Jesse Holmberg* have shed light on the importance of early intervention and therapy for autism. *E.T.T.M. Pasipandya, Yogesh K. Arya* and *Tushar Singh* have delved into the depression and its correlates and evaluated the imagery re-scripting treatment approach for depression. The multicultural counselling and therapy in the wake of globalization is inspected by *Dhananjay Kumar* and *Arpita Srivastava.* The efficacy and application of cognitive behavioural paradigm is evaluated by *Anita Sharma, Bhawana* and *Tushar Singh* has empirically examined the usefulness of cognitive rehabilitation for patients with acquired brain injury. In the next three chapters the theoretical orientation and research application and effectiveness of three types of therapies namely, online therapy, play therapy and existential therapy is scrutinized by *Smriti Sawhney Joshi, Neelam Verma* and *Radha Maddhesia* with *Anubhuti Dubey*, respectively. The holistic treatment approach of trauma with special reference to rape has been examined by *Narendra Singh Thagunna.* The chapter by *Shalini Mittal* and *Tushar Singh* have also dealt with violence against women and talked about its consequences and rehabilitation strategies. The effectiveness of reality therapy in multiple perspectives by *Nisha Kumari* and *Anubhuti Dubey* has appeared next in the volume. Lastly, *Anubhuti Dubey* has pen downed the concluding chapter emphasizing the need for culture specific mental health therapies.

We, the editors, have made genuine efforts to shed light on the theoretical orientation and application of different therapies for treating mental disorders as well as promotion of mental health by emphasizing the importance of the social context of the person. However, the available therapeutic applications are enormous and it is not possible to cover all of them in one volume. We solemnly ask our venerated readers to give constructive remarks on the volume to make it better in future. It will be greatly solicited.

Anubhuti Dubey
Aradhana Shukla

List of Contributors

Prof. Anita Sharma, Assistant Professor, Department of Psychology, Himachal Pradesh University, Shimla.

Prof. Anubhuti Dubey, Associate Professor, Department of Psychology, DDU Gorakhpur University, Gorakhpur, Uttar Pradesh, India.

Prof. Aradhana Shukla, Professor, Department of Psychology, SSJ Campus, Kumaun University, Almora, Uttrakhand, India.

Prof. Arun Pratap Singh, Assistant Professor, Department of Psychology, School of Humanities and Social Sciences, MG International Hindi University, Wardha, Maharashtra, India.

Bhawna, Research Scholar, Department of Psychology, B.H.U., Varanasi-221005, U.P.

Prof. Dhananjay Kumar, Associate Professor, Psychology Department, D.D.U. Gorakhpur University, Gorakhpur.

E.T.T.M. Pasipanodya, Research Scholar, Department of Psychology, Banaras Hindu University, Varanasi-221005, UP, India.

Gurjeet Sidhu, M.S., LMFTA, Antioch University Seattle, USA.

Jessie Holmberg, Executive Director, Cerebral Palsy Alliance, Singapore.

Mohammad Ali Khalid, Director, Academic Programmes Professional Institute of Business and Visiting Faculty, Ahsanullah University of Science and Technology, Bangladesh.

Narendra Singh Thagunna, Technical Adviser/Psychologist, Koshish, Kathmandu, Nepal.

Neelam Verma, Consultant Clinical Psychologist, Talk to Cure. www.talktocure.com

Nisha Kumari, Research Scholar, Department of Psychology, D.D.U. Gorakhpur University, Gorakhpur, U.P.

Piyali Chakrabarti, M.Phil., Head, Department of Psychology, Cerebral Palsy Alliance, Singapore.

Radha Maddhessia, Research Scholar, Department of Psychology, DDU Gorakhpur University, Gorakhpur, Uttar Pradesh, India.

Shalini Mittal, Research Scholar, Department of Psychology, Banaras Hindu University, Varanasi-221005, U.P., India,
Email: mittal.shalini2011@gmail.com

Prof. Smriti Sawhney Joshi, Assistant Professor, Department of Psychology, Amity Institute of Psychology and Allied Sciences, Amity University, Noida.

Tien Liang, ABPP, Dongbei University of Finance and Economics, Antioch University, Seattle, USA.

Prof. Tushar Singh, Assistant Professor, Department of Psychology, Banaras Hindu University, Varanasi-221005, U.P., India,
Email: tusharsinghalld@gmail.com

Prof. Yogesh Kumar Arya, Assistant Professor, Department of Psychology, Banaras Hindu University, Varanasi-221005, U.P., India.

1

Mental Health: Therapeutic Applications

Anubhuti Dubey and *Aradhana Shukla*

Mental health, vital and basic constituent of health is defined by World Health Organization (WHO) as a state of well-being in which an individual realizes his or her own abilities, can cope with the normal stresses of life, can work productively and is able to make a contribution to his or her community. In this positive sense, mental health is the foundation for individual well-being and the effective functioning of a community (WHO, 2001c). India, the second most populated country of the world, is a country of contrasts. Although characterized as one of the world's largest industrial nations, nonetheless the majority of the negative characteristics of poor and developing countries classify India too. According to various community based surveys, prevalence of mental disorders in India is 6-7 per cent for common mental disorders and 1-2 per cent for severe mental disorders and rate of psychiatric disorders in children aged between 4 to 16 years is about 12 per cent and nearly one-third of the population is less than 14 years of age. With such a magnitude of mental disorders, it becomes necessary to promote mental health services for the well-being of general population, in addition to provide treatment for mental illnesses. Here, only a diminutive percentage of the aggregate annual budget is spent on health which incorporates mental health also. Hence, mental health is fraction of the general health services, and contains no separate funds. At the time of Independence in 1947, the mental health infrastructure and specialist resources in India were scanty. In comparison to economically rich countries, the development of psychiatric services in India has occurred against the conditions of roughly no mental health services at the time of Independence (Thornicroft and Szmukler, 2001; Thornicroft, Tansella, and Law, 2008). At that time all people with mental disorders live in the community, largely do not have admittance to any organized services. Only their family provide care in whatever form it is able to do (ranging from isolation to going to traditional healers to committed care). In India, the National Mental Health Programme (NMHP) functions as the Mental Health Policy (MHP) which was formulated in 1982 with the objectives to ensure availability and accessibility of minimum mental health care for all to encourage mental health knowledge and skills and to promote community participation in mental health service development and to stimulate self-help in the community (Srinivasan, 2000). The District Mental Health Programme (DMHP) was initiated in 1996 during the Ninth Five Year Plan based on Bellary Model developed by the National Institute of Mental Health and Neuro Sciences (NIMHANS), Bangaluru. During the plan period, 27 districts were covered under DMHP. At present DMHP is covering 123 districts in 30 States and Union Territories. In addition to early identification and treatment of mentally ill, District Mental Health Programme has now incorporated promotive and preventive activities for positive mental health which include School Mental Health Services, College Counselling Services, Workplace Stress Management and Suicide Prevention Services. The issues of awareness regarding mental illness and availability of treatment are addressed through Information, Education and Communication (IEC) activities at District level by the DMHP (Ministry of Health and Family Welfare, Annual Report 2012-13).

All through these years, there have been a considerable number of community initiatives to deal with a varied mental health needs of the community through programmes on suicide prevention, care of the elderly, substance use and disaster mental health-care, and by setting up of day-care centres, half-way homes, long-stay homes and rehabilitation facilities (Patel and Thara, 2003; Ranganathan, 1996). The speedy expansion of psychiatry and clinical psychology in the private sector is another significant development which has taken place in recent years. Nevertheless, in the Tenth Five Year Plan (2002-2007), there was an eightfold increase in budget allocation for the National Mental Health Programme for the development of mental health services. The Eleventh Five Year Plan (2007-2012) had recognized the importance of mental health care and will concentrate on providing counselling, medical services, and establishing help lines for all, especially people affected by calamities, riots and violence. The Government has settled main concern especially to child and adolescent mental health care during the Twelfth Five Year Plan (2012-2017). The Government is also incorporating various components of National Mental Health Programme with the components of National Rural Health Mission, namely, School Health, Reproductive Child Health and Adolescent Friendly Clinics during the Twelfth Five Year Plan to straighten to the community in a more useful way. Moreover, at global level, the Director General, World Health Organization launched the Mental Health Action Plan 2013-2020 on 7 October, 2013. This action plan acknowledges the essential role of mental health in achieving health for all people. It aims to achieve equity through universal health coverage and stresses the importance of prevention. The four major objectives of the Action Plan are to: (1) Strengthen effective leadership and governance for mental health; (2) Provide comprehensive, integrated and responsive mental health and social care services in community-based settings; (3) Implement strategies for promotion and prevention in mental health; and (4) Strengthen information systems, evidence and research for mental health.

Training opportunities for various kinds of mental health personnel are gradually increasing in various academic institutions in the country and recently, there has been a major initiative in the growth of private psychiatric and clinical psychology and counselling services to fill a vacuum that the public mental health services have been slow to address. A number of non-governmental organizations have also initiated activities related to rehabilitation programmes, human rights of mentally ill people, and school mental health programmes. Despite all these efforts and progress, a lot has still to be done towards all aspects of mental health care in India in respect of training, research, and provision of clinical services to promote mental health in all sections of society.

Different types of therapies for mental disorders as well as mental health promotion are available. There are a variety of different kinds of psychotherapies which differ in intensity and duration. Three of the most common classifications are: individual, group, and pharmacological (drug). Different types of individual therapies include: psychoanalytical, behavioural, cognitive, and cognitive-behavioural. Different types of group therapies include family therapy and psychodrama. Quite recently, the types of pharmacological or drug treatments available to treat mental illnesses have resulted in four different classifications: antipsychotic agents, anti-manic or mood-stabilizing agents, antidepressants and anti-anxiety agents. It all depends on the counsellor or psychotherapist that which type or mode of therapy he/she finds appropriate for the specific mental disorder or suitable to client's need. Some counsellors or psychotherapists practice a form of '*integrative*' therapy, which means they draw on and blend specific types of techniques. Other practitioners work in an '*eclectic*' way, which means they take elements of several different models and combine them when working with clients. There are also a number of specific other therapies that can be used.

Recent reviews of the group psychotherapy literature indicate that group is a beneficial and cost-effective treatment format. However, collective findings on the differential efficacy of group when compared with individual therapy remain problematic, incomplete, or controversial. To remedy this problem, McRoberts, Burlingame, and Hoag (1998) had conducted a meta-analysis of 23 outcome studies that directly compared the effectiveness of the individual and group therapy formats when they were used within the same study. Results were consistent with previous reports that indicated no difference in outcome between the group and individual formats. These findings support past reports that group therapy can be used as an efficacious cost-effective alternative to individual therapy under many different conditions.

Psychoanalytical and Psychodynamic Therapies

These therapies are based on an individual's unconscious thoughts and perceptions that have developed throughout their childhood and how these affect current behaviour and thoughts. Major Psychoanalytical and Psychodynamic Therapies are:

- ***Jungian therapy*** proposed by leading psychotherapist, Carl Gustav Jung (1958, 1967) who believed that the personal unconscious is only the top layer of a much deeper, larger collective unconscious—the uncontrollable, inherited part of the human psyche which is made-up of patterns (archetypes) common to all humanity. Through the process of self-awareness, transformation and actualisation, Jungian therapy can help individuals see what is out of balance in their psyche. Since, the 1990s studies on Jungian Psychotherapy have been conducted mainly in Germany and Switzerland which showed that Jungian treatment moves patient from a level of severe symptoms to a level where one can speak of psychological health. These significant changes are reached by Jungian therapy with an average of 90 sessions, which makes Jungian psychotherapy an effective and cost-effective method (Roesler, 2013).
- ***Psychoanalysis*** is a therapeutic process that focuses on an

individual's unconscious and deep-rooted thoughts. It takes the view that our current behaviour, thoughts and feelings are directly influenced by our childhood and past experiences. Over time these can become repressed and may manifest themselves as depression or other negative symptoms. Developed by leading psychotherapist, Sigmund Freud (1916-17), psychoanalysis therapy is widely used to help clients recognise and understand how unconscious factors affect their current relationships and patterns of behaviour. Through techniques such as free association and dream analysis, clients can learn how to interpret deeply buried and complex memories or experiences that may be causing them distress and preventing them from living life to the fullest. Salzer *et al.* (2010) concluded that psychoanalytic psychotherapy was effective for treating people with depressive (77%), anxiety (45%), and personality (39%) disorders (Huber *et al.*, 2013).

- ***Psychodynamic therapy*** or psychodynamic counselling has its roots in Freud's psychoanalysis approach, but Carl G. Jung, Alfred Adler, Otto Rank and Melanie Klein are all widely recognised for further developing the concept and application of psychodynamics. The aim of psychodynamic therapy is to bring the unconscious mind into consciousness—helping individuals to unravel, experience and understand their true deep-rooted feelings in order to resolve them. It takes the view that our unconscious holds onto painful feelings and memories, which are too difficult for the conscious mind to process. In order to ensure these memories and experiences do not surface, many people will develop defences, such as denial and projections. The therapeutic relationship in contemporary psychodynamic counselling is based on acceptance, empathy and understanding, with an emphasis on developing a good working alliance that fosters trusts. A newly released meta-analysis examined the efficacy of short-term psychodynamic therapy for somatic disorders (Abbass, Kisely, and Kroenke, 2009). It included 23 studies involving 1,870 patients who suffered from a wide range of somatic conditions (e.g. dermatological, neurological, cardiovascular, respiratory, gastrointestinal, musculoskeletal, genitourinary, and immunological). The study reported effect sizes of 0.69 for improvement in general psychiatric symptoms and 0.59 for improvement in somatic symptoms.

Humanistic Therapies

These therapies focus on self-development, responsibilities and growth. They seek to help the individual to recognize their strength, creativity and choices in the "here and now".

- ***Existential Therapy*** is a unique form of psychotherapy that looks to explore difficulties from a philosophical perspective, rather than taking a technique-based approach. Focusing on the human condition as a whole, existential therapy applauds human capacities and encourages individuals to take responsibility for their successes. This therapy is discussed in detail in one of the chapters of this volume.
- ***Gestalt Therapy*** refers to a form of psychotherapy that derives from the Gestalt school of thought. It was developed in the late 1940s by Fritz Perls and is guided by the relational theory principle that every individual is a whole (mind, body and soul), and that they are best understood in relation to their current situation as he or she experiences it. The approach combines this relational theory with present state—focusing strongly on self-awareness and the here and now. In gestalt therapy, self-awareness is key to personal growth and developing full potential. It is the aim of a Gestalt therapist to promote a non-judgemental self-awareness that enables clients to develop a unique perspective on life (Pearl, 1968).
- ***Human givens Therapy*** is based on the premise that humans have a set of innate needs (or 'givens') and if these needs are not met, psychological distress can follow. Practitioners believe that these needs have been refined over thousands of years and that we have in-built resources to help us fulfil these needs (Griffin and Tyrrell, 2013).
- ***Person-centred Therapy*** also known as person-centred counselling or client-centred counselling deals with the ways in which individuals perceive themselves consciously rather than how a counsellor can interpret their unconscious thoughts or ideas. Created in the 1950s by American psychologist, Carl Rogers, the person-centred approach sees human beings as having an innate tendency to develop towards their full potential. However, this ability can become blocked or distorted by our life experiences—particularly those that affect our sense of value.

The counsellor or psychotherapist in this approach works to understand an individual's experience from their point of view.

- ***Psycho-Synthesis*** is a therapeutic approach that derives from psychoanalysis. It was developed in the early twentieth century by Italian psychiatrist, Roberto Assagioli. A key assumption of psycho-synthesis is that every human being has a vast potential for personal growth—a natural tendency to synthesise all aspects of their being to become the fullest realisation of themselves.
- ***Reality Therapy*** is a person-centred approach that focuses on the here and now rather than issues from the past. Developed by William Glasser in the 1960s, it promotes problem-solving and making better choices in order to achieve specific goals. There is a chapter in this volume devoted to reality therapy to be discussed in detail.
- ***Solution-focused Brief Therapy*** developed in America in the 1980s by husband and wife team Steve de Shazer and Insoo Kim Berg, along with their team at the Brief Family Centre, is an approach to psychotherapy based on solution-building rather than problem-solving. Although it acknowledges present problems and past causes, it predominantly explores an individual's current resources and future hopes—helping them to look forward and use their own strengths to achieve their goals. As its name suggests, solution-focused brief therapy is considered a time-limited approach, however, the technique is often incorporated into other long-term therapy types and effects can be long-lasting. The therapy is based on seven basic philosophies and assumptions such as—Change is both constant and certain; Emphasis on what is changeable and possible; Clients must want to change; Clients are the experts and outline their own goals; Clients have resources and their own strengths to solve and overcome their problems; Therapy is short-term; Focus on the future—history is not essential.
- ***Transactional Analysis (TA)*** is considered a fundamental therapy for well-being and for helping individuals to reach their full potential in all aspects of life. Though, it is commonly recognised as a brief and solution-focused approach, transactional analysis can also be applied as an effective long-term, in-depth therapy. Founded by Eric Berne in the late 1950s, TA therapy is based on the theory that each person has three ego states—parent, adult and child. These are used along with other

key transactional analysis concepts, tools and models to analyse how individuals communicate and identify what interaction is needed for a better outcome. Throughout therapy, the TA therapist will work directly on here and now problem solving behaviours, whilst helping clients to develop day-to-day tools for finding constructive creative solutions. The ultimate goal is to ensure clients regain absolute autonomy over their lives.

- ***Transpersonal Psychology*** developed by American psychologist, Abraham Maslow designate the term 'transpersonal' to 'beyond the personal', which in itself suggest the core aim of the therapy—to explore human growth and help people to discover a deep and more enduring essential self that exists beyond the conditioned ego. The methodology used to drive this therapeutic process is a combination of spiritual traditions from around the world, which are integrated with elements of contemporary psychology. This framework can help a wide range of individuals—including groups of people such as families and work colleagues. Clients of transpersonal psychology are expected to gain a complete understanding of themselves, their capacities, and their relationships, and will leave equipped with the skills to help them deal with these beyond therapy.

Cognitive Behavioural Therapies

These therapies are based on the way a person think (cognitive) and/or behave. These therapies recognize that it is possible to change or recondition a person's thoughts or behaviour to overcome specific problems.

- ***Acceptance and Commitment Therapy (ACT)*** uses acceptance and mindfulness strategies to help increase psychological flexibility. This therapy takes the view that by accepting negative thoughts and feelings, individuals can choose a valued direction in which to take action and make positive changes.
- ***Behavioural Therapy*** is directed to raze unwanted or maladaptive behaviour. Practitioners of behavioural therapy believe that behaviour is learned and can, therefore, be un-learned *via* therapy. This therapy is applied for those behavioural problems or mental health conditions that involve unwanted behaviour, like

addictions, anxiety, phobias and obsessive compulsive disorder (OCD). There are specific issues that counter exceptionally well to this type of therapy as well as the associated integrated forms, such as Cognitive Behavioural Therapy (CBT).

- ***Cognitive Analytic Therapy*** looks into the past events and experiences to be aware of why a person feels/thinks/behaves the way he do, before helping them problem solve and develop new ways of coping. Each programme of therapy is customized to the individual's needs, taking into consideration their present situation and problems they are dealing with. It is a time-limited therapy that can go on between four and 24 weeks depending on the characteristics of the problem being investigated, but an average of 16 weeks is regarded as the norm.
- ***Cognitive Behavioural Therapy (CBT)*** is a talking therapy that looks to help a person to manage problems by enabling him/her to recognise, and ultimately change, the way she/he thinks and behaves. The chapter in the volume is devoted to CBT, hence I am going into the details of it.
- ***Cognitive Therapy*** is based on the principle that thoughts and perceptions can impact our feelings and behaviour, and looks at ways to reassess negative thoughts so individuals can learn more flexible, positive ways of thinking that will subsequently influence behaviours. It covers traditional Cognitive Therapy (CT), Rational Emotive Behaviour Therapy (REBT) and Mindfulness-Based Cognitive Therapy (MBCT).

Art Therapies

Art therapies require the application of creative art forms like music, art, drama and dance into a therapeutic environment. In his seminal work *The Arts and Psychotherapy*, McNiff (1981) observes that expressive therapies are those that introduce action to psychotherapy and that "action within therapy and life is rarely limited to a specific mode of expression" (p. viii). While talk is still the traditional method of exchange in therapy and counselling, practitioners of expressive therapies know that people also have different expressive styles—one individual may be more visual, another more tactile, and so forth. When therapists are able to include these various expressive capacities in their work with clients, they can more fully enhance each person's abilities to communicate effectively and authentically. The other versions of expressive therapies are talking therapy, therapeutic story-telling, biblio-therapy and poetry therapy. Art therapy is a type of psychotherapy that utilises art and artistic mediums to help people explore their thoughts and emotions in a unique way. Drama therapy and psychodrama often capture our imagination because they take us away from our reality, transporting us to different times, places—even planets. The fiction element of this type of therapy acts like a filter, so that the feelings encountered do not engulf those taking part, instead allowing them to acknowledge and deal with what comes up as and when it surfaces. Enabling participants to experience and explore difficult emotions in this indirect way often triggers a sense of catharsis. A piece of music can bring back memories, lift our spirits and soothe our soul—helping us to express emotions when words fail us. Music is one of the few things in life that has the power to move us emotionally. It is this power that music therapy harnesses, using the various musical components to provide a way of relating within a therapeutic relationship. A chapter in this volume is also dealing in detail with Music Therapy.

Other Therapies

Although psychological therapies generally fall into the categories mentioned above, there are also a number of other specific therapies too.

- ***Family/Systemic Therapy*** is an approach that acts with families and those who are in close relationships to promote modification and change. These changes are vision analysed in terms of the systems of interaction between each person in the family or relationship. It is explainable that families and those in relationships occasionally get into difficulties because of their dissimilarity, or undergo the pressure when loved ones have dilemma. The therapy is aimed to work on these problems by giving confidence to the family members and nearest and dearest to lend a hand and empathise with each other. They are provided the chance to realize and acknowledge each other's needs and wishes; foster on family strengths and eventually render constructive changes in their lives and relationships.
- ***Integrative Therapy or Integrative Counselling*** is a combined approach that brings together different elements of specific therapies with a view that there is no single approach that can treat each client in all situations. Each person needs to be considered as a whole and counselling techniques must be

tailored to their individual needs and personal circumstances. The integrative approach refers to the infusion of a person's personality and needs—integrating the effective, behavioural, cognitive, and physiological systems within one person, as well as addressing social and spiritual aspects. Essentially, integrative counsellors are not only concerned with what works, but why it works—tailoring therapy to their clients and not the client to the therapy.

- ***Mindfulness*** aims to reconnect us with ourselves to alleviate stress. It also helps us to feel more attuned with our emotions and generally more aware of ourselves both mentally and physically.
- ***Play Therapy*** enables children to be aware of confused feelings and upsetting experiences that they have not yet had a chance to process. At times a child starts to develop patterns of behaviour that may be causing disruption to his life and to the lives of those around him/her. Parents, carers and teachers may be acquainted with signs such as excessive anger, fear or worry that may be disturbing a child's development and their ability to manage with their family and friends at school. While adults experiencing emotional and behavioural difficulties can seek help in the form of talking therapies, children tend to find this therapeutic setting threatening and almost like an interrogation. Thus, play therapy is exercised to facilitate children communicate at their own level and at their own pace. A chapter in this volume is offered to Play Therapy.
- ***Psychosexual Therapy*** is a specialised therapeutic technique carried out by professionals with background of counselling, nursing or medicine. It is specifically designed to help people living with difficulties that are of a psychological, sexual nature and that are too difficult or complex to be resolved on their own. It incorporates the key behavioural and cognitive principles and has proven successful in helping people of all ages, health and sexuality to overcome their sexual problems.
- ***Hypnosis or Hypnotherapy*** uses guided relaxation, intense concentration, and focused attention to achieve a heightened state of awareness that is sometimes called a trance. The person's attention is so focused while in this state that anything going on around the person is temporarily blocked out or ignored—with the help of a trained therapist. Hypnosis is usually considered

an aid to psychotherapy, because the hypnotic state allows people to explore painful thoughts, feelings, and memories they might have hidden in their conscious minds.

- Online therapeutic interventions and use of offline video games have also been utilized for therapeutic purposes in recent times, particularly for the treatment of special-needs groups such as the young, the elderly and people with various conditions such as Attention Deficit and Hyperactivity Disorders (ADHD), anxiety and autism spectrum disorders. A chapter on online mental health intervention is given in the present volume.

Besides these alternative therapies, there is a list of culture specific mental health therapies for culture specific syndromes as well as for other mental health problems. Attitudes towards mental illness vary among individuals, families, ethnicities, cultures, and countries. Cultural and religious teachings often influence beliefs about the origins and nature of mental illness, and shape attitudes towards the mentally ill. Cultural values and beliefs affect the patterns of help-seeking behaviour also. The orientation of traditional healers and their healing approaches are governed by attribution beliefs, and their practices differ greatly from those of the professional establishment (ceremonies/rituals, incantations, prayers, herbal remedies, sweat lodges, spiritual counselling etc. (Rogler and Cortes, 1993).

Conclusion

Counselling requirements in the Indian context transpire alongside the backdrop of immense social change. Additionally, the previous two decades of economic reforms have supplemented the tempo of these changes and foster transformation in way of life. Mental health providers need to understand how to win confidence and collect information from the patient, the patient's family, friends and significant social relations, and to engage them in a treatment scheme. However, existing counselling services are mostly rooted in Western approaches to psychology. These approaches have been extensively criticised as not being relevant to the Indian cultural context. A relevant and culturally valid counselling psychology, therefore, has remained a fledgling discipline. Psychological thought is not new to India, and ancient traditions, present ideas and constructs that are rich in possibilities for application (Arulmani, 2007) can be developed.

References

Abbass, A., Kisely, S., and Kroenke, K. (2009). Short-term psychodynamic psychotherapy for somatic disorders: Systematic review and meta-analysis of clinical trials. *Psychotherapy and Psychosomatics,* 78, 265-274.

Arulmani, G. (2007). Counselling Psychology in India: At the Confluence of Two Traditions. *Applied Psychology: An International Review*, 56, 69-82.

Freud, S. (1916-1917). *Introductory Lectures on Psychoanalysis*. SE, 22, 1-182.

Griffin, J. and Tyrrell, I. (2013). *Human Givens: The New Approach to Emotional Health and Clear Thinking.* Human Givens Publishing.

Huber, D., Henrich, G., Clarkin, J., and Klug, G. (2013). Psychoanalytic *versus* psychodynamic therapy for depression: A three-year follow-up study. *Psychiatry: Interpersonal and Biological Processes,* 76, 132-149.

Jung, C.G. (1958-1967). *Psyche and Symbol* (R.F.C. Hull, Trans.). Princeton, New Jersey: Princeton University Press (Published in 1991).

McNiff, S. (1981). *The Arts and Psychotherapy*. Springfield, IL: Thomas.

McRoberts, C., Burlingame, G.M., and Hoag, M.J. (1998). Comparative efficacy of individual and group psychotherapy: A meta-analytic perspective. *Group Dynamics: Theory, Research, and Practice*, 2(2), 101.

Ministry of Health and Family Welfare, *Annual Report 2012-13*, p. 161.

Patel, V. and Thara, R. (eds.) (2003). *Meeting Mental Health Needs in Developing Countries: NGO Innovations in India*. New Delhi: Sage (India).

Perls, F. (1968). *Gestalt Therapy Verbatim*. Moab, UT: Real People Press.

Ranganathan, S. (1996). *The Empowered Community: A Paradigm Shift in the Treatment of Alcoholism*. Madras: TTR Clinical Research Foundation.

Rogler, L., and Cortes, D. (1993). Help-seeking pathways: A unifying concept in mental health care. *American Journal of Psychiatry*, 150(4), 554-561.

Salzer, S., Leibing, E., Jakobsen, T., Rudolf, G., Brockmann, J., Eckert, J., Leichsenring, F. (2010). Patterns of interpersonal problems and their improvement in depressive and anxious patients treated with psychoanalytic therapy. *Bulletin of the Menninger Clinic,* 74, 283-300. doi: 10.1521/bumc.2010.74.4.283

Srinivasa, M.R. (2000). Community mental health in India. In *Mental Health in India*—Essays in honour of Prof. N.N. Wig. Bangalore: Peoples Action for Mental Health, 150-76.

Thornicroft, G.J., and Szmukler, G. (2001). *Textbook of Community Psychiatry*. Oxford: Oxford University Press.

Thornicroft, G., Tansella, M., and Law, A. (2008). Steps, Challenges and Lessons in Developing Community Mental Health Care. *World Psychiatry*, 7, 87-92.

WHO (2001c). *Mental Health: New Understanding, New Hope.* The World Health Report. Geneva, World Health Organization.

2
Role of Psychotherapy in Stress Management

Mohammad Ali Khalid

In the modern world scenario, life brings along many leaps and bounds that call for stress. Stress may not be only related to specific events, but may develop in early childhood as an anxiety response to difficult situations and carried into adult life as the characteristic way of dealing with difficulties. Surveys report that one out of every four people, seeks treatment for stress at some time or other in his life. According to Baum (1990), stress is a negative emotional experience accompanied by predictable biochemical, physiological, cognitive, and behavioural changes that are directed either towards altering the stressful event or accommodating to its effects.

Stress is supposed by some to be a good thing, for themselves or others, in that it stimulates excitement and positive feelings. If these are the effects then it is not stress as defined here. It is the excitement and stimulus derived (by one who wants these feelings and can handle them) from working hard in a controlled and manageable way towards an achievable and realistic aim, which for sure, can be very exciting, but it is not stress. Stress is bad for people and organizations, it is a threat and a health risk, and it needs to be recognized and dealt with, not dismissed as something good, or welcomed as a badge of boldness.

Though, stress is not always a bad thing. It is simply the body's response to changes that create taxing demands. There is a difference between eustress (which is a term for positive stress) and distress (which refers to negative stress). In daily life, we often use the term "stress" to describe negative situations. This leads many people to believe that all stresses are bad for them, which is not true. Eustress, or positive stress motivates, focuses energy, is short-termed, perceived as within our coping abilities and improves performance. While, distress or negative stress causes anxiety or concern, can be short or long-term, perceived as outside of our coping abilities, feels unpleasant, decreases performance and may even lead to mental and physical problems.

It is difficult to group stressors into objective lists of those that cause eustress and those that cause distress, because different people will have different reactions to particular situations. However, by generalizing, we can predict certain stressors that are typically experienced as negative or those that seem positive to most people, most of the time. Some of the examples of negative personal stressors include: the death of a spouse, filing for divorce, losing contact with loved ones, the death of a family member, hospitalization (oneself or a family member), injury or illness (oneself or a family member), being abused or neglected, conflict in interpersonal relationships, bankruptcy or financial problems, unemployment, children's problems at school, legal problems and many more. While, some of the positive personal stressors include receiving a promotion or raise at work, starting a new job, marriage, buying a home, having a child, shifting to another place, taking a vacation, retirement, taking educational classes or learning a new hobby.

Stressors are not always limited to situations where some external situation is creating a problem. Internal events such as feelings and thoughts and habitual behaviours can also cause negative stress. Some common internally caused sources of distress include fears: (e.g. fears of flying, heights, public speaking, chatting with strangers at a party), repetitive thought patterns, worrying about future events (e.g. waiting for medical test results or job restructuring), perfectionist expectations etc. Few habitual behaviour patterns that can lead to stress include over-scheduling, failing to be assertive, procrastination and/or failing to plan ahead.

An individual's personality and temperament, and apart from the situation, also decide whether stress is felt or not. A person's susceptibility to stress can be affected by any or all of these factors, which means that everyone has a different tolerance to stressors. And in respect of some of these factors, stress susceptibility is not fixed, so each person's stress tolerance level changes over time. Stress susceptibility is altered by childhood experience (abuse can increase stress susceptibility), personality (certain personalities are more stress-prone than others), genetics (particularly inherited 'relaxation response', connected with serotonin levels, the brain's 'well-being chemical'), immunity abnormality (as might be caused by certain diseases such as arthritis and eczema, which weaken stress resilience), lifestyle (principally poor diet and lack of exercise), duration and intensity of stressors.

Stress is non-specific response of the body to any demand made upon it. Although it seems easy to comprehend stress, but there are various complications and confusions as there are different types of stresses—acute stress, episodic acute stress, and chronic stress. Each type of stress has its own characteristics, symptoms, duration and treatment approaches.

Acute Stress: Acute stress is the most common form of stress. It comes from demands and pressures of the recent past and anticipated demands and pressures of the near future. Acute stress is thrilling and exciting in small doses, but excess of it is exhausting. Exaggeration on short-term stress can lead to psychological distress, tension, headaches, upset stomach and other symptoms. Fortunately, the symptoms of acute stress are known by most people. As it is short-term, acute stress does not has much time to do the widespread damage as accompanying long-term stress. The most common symptoms include:

- *Emotional distress*—some combination of anger or irritability, anxiety and depression, the three stress emotions.
- *Muscular problems* including tension, headache, back pain, jaw pain and the muscular tensions that lead to pulled muscles and tendon and ligament problems.
- *Stomach, gut and bowel problems* such as heartburn, acid stomach, flatulence, diarrhoea, constipation and irritable bowel syndrome.
- *Transient over arousal* leads to elevation in blood pressure, rapid heartbeat, sweaty palms, heart palpitations, dizziness, migraine headaches, cold hands or feet, shortness of breath and chest pain.

Acute stress can crop up in anyone's life, and it is highly treatable and manageable.

Episodic Acute Stress: Some people, however, suffer acute stress frequently and thus their lives are so disordered that they are in total chaos and crisis. They are unable to organize the swing of self-inflicted demands and pressures calling out for their attention. They seem continuously in the grasps of acute stress. People with acute stress are usually over-aroused, short-tempered, irritable, anxious and tense. They are always in rush, they are likely to be hasty, and sometimes their irritability comes through as hostility. Interpersonal relationships get worsen rapidly when others respond with real hostility. The workplace becomes a very stressful place for them. The cardiac prone, "Type A" personality described by cardiologists is similar to an extreme case of episodic acute stress. "Type A" have an "excessive competitive drive, aggressiveness, impatience, and a harrying sense of time urgency." In addition there is a "free-floating, but well-rationalized form of hostility, and almost always a deep-seated insecurity." Such personality characteristics would seem to create frequent episodes of acute stress for the "Type A" individual.

An additional form of episodic acute stress comes from continual worry. "Worry warts" see disaster around every corner and pessimistically forecast catastrophe in every situation. The world is a dangerous, unrewarding, punitive place where something awful is always about to happen. They also tend to be over-aroused and tense, but are more anxious and depressed than angry and hostile.

The symptoms of episodic acute stress are the symptoms of extended over-arousal, like persistent tension, headaches, migraines, hypertension, chest pain and heart disease. Treating episodic acute stress requires intervention on a number of levels, generally requiring professional help, which may take many months.

Often, lifestyle and personality issues are so ingrained and habitual with these individuals that they see nothing wrong with the way they conduct their lives. They blame their despairs on other people and external events. Frequently, they see their lifestyle, their patterns of interacting with others, and their ways of perceiving the world as part and parcel of who and what they are.

Chronic Stress: Chronic stress is not thrilling and exciting. This is the relentless stress that wears people away day after day, year after year. Chronic stress destroys bodies, minds and lives. It is the stress of poverty, of dysfunctional families, of being trapped in an unhappy marriage or in a shunned job or career. Chronic stress comes when a person never sees a way out of a miserable situation. It is the stress of hammering demands and burdens for apparently perpetual periods of time. With no hope, the individual gives up searching for solutions. Some chronic stresses stem from traumatic, early childhood experiences that become internalized and remain for ever painful and present. Some experiences extremely affect personality. A view of the world, or a belief system, is created that causes unending stress for the individual.

The worst aspect of chronic stress is that people get used to it. They forget it is there. People are immediately aware of acute stress because it is new; they ignore chronic stress because it is old, familiar, and sometimes, almost comfortable.

Chronic stress kills through suicide, violence, heart attack, stroke and, perhaps, even cancer. People wear down to a final, fatal breakdown. Because physical and mental resources are depleted through long-term attrition, the symptoms of chronic stress are difficult to treat and may require extended medical as well as behavioural treatment and stress management.

The Biology behind Stress

Our stress response is profoundly connected to our biological mechanism. According to Hans Selye (1956), there are three phases in our stress response, called alarm, resistance, and exhaustion. The biological mechanism behind stress can be divided into two parts: Hypothalamic Pituitary Adrenal (HPA), Axis Activation and Sympathetic Adreno Medulory (SAM) system.

Whenever we face a stressor, it activates the cerebral cortex which further triggers the hypothalamus for arousal of the sympathetic nervous system. The aroused sympathetic nervous system results in flight or fight response, also this stimulates the medulla of adrenal glands that thereby secretes catechol-amines, epinephrine and non-epinephrine. The secretion of the catechol-amines leads in the cranked-up feeling in response to stress. This chain of events is referred to as Sympathetic Adreno Medulory (SAM) system. Facing stress leads to activation of hypothalamus which triggers pituitary gland for release of adreno-cortico-tropic hormone (ACTH), this hormone stimulates adrenal cortex for release of glucosecorticoids. Thus, the stress response occurs.

The term "stress" has appeared in medical and medical-related literature since 1956, when Hans Selye developed the concept of stress to explain the physiological response of people to various environmental stimuli. Considerable research was conducted in the area of epidemiology in public health departments throughout the country. A later development in stress research concerns the personality type and other psychological characteristics of individuals, particularly men, who respond to stress situations with physiological breakdown, e.g. cardiac disease, peptic ulcers, and other psychosomatic disorders.

In the last decade or so, we find researchers have looked more at psychological variables in an effort to understand the stress response. Appley and Trumbel (1967) define stress as the "affective, behavioural, and physiological response to aversive stimuli." At approximately the same time, Lazarus (1966) preferred to talk almost exclusively about psychological stress and defined the term as "the threat or anticipation of future harm."

Stress Management

Stress Management refers to the wide spectrum of techniques and psychotherapies aimed at controlling a person's levels of stress, especially chronic stress, usually for the purpose of improving everyday functioning. In this context, the term 'stress' refers only to a stress with significant negative consequences or distress, rather than eustress, a stress whose consequences are helpful or otherwise positive. Stress management has been in common use by the lay public and mental health professionals for many years. The emphasis in stress management is on the client taking individual responsibility for his or her care and treatment within the context of psychological consultation and guidance. Although stress management programmes vary somewhat in format and content, most of them contain several important components:

- **A.** A survey or assessment of specific stressful problem areas for each participant.
- **B.** The specific stress management training, focusing on cognitive restructuring and de-stressing skills.
- **C.** Homework assignments.
- **D.** The development of an "action plan" by each participant which is individual, operational, and specific.

Stress produces numerous physical and mental symptoms which vary according to each individual's situational factors. These can include physical health decline as well as depression. The process of stress management is named as one of the keys to a happy and successful life in modern society. Although life provides numerous demands that can prove difficult to handle, stress management provides a number of ways to manage anxiety and maintain overall well-being.

Despite stress often being thought of as a subjective experience, levels of stress are readily measurable, using various physiological tests. Many practical stress management techniques are available which may help an individual reduce their levels of stress, provide positive feelings of control over one's life and promote general well-being.

Since there is a limited research in the area, evaluating the effectiveness of various stress management techniques can be difficult. There are several models of stress management, each with distinctive explanations of mechanisms for controlling stress. Much more research is necessary to provide a better understanding of which mechanisms actually operate and are effective in practice.

Model of Stress Management

Transactional model: Richard Lazarus and Susan Folkman (1984) suggested that stress can be thought of as resulting from an "imbalance between demands and resources" or as occurring when "pressure exceeds one's perceived ability to cope". Stress management was developed and premised on the idea that stress is not a direct response to a stressor, but rather one's resources and ability to cope mediate the stress response and are amenable to change, thus allowing stress to be controllable.

In order to develop an effective stress management programme, firstly it is necessary to identify the factors that are central to a person controlling his/her stress, and to identify the intervention methods which effectively target these factors. Lazarus and Folkman's interpretation of stress focuses on the transaction between people and their external environment. The model contends that an event, thing, situation or person may not be a stressor, if the person does not perceive the stressor as a threat, but rather as positive or even challenging. Also, if the person possesses or can use adequate coping skills, then stress may not actually be a result or develop because of the stressor. The model proposes that people can be taught to manage their stress and cope with their stressors. They may learn to change their perspective of the stressor and provide them with the ability and confidence to improve their lives and handle all types of stressors.

Health realization/innate health model: This model is based on the idea that stress does not necessarily follow the presence of a potential stressor. Instead of focusing on the individual's appraisal of so-called stressors in relation to his or her own coping skills, the health realization model focuses on the nature of thought. The model suggests that ultimately a person's thought processes determine the response to potentially stressful external circumstances. In this model, stress results from appraising oneself and one's circumstances through a mental filter of insecurity and negativity, while a feeling of well-being trigger off from dealing with the world with a "quiet mind". This model recommends that helping stressed individuals to be aware of the nature of thought, particularly conferring them with the ability to identify when they are in the clutch of insecure thinking, disengage from it, and access natural positive feelings, will reduce their stress.

Role of Psychotherapy in Stress Management

Psychotherapy, as thought of, is a practical method that promotes mental health and overall well-being. It helps in attaining competences that are crucial for managing stress and reducing our inefficiency in every life settings. Psychotherapy when used in stress management plays a role to in-built in us the effective emotional responses to bombarding stressful events of daily life. It pursues to recalibrate the nervous system so as to yield more refined, more sophisticated neuro-chemical responses to stress than the disturbing adrenalin-based responses. Psychotherapy is helpful in all conditions of past, present and future; develops understanding of the past stressful instances so that it may not distort our perception of the present, shifts focus to manage present stressors conveniently and reflects into recognition of future novel prospects. Psychotherapy in stress management focuses on developing such skills in individual so as to enhance their relationships and experiences. These basic skills though can be complicated and confusing, but are easy to learn and monitor. They may be simplified for comprehending four key behaviours: conscious recognition of anxiety-based behaviour, tolerating the presence of distressed feelings without becoming reactive, responding to our distress from the perspective of positive intent, and responding with more interpersonally attuned behaviours.

Anxiety is an omnipresent experience related to individuals due to which the personal and professional lives are spent in a state of sustained hyper vigilance and people find themselves caught up in the adrenalin rich fight or flight response of the sympathetic nervous system. The use of flight or fight response is only limited to restriction of danger, while we allow it and thus the adrenalin rush to dominate our environment. Until and unless we recognize our anxiety-based responses and learn to master them, the adrenalin would continue to bring snags in life and thereby compromises in health.

Another skill of psychotherapy required to manage stress is learning to tolerate anxiety-based emotions. Generally, people are unable to put up with the physical sensations attached to the negative emotions and thus indulge in combative compensatory behaviours like overeating, substance abuse, physical illness, etc. Once people learn to master over such physical or emotional distress their reliance on dysfunctional responses would diminish.

Being able to make an individual practice positive intent is another key skill. People should learn to be open to situations hoping that even when problem arises there would be a prospect of things getting better and even if not, would overcome it. Positive intent is not the hope for the best, but an acceptance to whatever comes along. One can easily learn to practice positive intent, but would find it challenging to master it, although this would be the most practical thing that one can do easily in any problematic situation.

If a person becomes aware of anxiety-related behaviours learns to tolerate negative emotions and get attuned to the art of positive intent, his/her sentiments travel from the flight/fight response to energy-saving, and healing and serene parasympathetic nervous system response. Thus, one can practice interpersonally attuned behaviour. Psychotherapy can speed up a lifetime learning process which alters stress-response from harmful, avoidant behaviours to enriching, helping behavioural responses. Once a person learns the basic skills involved in psychotherapy, it is solely his/her mastery by continual practice.

References

AHA and ACS (1996). *Living Well, Staying Well.* Times Books, New York.

Bower, J.E. and Segerstrom, S.C. (2004). "Stress management, finding benefit, and immune function: positive mechanisms for intervention effects on physiology". *Journal of Psychosomatic Research,* 56 (1), 9-11.

Bowman, Rachel; Beck, Kevin D.; Luine, Victoria N. (January 2003). "Chronic Stress Effects on Memory: Sex differences in performance". *Hormones and Behaviour*, 43 (1), 48-59.

Caplan, R.P. (November 1994). Stress, Anxiety, and Depression in Hospital Consultants, General Practitioners, and Senior Health Managers. *BMJ Journal,* 309 (6964), 1261-1269.

Hardy, Sally (1998). *Occupational Stress: Personal and Professional Approaches*. United Kingdom, Stanley Thornes, 18-43.

Hogh, A., Hansen, Å.M., Mikkelsen, E.G., and Persson, R. (2012). Exposure to negative acts at work, psychological stress reactions and physiological stress response. *Journal of Psychosomatic Research*, 73(1), 47-52.

Katherine, M.G., and Kessler, R. (1990). Chronic Stress, Acute Stress, Depressive Symptoms. *American Journal of Community Psychology*, 18 (5), 681-706.

Lazarus, R.S., and Folkman, S. (1984). *Stress, Appraisal and Coping*. New York: Springer.

Lehrer, P.M., David, H., Woolfolk, R.L., and Wesley, E.S. (2007). *Principles and Practice of Stress Management, Third Edition*, 46-47.

Monahar, J. (2001). *Stress Management and Psychotherapy*. Mercer Business.

Parrott, A.C. (1999). Does Cigarette Smoking Cause Stress? *American Psychologist*, 54(10), 817-820.

Petersen, H., Kecklund, G., D'Onofrio, P., Nilsson, J., and Åkerstedt, T. (2013). Stress vulnerability and the effects of moderate daily stress on sleep polysonography and subjective sleepiness. *Journal of Sleep Research*, 22(1), 50-57.

Posen, D.B. (1995). Stress management for patient and physician. *The Canadian Journal of Continuing Medical Education*, 7(1), 65-82.

Schultz, S.E. and Schultz, D. (2010). *Psychology and Work Today*. New York: Prentice Hall, p. 374.

3

Mansik Psychotherapy

A Theoretical Orientation and Treatment Approach

Tien Liang, Narendra Singh Thagunna and *Gurjeet Sidhu*

Approaches towards culture and mental health usually focus on one of the two orientations: the Universalist and Cultural relativist. The Universalist view holds that there exists similarities in mental disorders across all cultures, but the expression of these disorders varies from culture to culture. The cultural relativist approach holds that some disorders are unique to a culture and may only be understood from a cultural perspective (Kirmayer, 1991). Many South Asian psychologists hold to the universal view of mental illness and are convinced of the global applicability of Western psychology. Western psychology is regarded as ready-made imports (Sinha, 1986). If there are deviations, then South Asian psychology is considered a "Pale Copy of Western Psychology" (Sinha, 1993). Keeping the discipline free of South Asian traditions, published scholarly material are kept to a Western framework, despite the fact that such a pattern does not reflect the social and cultural reality of the Indian or Nepalese people (Subba, 1994). To accommodate the cultural differences, Indian and Nepalese psychology has imported Western psychology's tripartite model of multicultural competency training. The tripartite model for culturally sensitive psychotherapy typically addresses attitudes, knowledge, and skills (Betancourt, 2003). In the attitudes portion, this multicultural approach typically includes self-reflection on one's own biases and stereotypical thinking, with instruction to appreciate diversity (Betancourt, 2003). The knowledge portion emphasizes essential characteristics of different groups (Betancourt, 2003). The skills portion focus on communication skills and interviewing techniques that can be universally generalized across various cultural groups (Betancourt, 2003). Most commonly cited approaches are a combination of information on a specific cultural group with enhancements to communication and assessment skills. Some widely used therapy models which are based on the tripartite model are listed herein. The first is the LEARN model (Berlin and Fowkes, 1983), which stands for Listen with sympathy and understanding to the patient's perception of the problem; Explain your perceptions of the problem; Acknowledge and discuss the differences and similarities; Recommend treatment; and finally Negotiate agreement. Second is the HEARTS Model (Hanscome, 2001). The HEARTS acronym stands for listening history focusing on emotions and reactions, asking questions about symptoms, Explaining reasons for symptoms, teaching relaxation and coping strategies, and Helping with self-change. Third is the ETHNICS framework, which stands for Explanation Treatment Healers Negotiate Intervention Collaborate Spirituality (Levin and Gottlieb, 2000). Research publications in the *Indian Journal of Psychiatry* (*IJP*) continue this Western focus with recent focus in evidence-based treatment (Nand, 1959, 1961; Thomas and Kumar S., 2007). Despite Dhairyam's (1945) and Neki (1977, 1992) call for psychotherapy outcome research in India and Nepal, there is a dearth of published literature on this topic.

Treatment based on this kind of universal multicultural approach leads to misunderstandings when exported to India and Nepal. Western cultural emphasis on independence, for instance, is at odds with Indian and Nepalese collectivistic cultural notions that individuals exist within the enclosure of extended families and community. As early as 1961, there were attempts to integrate indigenous concepts into the application of psychotherapy. Psychiatrists practicing psychotherapy in India have published the influence of religion as an essential ingredient of psychotherapy from the very early days (Hoch, 1974; Hosseini, 1983; Nand, 1961; Neki, 1977, 1992; Surya and Jayaram, 1968; Verma, 1982; Wig, 2004).

Paradoxically, Western psychology has been experimenting with Indian and Nepalese cultural approaches. Emerging new psychotherapeutic treatments in Western psychology, such as narrative therapy and positive psychotherapy, incorporate Buddhist tenets of mindfulness and acceptance. Similarly, there has been experimentation with non-Western Buddhist model of psychotherapy in the East. Daya (2000) claims that Buddhist Psychology offer a positive therapeutic approach that emphasizes the development of human potential. Balakrishna *et al.* (1977) and Vahia (1966) studied the effect of *Patanjali Yoga* on 'psycho neuroses' and found it useful in stress induced psychological disorders. Though, neither from India nor Nepal, another example of psychotherapy that is not based on the Western model, but on Eastern Buddhism, is the Japanese Morita Therapy. Yet others have developed relaxation technique that combines four yogic postures and repetition of a religious word. The technique appears to be effective for everything from depression to panic disorder to stress management, in part because *yoga* is so culturally congruent and familiar to Indians. Psychologists incorporating indigenous practices prescribe various forms of meditation to help clients enhance their potential or overcome depression, anxiety and other problems. To lay the groundwork for therapy, therapists often recommend that patients spend a few weeks beforehand learning to relax at a meditation or yoga camp. In an extensive series of studies, therapists have found that spending time in such camps improved positive measures and decreased negative symptoms when compared with those in control groups (Balakrishna *et al.*, 1977; Daya, 2000; Hoch, 1974; Hosseini, 1983; Manickam, 1985, 1986, 1990, 1991, 1995, 1997; Nand, 1961; Neki, 1977, 1992; Surya and Jayaram, 1968; Verma, 1982; Vahia 1966; Wig, 2004).

Continuing this tradition of developing psychotherapy approaches that emphasizes and is based on cultural concepts indigenous to India and Nepal, we offer the Mansik Psychotherapy approach.

Mansik Psychotherapy

This chapter introduces the core ideas and techniques used in Mansik psychotherapy. Mansik health means the health that can be maintained by taking care of mind. These ideas are based upon and derived from source text of Buddhist teachings. Mansik Psychotherapy rests primarily on the worldview reflected in the *Abhidhamma* texts, while the psychotherapy techniques borrow primarily from the *Satipatthana Sutta*. This section starts with introduction and discussion of the basic core ideas of Self, Suffering, Impermanence and Karma. Through the use of applied relaxation and attending to the body, the patients are invited to first discern, and then to understand their own emotional state as exhibited in their body and their feelings. When a patient is able to discern the connection between the state of his/her body and the subjective feelings; then the therapist comments on these feelings in the context of suffering and impermanence. Once insight into the impermanent nature of their own discomfort is realized, the patient will be able to increase their tolerance for discomfort sufficiently to implement psychotherapeutic interventions. The final step in the psychotherapeutic encounter is imparting the knowledge to the patient that what they choose to do have consequences to themselves and to others around them. Through the joint analysis with the counsellor, the patient is invited to make personal changes.

We first provide a very brief discussion of a few basic ideas from the Indian cultural worldview, followed by application of these culturally based ideas and techniques used in Mansik Psychotherapy.

Core Concepts

Self

- The body is not self,
- Feeling is not self,
- Perception is not self,
- Volition is not self,
- Consciousness is not self,
- All conditions are transient, and
- There is no self in the created or the uncreated. (Salutations of the triple gem, morning chants, English)

Our patients come seeking ways to reduce their emotional or psychological pains. They often come saying things like: "I worry that ..." or "I feel bad because ..." or "A bad thing happened to me..." or a variety of other "I" statements that reference the self in an unhappy state. In making these comments, or feeling these discomforts, the person conceptualizes the existence of a "self". Concepts of self in the context of the family or community and psycho-emotional functions of the self are central to a person's ideas of what makes them uncomfortable. By extension, the self is necessarily involved in the application of mental health interventions.

Who and what is the self that experiences emotional discomforts or psychological pain? What is this self? In medicine, a person is not considered deceased until all brain activities have ceased. By extension, it can be said that the person resides in the brain. However, the brain is not equivalent to the self. The *Abhidhamma* texts refer to the self as a label that is applied to a collection of parts. A general way of understanding the self as a label applied to parts can be understood in this interchange found in the *Abhidhamma* between King Milinda and the Arahat Ven. Nagasena (Mon, 1995: 29).

The King asked, "By what name shall I know you, Sir?"

Venerable Nagasena answered, "My companions call me Nagasena, but the name and the person whom the name refers to do not really exist."

The King commented, "If Nagasena and the person do not exist, to whom do people offer alms and who receive these offerings? Since you receive them, you really exist. Why did you tell a lie in spite of your higher nobility?"

Ven. Nagasena enquired, "Your Majesty, did you come to this monastery on foot or by chariot?"

The King replied, "I came by chariot."

Ven. Nagasena enquired further, "Well then, please show me your chariot? Is the horse the chariot? Is the wheel the chariot? Is the axle the chariot? Is the carriage the chariot?"

The King answered, "No" to all these questions.

Ven. Nagasena remarked, "Is there a chariot beside the horse, the wheel, the axle, the carriage etc.?"

The King again said "No".

Ven. Nagasena commented, "Your Majesty, you said you came here by chariot; yet you could not show me the chariot! Why did you tell a lie in spite of your high honour?"

The King consented, "There is no chariot beside the horse, the wheels, the axle and the carriage. Just a combination of these things has been named the chariot."

Ven. Nagasena remarked, "Very well, your Majesty, you should understand Nagasena as you understood the chariot."

Like the example of the chariot, the self consists of parts. At a minimum, the self consists of the body and the mind. The body contains six (6) sense organs: eye, ear, nose, tongue, skin, and mind. The eye perceives sight; the ear perceives sound; the nose perceives smell; the tongue perceives tastes, the skin perceives touch, and the mind perceives ideas. The person experiences the world through the sense; based on these senses, there is an accompanying feelings; based on these feelings, the mind perceives the world; from the mind's perceptions, consciousness of reality is generated. These sequences of events constitute the parts in the construction of the self.

Mansik psychotherapy rests on this construct of the self; it rests on the idea that the self is made up of parts. The mind, Mansik, is a vital part of the self. Like the parts of the chariot, this mind needs to be maintained to keep it healthy and functioning. The mind is much like water in that a healthy mind allows thoughts to flow freely, much like the water that flows in a river. In contrast, the unhealthy mind is similar to still and foul water where the thoughts are dammed and stuck, as in obsessive rumination. Grasping at thoughts, or ruminations, are the equivalent of damming a flowing river. Thoughts need to be invited to flow freely, to come into the mind and then, on their own accord, to exit the mind. In this way, like the fresh water, new thoughts enter the mind. With new thoughts, the possibility of new perspective on one's own problems is born. Knowing these parts leads a person to sufficient knowledge of the self to make changes.

The first act in maintaining the mind is to notice the mind. Similar to trying to work on the chariot, one cannot do maintenance work on the chariot without knowing where to locate the chariot. One cannot maintain a healthy mind without first being aware of the mind; without first knowing where to find the mind. In Mansik psychotherapy, the patient is introduced to the mind through the learning of applied relaxation and later meditation. However, first are the core cultural concepts used in Mansik Psychotherapy.

Suffering/Dukkha

"*Birth* is *dukkha* (suffering), *ageing* is *dukkha* (suffering), *death* is *dukkha* (suffering); sorrow, lamentation, pain, grief, and despair are *dukkha* (suffering); association with the dislike is *dukkha* (suffering); separation from the liked is *dukkha* (suffering); not getting what is wanted is *dukkha* (suffering)" (SN 56.11).

Birth, ageing and death: One fate common to all who are born is death. On the way to death, humans experience illness, ageing, and the process of dying. The struggle against the inevitability of illness, ageing and death is futile. To believe one can change the inevitable, like preventing the death of a loved one, is arrogant. The struggle against, the attempts to ward off, and/or the denial of the existence of these neutral events cause the emotional and psychological suffering.

Seeking pleasant and avoiding unpleasant: We humans live in continuous contact with the world through our six senses (Bodhi, 2010). Each of the senses give us pleasantries and discomforts; for example: for eyes—things that are beautiful to behold, like a crimson sunset; for ear—things a pleasure to hear, like the song of a lark; for nose—things scrumptious to smell, like fresh baked bread; for tongue—things delicious to taste like fresh fruit; for skin—things luxurious to touch, like silk blanket; and for mind—the idea that pleasant experiences will continue without end. The endless toil to prolong the pleasant sensations drives many of our daily activities. The fear of losing the possibility of acquiring these pleasant sensations, like having enough money to purchase silk blankets, populates many obsessive thoughts. The struggle to keep or acquire pleasing sense experiences causes many emotional and psychological sufferings.

Human Contact

We humans live in contact with other humans. Even those who live in isolation from other humans from day-to-day cannot avoid human contact. For example, the process needed for the construction of one's residence, the provision of food, or even the isolated task of reading a book requires contact with other humans. To get the material, like concrete, necessary for construction of a house, one has to rely on those who mix the concrete. To get the food one consumes daily, one has to rely on the farmer who grows the food. To sit quietly reading a book, one has to rely on the existence of a person who wrote the book. In short, humans are in constant contact with other humans. In this mix of human negotiations, it is inevitable to interact with someone one does or does not like. It seems natural to gravitate towards those who are friends, and shy away from those who are disliked enemies. However, the world is not so accommodating nor is any person so powerful that he/she can avoid to have contact with a disliked person. Therefore, having to interact with those disliked people is inevitable. The emotional agony that often accompanies interactions with distasteful people is self-induced, thus not inevitable. While it is inevitable to interact with someone whom one does not like, the emotional reaction is not inevitable. It is the self-induced emotional discomfort in reaction to the inevitable association with disliked people that causes many emotional and psychological sufferings. Inasmuch as the emotional reaction is self-induced, such negative emotional experiences are within one's control and, therefore, are unnecessary.

In Mansik psychotherapy, the patient is invited to differentiate between natural events, such as ageing or having to associate with unpleasant people, and their self-generated emotional reactions to natural/

neutral events. In the realization that the emotional and psychological reaction is self-generated, the idea that the patient can thus change their emotional and psychological reaction is introduced. With new emotional reactions, the possibility of new perspective on one's own problems is born. Knowledge of this self-induced nature of suffering may give a person sufficient knowledge of the self to make changes.

Impermanence/Anichchha

It would be better... if an uninstructed ordinary person regarded this body, ... as himself rather than the mind. ... This body is seen to continue for a year, for two years, five years, ten years, twenty years, fifty years, a hundred years, and even more. But of that which is called mind, is called thought, is called consciousness, one moment arises and ceases as another continually both day and night (SN 12.61).

That change occurs in the physical realm is undeniable. Newly built houses deteriorate over time; plants grow and decay; the human body changes from childhood to adulthood then to old age. As ageing and death is inevitable, so is change. To the extent that change is inevitable, it is inevitable that pleasant events come to an end. The end of pleasantness may be cause for sadness. Conversely, it is also inevitable that unpleasant events come to an end. The thought and knowledge that whatever unpleasant event is occurring will cease to exist may be cause for human endurance and optimism. Change is so ever present that *the only constant in life seems to be change.*

Events in the mind change even more quickly than what can be perceived in the physical world. Ideas enter into and move out of the mind so quickly it appears to be continuous; like a video, though it is comprised numerous still images, when played they appear to be continuous. Likewise the mind, and by extension, the self, appears to be continuous.

In reality, the person that I am at this very moment is not the person I was a moment ago, nor will I be the same person the next moment in time. An analogy is that the seed is not the tree; the tree is not the fruit, though seed, tree and fruit are derived from each other. The person I was a moment ago is like the seed that will generate the tree. The person I will be in the next moment is like the fruit that is produced by the tree. This continuous change also gives hope for the human capacity to make changes so as to ease the emotional and psychological experience of distress.

Karma and Vipaka: Action has Consequences

A pebble thrown into a pond generates ripples in the water. If a grain of rice is dropped into a small bowl of water, the ripples are distinct and easily seen. If 10 pebbles are successively thrown into a small pond of still water, the interacting effects of the ripples from each pebble thrown are sufficiently distinct to be seen. It is clear to see that the wake from each pebble effect the ripples generated from each successive pebbles. If one thousand pebbles are thrown into a sea, there still are ripples from each pebble. The wake from each pebble thrown will still have effect on ripples from other pebble. However, the interactive effects are much more complex and much less discernible to the casual observer.

Likewise, each action taken by a person is like a pebble thrown into water. Each action taken generates ripples of effects into the complex interactions of humanity. The action taken, be it in body, speech or mind, is a pebble thrown; this is called *Karma*. Each action taken, like a pebble thrown in water, generates its own consequence; the consequence is called *Vipaka*. Like a thousand pebbles thrown into a large ocean, the consequences are almost impossible to discern. Nonetheless, *Karma* and *Vipaka* are as inevitable as ripples generated from pebbles thrown into water.

Karma is action and *Vipaka* the result of action. A person living is in continuous action either through their body, their speech and/or their mind. Each action taken will generate its own consequence. Ill-intentioned actions in body, speech or mind will eventually generate unpleasant consequence. Actions of body, speech or mind taken with wholesome intent will eventually generate pleasant consequence. Thus, it is understood that a person in living creates his own life. In Mansik Psychotherapy intervention, the focus is first on identifying action taken and then eventually to give realizations that there are effects of actions taken; some identifiable, many not identifiable by the individual.

Procedure of Mansik Psychotherapy

When experiencing the mind, one has a tendency to sink in the suffering. The task and goal of the psychotherapy intervention is to help the patient swim instead of sinking into the suffering. Mansik psychotherapy interventions are designed to help the patient note what his/her body needs, understand how he/she is interpreting his/her current life circumstances, and to know what of his/her life situation is impermanent. Eventually, to help the patient discern what part of the suffering is of his/her own making, and then ultimately, what type of choices he/she has to change her experience and life phenomenon.

Because each manifestation of suffering is idiosyncratic to a specific patient, it is difficult to have a general discussion of how Mansik psychotherapist should function with patients. Such discussion would be so general to render it almost useless. Instead, we are choosing to demonstrate the working of Mansik psychotherapy through the analysis of a case. This case is a composite of many cases, the authors have treated. There may be elements that appear to be recognizable to anyone specific case. Such appearance may be a reflection of the wide-ranging experience of the authors, not a faithful reporting of anyone case.

Discussion of general technique and application of Mansik Psychotherapy are covered in this order below, the first section is on how to notice the body; the second section on applying core ideas listed above to a patient's life story; third on analyzing the workings of the mind; and finally on making choices for change.

Attending to the Body: Applied Relaxation

Meena was referred for treatment by a very concerned neighbour because of possible neglect of two young children. On initial visit, her 4 year-old daughter and 2 month-old son accompanied Meena. The two children were clean and well groomed. The 4 year-old clung to Meena, wide-eyed and silent. Meena herself was clean while her clothing was a bit wrinkled and shabby. Meena reports that she has been having some problems taking care of the two children alone in the last month. She feels empty and tearful most of the time; she has not been able to sleep well because of the new baby; and she has no appetite though she knows she should eat for the health of the baby. She has been experiencing suicidal ideations since her husband left the house to work on a construction site in another city. Her mother-in-law also moved out about the same time when her husband left for work last month, leaving her to tend to the child by herself without help.

Reduction of physical tension can be tremendously helpful to the well-being of our mansik health. Relaxation is highly valuable if practiced regularly in daily life. Applied relaxation techniques were first described by Jacobson (1938). These techniques are now widely used to reduce anxiety and cope with stress-related problems. There are countless methods used to achieve relaxation, but the procedures that are most commonly practiced in the clinical setting are related to Jacobson's (1938) Progressive Muscle Relaxation. A meta-analysis of 27 studies during 1997-2007 supports the efficacy of relaxation training for reducing anxiety in psychological and medical patients (Manzoni *et al.*, 2008). Öst's (1987) studies also reported the efficacy of relaxation techniques. Overall, relaxation techniques have garnered consistent empirical support and can be generalized to support one's health.

Through focused practice one can begin to see the difference between relaxed body and tense body. Jacobson's (1938) technique involved first tensing and then releasing major muscle groups in a two-step order. To get ready for relaxation, invite the patient to wear comfortable clothing that does not interfere with free movement. Then have the patient sit comfortably in a quiet place. An armchair or other comfortable seating is ideal. It is not recommended that the patient lie down since there is the chance that the patient will fall asleep while lying down. If this is done before bed, it can improve sleep, but it is important for one to learn to relax while awake.

Once comfortably sitting, invite the patient to take five slow deep breaths while thinking of filling the belly with air on the inhaling, and slowly release like air coming out of a balloon on the exhaling. After 5 deep breaths, instruct the patient to first, tense the muscles, and then relax the tense muscles for approximately 5 seconds, followed by letting go of all the tenseness of the body. In addition, the accompanying breathing is to inhale when tensing the muscles and exhale when releasing the tension, paying attending to each breath. Instruct the patient to tense and relax each muscle group in the following order:

- Foot (to tense the foot one needs to curl their toes downward and then release it)
- Lower leg (for lower leg one need to tighten their calf muscle by pulling toes towards them and then slowly releasing it)
- Entire leg (one needs to squeeze their thigh muscles and then releasing it)
- Hand (for hands one needs to clench their fist and then release it)
- Entire arms (to tighten biceps one needs to draw their forearm up towards their shoulder and to make a muscle while clenching fist and then release it)

- Buttocks (to tighten buttocks one needs to pull their buttocks together and release it)
- Stomach (to tense the stomach one needs to suck their stomach in then release it)
- Chest (to tighten chest one needs to take a deep breath hold the breath and then release it)
- Neck and shoulders (to tense the shoulder one needs to raise their shoulders up to touch their ears and release it)
- Mouth (to tense one's mouth one needs to open their mouth wide enough to stretch the hinges of their jaw and then release it)
- Eyes (to tense one's eyes one needs to clench their eyelids tightly shut and then open it or release it)
- Forehead (to tense one's forehead raise ones eyebrows as far as they can and then release it)

Teach some form of applied relaxation technique in the first session. The Mansik psychotherapist may use Jacobson's technique described above, or any other relaxation technique. Allowing a good amount of time in the first session to go through the relaxation techniques is extremely helpful to provide appropriate training so as to enable the patient to repeat the necessary relaxation exercise at home. It may be helpful to let the patient know that at first, it can feel awkward or discomforting like a chore; however, in time this exercise can be gratifying. Instruct the patient to do this applied relaxation technique at least once a day at home or in their workplace. Many patients claim that their lives are very busy and do not have time to do daily relaxation. Point out that this can take as little as 10-15 minutes a day, so such small amount of time can easily be found some time during the day.

To individualize the exercise, the therapist can make special instructions for specific patient. For example, Meena would be given an additional task of attending to areas around her abdomen for this is where the first hint of hunger will manifest. This can be done by asking Meena to do one round of relaxation for her whole body, and then to repeat the relaxation around her abdomen after the full body relaxation. To individualize the treatment, patients may be instructed to repeat that section of the body that is specially affected by their emotional discomfort. Since Meena's mind is having difficulty feeling the body's experience of hunger, treatment should call special attention to the stomach digestive areas of the body.

Attending to the Body: Breathing

"Experiencing the whole (breath-) body, I shall breathe in", thus he trains himself. "Experiencing the whole (breath-) body, I shall breathe out", thus he trains himself. "Calming the activity of the (breath-) body, I shall breathe in", thus he trains himself. "Calming the activity of the (breath-) body, I shall breathe out", thus he trains himself (Bodhi, 2010).

In the next session, ask the patient what was noticed about the body while doing the relaxation. Inquire if he/she felt her body being warmer or colder, more relaxed or tense, more agitated or tired? Also inquire if she notices any change in her thoughts as she performed the full body relaxation between previous session and current session. Repeat this type of inquiry till the patient has reported success in being more relaxed.

When the patient reports feeling more physically relaxed and sleeping better, then introduce the method to notice the mind. As part of the study of the mind, we have to first train for finding and observing the mind. Just as people are trained on how to do reading or math in school, we provide training to the patient on the mind. One of the easiest and the most time-honoured way to study the mind is first through the observation of the breath.

Instead of Jacobson's relaxation technique in the treatment session; ask the patient to sit comfortably in a relaxed position with their eyes closed. Instruct the patient to focus on the breath while breathing in and breathing out. After the patient has sat for about 2 minutes (depending on the patient, if there is no agitation, he/she can be allowed to sit for up to 5 minutes), ask the patient to open his/her eyes. Asking the patient questions about his/her experience of the breath is the first step in guiding his/her attention; a way of guiding the mind. Ask the following questions about his/her breathing (Nissanka, 1993).

(1) What happens to your chest when you breathe in?
  (a) Does the chest expand when you breath in?
(2) What happens to your stomach when you do not breath in?
  (a) Does your stomach expand when you do not breath in?
(3) Which parts of your body are affected by breathing?

(a) Chest	(b) Neck
(c) Stomach	(d) Heart
(e) Nostrils	(f) Lungs
(g) Ears	(h) Hand

(i) Shoulders
(j) Heart
(k) Eyes
(l) Legs

Ask the patient to perform the attending-to-the-breath exercise daily at home. Have the patient first sit for 5 minutes attending to the breath and then perform the applied relaxation exercise. On return to session, repeat the inquiry with the same set of questions as outlined above. It is not unusual for the patient to start reporting the content of his/her thoughts during attending-to-the-breath and relaxation session. In noticing and reporting the content of their thoughts, the patient has started to notice the mind.

Discuss with the patient that those thoughts may sometimes produce pleasant experiences, or sometimes violent unpleasant experiences. Invite the patient to note these thoughts at home and then bring them into the psychotherapy session for discussion. In the meantime, while practicing at home, invite the patient to consider these thoughts as boats going down the river—some are fast and some are slow, but they all pass. To picture him/her self as sitting on the bank of the river watching the boats go by, noticing the different kinds of boats, but to remain aware of the fact that he/she is not on the boat, thus not to follow the thoughts. Be sure to enquire as to the nature of the thoughts that surfaces during the home sessions of attending-to-the-breath and relaxation exercises.

Listening to the Client's Story

Meena is 24 year-old. She grew up in a poor farming family on the north-eastern border of India. She remembers a happy childhood with her parents and two sisters. She attended school till the end of primary education. She then worked at home and helped her mother with selling their farm products in the markets. Her parents arranged for her marriage to a young man in their village. Meena reported a happy marriage, living close to both her husband and his family. The only difficulty in their marriage was her two miscarriages. He was killed in a car accident when their only child was still an infant. She continued living close to both families after his death. Last year, she met her current husband while selling in the market. He was a construction worker who came out of the worksite for lunch and always made a point to purchase something from her vegetable stall daily. After 6 months, at the end of that construction project, he asked her to marry him, to which she consented. Meena then moved to join him in his native village that was of significant distance from her home village. From the very beginning, her mother-in-law was unhappy with the marriage. She considered her son to be too good for a widow, too good to be raising someone else's child. Meena felt mistreated by her mother-in-law and unsupported by her husband. Constant arguments ensued between all three of them in various combinations about any number of daily activities. He started to drink alcohol in excess. She started to cry constantly. When she became pregnant, her mother-in-law started to pressure her husband to move out and marry someone else. Instead, he signed up for another long-term construction project in a distant city; the mother-in-law moved out to live with her sister; and Meena was left to herself with the young infant and her daughter.

It is the combined parts of the mind that produces consciousness. This consciousness is what patients report to the psychotherapist. Mansik psychotherapy identifies two things: (1) the natural order of things and (2) the workings of the mind. For the first, the Mansik psychotherapist simply labels. Through identifying core ideas by applying labels, the Mansik psychotherapist brings the patient's attention to those parts of his/her life circumstances that are the natural order of things. The elements to identify in the details of the patient's story are those basic concepts listed above—of the types of *dukkha* and of impermanence.

As Meena tells of her life, the Mansik psychotherapist notes the many incidences of inevitable natural order of things in Meena's story. Just as life appears with the birth of her two children; life disappears with the death of her two unborn children through miscarriage and the death of her first husband. The inevitability of illness must have been evident as Meena witnessed her husband's physical pain after the car accident. The inevitability of death is evident in her life circumstances. Using basic counselling skills, the Mansik psychotherapist finds the appropriate times to gently comment on the inevitability of the big life events like birth, illness, ageing and death. In the gentle comments, the Mansik psychotherapist draws Meena's attention to the simple life fact of birth, ageing and death.

The impermanent nature of life circumstances is abundant in Meena's life. The Mansik psychotherapist makes note and comments in a neutral tone on the changing nature of Meena's life. Her early happy childhood with her parents and siblings came to an end when she married. The ending of her childhood changed to the happiness of her first marriage. The unhappiness of the miscarriages came to an end with the birth of her first child. The happiness of her first marriage ended with her husband's death. The sadness of widowhood ended when she married her second husband. The comforts of associating with her parents ended with moving away with her second husband. The daily discomfort of associating with her mother-in-law ended when she moved out of the house. That happy and unhappy events' end is the nature of impermanence. The Mansik psychotherapist comments are not to be accompanied by judgements of desirability or avoidance of each incident, but neutral noticing of the changing nature of life, thus the impermanence of life situations.

Listening to the Client's Mind

Meena's thoughts are like a stream flowing from one topic to another:

1. She *thought* it was unfair of her mother-in-law to think Meena is not good enough for her son.
2. She *thought* her mother-in-law was incorrectly grouping young widows and divorcees together, thus rendering widows as loose women, which Meena is not.
3. She *thought* her mother-in-law to be a bad person to have such evil thoughts about her son's wife.
4. She *thought* her husband was a very weak person not to defend her honour against his mother's accusations of Meena seducing her mother-in-law's son, whom the mother thought was an innocent when he met Meena.
5. She *regretted* ever agreeing to a love marriage; condemning herself as a weak person for not being able to resist the romantic pursuit of such a handsome man as her husband.
6. She now *thinks* she is not pretty enough to keep his love since he has decided to work on another construction site.
7. She is *sure* that he will fall in love with someone else at this new construction site, just as he fell in love with her at his previous construction site.
8. She *disbelieves* his attestation of disinterest in any other woman except her.
9. She *believes* he is lying to her so as to get her to stay in his house to take care of his child.
10. She *wishes* he would just come home and stay with her instead of going off to work.
11. She *resents* his ruin of her beauty by begetting her with a child,

thus ruining any future chances of a happy marriage with someone else.

12. She *berates* herself for not listing and waiting for her parents to find her another husband.
13. She *misses* her parents and her home village so much that she does not want to leave the house since to leave the house is to be reminded of the reality that where she lives is not her home village.
14. She *fears* her mother-in-law is right that Meena is so evil that she has driven her husband to drink and thus will ruin any chance of future fidelity and happiness.

After bringing the patient's attention to the body and teaching the patient how to notice the condition of the body, the second focus of the Mansik psychotherapy approach is to bring the patient's attention to the workings of the mind. As patients progress in their daily home practice sessions, their reports of those thoughts that float through their mind will become ever more rich and complex. It is the Mansik psychotherapist's opportunity to notice and make comment on the state of their mind. It is not the aim or the ultimate goal of Mansik psychotherapy to develop a trained meditator or a *yogi*, but to provide psychotherapy within the framework of the Indian and Nepalese worldview. Thus, the treatment technique is for the Mansik psychotherapist to notice, note and comment on the identified parts of the mind as it manifests during the patient's reporting of their life circumstances or their continuous and newly noticed thoughts. In Meena's reported thoughts are evidence of the construction of a self and the emotions/notions that befuddle the mind. As categorized in the *Vatthupama Sutta*, there are sixteen types of befuddled mind states. These mind states are: (1) Covetousness and unrighteous greed, (2) ill-will, (3) anger, (4) hostility or malice, (5) denigration or contempt, (6) domineering or presumption, (7) envy, (8) jealousy or selfishness, (9) hypocrisy or deceit, (10) fraud, (11) obstinacy, (12) presumption or rivalry, (13) conceit, (14) arrogance, (15) vanity, and (16) negligence in social behaviour or lack of consideration (Thera, 2013). Chief among the 16 listed in the *Vatthupama Sutta* are the three common states of greed, anger, delusion (or misapprehension of reality) (Bodhi, 2010). Each of these mind states can and do produce emotional and psychological pain. Categorizing Meena's mind states and noted by the Mansik Psychotherapist may be thus:

She thought it was unfair of her mother-in-law to think Meena is not good enough for her son.	This is an angry mind in which the thoughts manifest.	Anger
She thought her mother-in-law was incorrectly grouping young widows and divorcees together, thus rendering widows as loose women, which Meena is not.	This is an angry mind in which the thoughts manifest.	Anger
She thought her mother-in-law to be a bad person to have such evil thoughts about her son's wife.	This is an angry mind filled with hatred in which the thoughts manifest.	Anger
She thought her husband was a very weak person not to defend her honour against his mother's accusations of her seducing her husband, who was an innocent when he met Meena.	This is an angry mind filled with hatred and ill-will in which the thoughts manifest.	Anger
She regretted ever agreeing to a love marriage; condemning herself also as a weak person not being able to resist the romantic pursuit of such a handsome man as her husband.	This is an angry mind against herself in which the thoughts manifest.	Anger
She now thinks she is not pretty enough to keep his love since he decided to go on another construction site.	This is a diluted misguided mind in which the thoughts manifest since she has not significantly changed her physical appearance in the last year.	Diluted mind (Misapprehension of reality)
She is sure that he will fall in love with someone else at this new construction site, just as he fell in love with her at his previous construction site.	This is a diluted misguided mind in which the thoughts manifest since she cannot know what the future will bring.	Diluted mind (Misapprehension of reality)
She disbelieves his attestation of disinterest in any other woman except her. She believes he is lying to her so as to get her to stay in his house to take care of his child.	This is a diluted misguided mind in which the thoughts manifest since she cannot know whether he is speaking truth.	Diluted mind (Misapprehension of reality)
She wishes he would just come home and stay with her instead of going off to work.	This is a greedy mind in which the thoughts manifest.	Greed
She resents his ruin of her beauty by begetting her with child, thus ruining any future chances of a happy marriage.	This is an angry mind in which the thoughts manifest.	Anger
She berates herself for not listing and waiting for her parents to find her another husband.	This is an angry mind in which the thoughts manifest.	Anger
She misses her parents and her home village so much that she does not want to leave the house to be reminded of the reality that where she lives is not her home village.	This is an angry and a greedy mind filled with desire and hatred in which the thoughts manifest. This is greed because she is filled with want.	Anger and Greed
She fears her mother-in-law is right that Meena is so evil that she has driven her husband to drink and thus will ruin any chance of future fidelity and happiness.	This is an angry mind filled with hatred and misapprehension in which the thoughts manifest.	Anger

The Mansik Psychotherapist noting and making comment might sound like "hmmm, that mind seemed to be full of regret when you think about now living in this village" or "I wonder if you experience anger when you think about your husband leaving to work on another construction site?" In calling attention to the mind state of greed, hatred and/or misapprehension of reality, the Mansik psychotherapist introduces Meena to her mind.

Once introduced to her mind, the Mansik Psychotherapist is then able to talk to Meena about her mind and mind states. Inquiries such as, "do you like it when your mind is filled with anger?" becomes possible. A discussion about anger can then be had. Psychotherapeutic dialogue is able to move away from things that are beyond Meena's control, such as mother-in-law's opinion of Meena, and move into a realm in which Meena does have some control, such as her angry reaction to her mother-in-law. Having identified the anger, it is an easy step to invite Meena to discuss her anger as a condition outside of her 'self', not as the self that is buffeted by the ill winds of fortune, such as an un-loving mother-in-law.

The interventions of Mansik Psychotherapy at this stage of treatment are focused on holding exhaustive discussions of each of the mind state that populate Meena's thoughts. Exhaustive discussions might include such topics as: how Meena's body feels when in the mind state of, for example anger; the rhythms of Meena's breath when the mind is angry; whether anger is a long time familiar state or a new state introduced since her second marriage; whether Meena likes the state of anger because it might give her energy to sustain self-pride; whether Meena dislikes the state of anger because it might keep her from talking to her husband; whether Meena thought herself to be sharper of mind and tongue when angry; whether Meena thought herself a better mother when angry; and any other aspects of anger that may be relevance for Meena.

The questions explored by the Mansik Psychotherapist and the patient would depend on the specifications of each patient. In general, the lines of inquiry would include the breath, the tension location in the body, the history and familiarity of the patient with each mind state, the accompanying opinion of the patient for each mind state exhibited in the thoughts manifest during her daily practice of attending to the body and applied relaxation and finally, whether she wishes to keep each of the mind states or whether she likes to work towards greater self-determination in responding to each of the mind states.

Decision for Change

After noticing and identifying mind states, and knowing the nature of suffering, the treatment interventions can focus on changing action, be it in body, speech or mind. Discussions between the Mansik Psychotherapist and the patient at this stage of treatment turns to the patient's capacity for change through his/her ability to decide or to change, emphasizing that making positively intended actions (*Karma*) will elicit positive consequences (*vipaka*).

Meena's mind is often in an anger state. The counter for anger, as explicated in many of the *suttas*, is loving-kindness. The first person towards whom one is to extend loving kindness is to one self. The Mansik Psychotherapy interventions would, therefore, focus on having Meena incorporate acts of loving kindness towards herself in her daily life, first towards the body and then towards the mind. The first area to target for intervention would be Meena's physical condition. Such an action for change to loving kindness towards her own situation may take the form of an invitation for Meena to heed her body's need for un-interrupted sleep. Meena and the Mansik psychotherapist could discuss ways for Meena to show loving-kindness towards her physical situation by acknowledging her need for help in the care of her baby in order to obtain un-interrupted sleep. To that aim, Meena might reach out to her neighbour, asking for temporary help to care for her baby. Alternatively, Meena might contact her mother to come temporarily live with Meena until she is physically better. The focus of discussion at this stage of Mansik Psychotherapy is to help Meena decide to turn towards loving kindness in her actions in regard to her own physical distress. By Meena taking care of her own physical needs, she then extends this loving-kindness to her children in the form of being more present and responsive to the needs of her two young children.

The second area of intervention is in taking care of the mind. The mind can be thought of as a city, and one's attention is the guard standing at the city gate. The primary duties of a guard are to protect the city through allowing entry to friends and shutting out enemies, as well as giving early alarm for approaching dangers. An attentive guard notices every person who seeks entry; knows the identity of those who are enemies and those who are friends; keeps out those who are enemies while opening the city gates for those who are friends; recognizes potential threatening conditions approaching the city and give early alarm so that those inside have time to mount a good defence against the approaching danger.

The Mansik Psychotherapist might suggest Meena to guard the mind against temptations to anger by shutting the mind's gate, as in not giving mind-thinking time, to enemies. This could take on the form of a discussion inviting Meena not to obsessively replay in her mind, thus giving thought time, to the spiteful words spoken by her mother-in-law. Concurrently, the Mansik psychotherapist might suggest Meena open wide the city gate, as in giving mind attention time, to friendly thoughts. For example, Meena might think about acts of kindness by her neighbour who referred Meena for treatment, or by her husband when he spends time at home on the weekends.

Meena's self-incriminating thoughts are a special virulent type of anger. This is an anger that is directed at the self. Her thinking that she is a weak person for loving her husband is an example of self-hatred. The counter to this type of self-hatred is still loving-kindness. This might include in-session dialogue regarding forgiveness and compassion. The Mansik psychotherapist might suggest that Meena could not have known the character of her mother-in-law when she and her husband were first getting to know each other; that it is misapprehension of reality to think she could have predicted the problems generated from her mother-in-law. In addition, the Mansik psychotherapist might remind Meena to be especially protective of her mind by guarding against angry thoughts from herself to herself.

Her desire to have her husband home with her is a form of greed. The counter to greed is generosity. The Mansik psychotherapist might explore her mental clutching at her husband to stay with her in their home instead of going to work. By Meena focusing on his absence, she reinforces her sense of desperation. Meena might be invited to consider focusing instead on the pleasant times they share when he is home. From attending to the times he is a loving husband, she is able to give generously of her enjoyment of his presence, may be her sense of deprivation would then recedes somewhat.

Finally, the Mansik psychotherapist could point out Meena's thoughts that do not accurately reflect reality. Thoughts like she is not pretty, that her mother-in-law looks down on widows, that widows are loose women, or that her husband lies to her are not based on verifiable reality. It is doubtful that her husband would endorse any of those ideas should Meena ask him. Meena might be reminded not to give credence to misapprehensions of reality.

By suggesting any and all of the above listed interventions, the Mansik psychotherapist is either implicitly or explicitly reminding Meena that she has a choice to act differently. In the act of choosing a different behaviour, or a different attitude, or an alternative thought, Meena is altering her *Karma*—for a more positive pleasant future situation.

Concluding Thoughts

Mansik psychotherapy is therapy of mind. A part of the construction of a person's mind is his/her experience with his/her family, community, and his/her life journey. During this journey, natural and normal events occur, such as birth, ageing and death. Suffering occurs when the mind construes such natural and normal events to be undesirable and cling to the desire for pleasant experiences to replace and overcome unpleasant experiences. Most importantly, humans crave and thrive upon contact with others in a manner that produces happiness and growth. However, life's events are impermanent like changing seasons or night after day and conditions of emotional pain and hurt are fleeting. One's *Karma*, the actions he/she takes and chooses in daily life, decides what *Vipaka* or results will be. In other words, the consequences of actions taken and decisions made in an attempt to reduce the subjective experience of negative emotional and psychological mind states can strongly impact one's life's circumstances. In order to facilitate change and bring solace and understanding, the Mansik psychotherapist begins with acceptance of one's situation that cannot be changed, such as an unpleasant mother-in-law. Through relaxation, the Mansik psychotherapist creates awareness and understanding of the body. Listening to the client's story of suffering is merely part of a total story where suffering has originated yet is not a permanent state. The psychotherapist continues to listen to the client's mind, especially the part of the mind that is resonant with all the negative emotions and suffering state (i.e. anger, guilt, shame, hatred and tempered/ worried mind). Overall, the Mansik psychotherapist supports the client to navigate through the suffering created by the mind in order to heal and tolerate life's changes.

References

Balkrishna, V., Sanghvi, L., Rana, K., Doongaji, D., and Vahia, N. (1977). The comparison of psychophysiological therapy with drug therapy. *Indian Journal of Psychiatry*, 19(2), 87.

Berlin, E.A., and Fowkes Jr., W.C. (1983). A teaching framework for cross-cultural healthcare—application in family practice. *Western Journal of Medicine*, 139(6), 934.

Betancourt, J.R. (2003). Cross-cultural medical education: Conceptual approaches and frameworks of evaluation. *Academic Medicine,* 78(6), 560-565.

Bodhi, B. (2010) "Purification of Mind": Access to Insight (Legacy Edition) Retrieved from http://www.accesstoinsight.org/lib/authors/bodhi/bps-essay_04.html

Borkovec, T.D., and Sides, J.K. (1979). Critical procedural variables related to the physiological effects of progressive relaxation: A Review. *Behaviour Research and Therapy,* 17(2), 119-125.

Daya, R. (2002). Buddhist Psychology, a theory of change process: Implications for counsellors. *International Journal for the Advancement of Counselling,* 22(4), 257-271.

Dhairyam, D. (1961). *Research need for development of psychotherapy. Recent Trends in Psychology*. New Delhi, India: Orient Longmans.

Harkness, S. and Super, C.M. (2002). Culture and parenting, In M.H. Bornstein (ed.), *Handbook of Parenting*, 2, 253-280.

Hanscom, K.L. (2001). Treating survivors of war trauma and torture. *American Psychologist*, 56(11), 1032-1039.

Hoch, E.M. (1974). Pir, faquir and psychotherapists. *The Human Context*, 6.

Hosseini, S.A. (1983). An elementary study of the principles of individual and group psychotherapy and mental health in Islam. *Indian Journal of Psychiatry*, 25(4), 335.

Kirmayer, L.J. (1991). The place of culture in psychiatric nosology: Taijin kyofusho and DSM-III-R. *The Journal of Nervous and Mental Disease*, 179(1), 19-28.

Kumar, P.S. and Thomas, B. (2007). Family intervention therapy in alcohol dependence syndrome: One-year follow-up study. *Indian Journal of Psychiatry*, 49(3), 200.

Levin, S.J., Like, R.C. and Gottlieb, J.E. (2000). ETHNIC : A framework for culturally competent clinical practice. *Appendix: Useful Clinical Interviewing Mnemonics. Patient Care,* 34 (9), 188-189.

Manickam, L.S.S. and Kapur, M. (1985). Empathy in professionals and trained lay counsellors: A comparison. *Indian Journal of Psychiatry*, 27(4), 297.

Manickam L.S. S. (1990). Empathy: A comparative study of professionals and lay counsellors using hypothetical situations. *Indian Journal of Psychiatry*, 32(1), 83.

Manzoni, G.M., Pagnini, F., Castelnuovo, G., and Molinari, E. (2008). Relaxation training for anxiety: a ten-years applied review with meta-analysis. *BMC Psychiatry,* 8(1), 41.

Mon, T.M. (1995). *Buddha Abhidhamma: Ultimate Science*. Yongon Myanmar, China: Buddanet's Book Library.

Nand, S.D. (1959). Analytic psychotherapy is applied biology. *Indian Journal of Psychiatry,* 1, 5.

Nand, S.D. (1961). A comparative study of scientific and religious psychotherapy with a special study of the role of the commonest Shivite symbolic model in total psychoanalysis. *Indian Journal of Psychiatry,* 3, 73.

Neki, J.S. (1977). Psychotherapy in India. *Indian Journal of Psychiatry,* 19(1), 10.

Neki, J.S. (1992). Editorial: Confidentiality, secrecy and privacy in psychotherapy: Socio-dynamic considerations. *Indian Journal of Psychiatry,* 34 (3), 171.

Öst, L.G (1987). Applied relaxation: description of a coping technique and review of controlled studies. *Behaviour Research and Therapy*, 25(5), 397-409.

Sinha, D. (1986). *Psychology in a Third Would Country: The Indian Experience.* New Delhi: Sage Publications.

Sinha, D. (1993). *Indigenization of psychology in India and its relevance.* Based on a paper presented at the Symposium on Indigenous Psychologies during the Eighth International Conference of Cross-Cultural Psychology, Istanbul, Turkey, July 1986. Sage Publications, Inc.

Subba, S. (1994). Review of psychology text-book. *Manas: Journal of Central Association of Psychology*, Kathmandu, Nepal.

Sue, D. and Sue, D. (1999). *Counselling the Culturally Different: Theory and Practice,* (3) New York: John Wiley & Sons.

Surya, N.C. and Jayaram, S.S. (1968). Some basic considerations in the practice of psychotherapy in the Indian setting. *Indian Journal of Psychiatry,* 46, 153.

Thera, Nyanaponika. (2013). *Vatthupama Sutta: The Simile of the Cloth* (MN 7), translated from the Pali. Access to Insight (Legacy Edition). Retrieved from http://www.accesstoinsight.org/tipitaka/mn/mn.007.nypo.html.

Verma, V.K. (1982). Present state of psychotherapy in India. *Indian Journal of Psychiatry*, 24(3), 209.

Vahia, N.S., Vinekar, S.L., and Doongaji, D.R. (1966). Some ancient Indian concepts in the treatment of psychiatric disorders. *The British Journal of Psychiatry*, 112(492), 1089-1096.

Wig, N.N. (2004). Hanuman complex and its resolution: An illustration of psychotherapy from Indian mythology. *Indian Journal of Psychiatry,* 46(1), 25.

4

Effectiveness of Yogic Lifestyle for Promoting Mental Health and Well-being

Implications for Therapeutic Value and School Healthcare Policy

Arun Pratap Singh

This chapter was conducted against the backdrop of sparse research on health-promotive value of Yogic Lifestyle (YLS), in particular among adolescents and rudimentary objective and coverage in and also inadequacy in research design of available studies to account for relationship between Yogic lifestyle and comprehensive aspects of mental health and wellness among adolescents. The study was conducted in a residential school using Between-Within Group Design. The students were divided into two groups—one serving as a control group (N=50) and the other intervention group (N=50). The participants in the intervention group were persuaded to adopt Yogic lifestyle through a theory-guided psycho-education programme. The data, analyzed by using SPSS 16.0 indicated that the adolescents who underwent positive changes in lifestyle behaviours (i.e. dietary habits, food intake, sleep habits, and practicing yoga) reported increase in self-reported health across physical, social, psychological and spiritual domains. In view of above findings, this chapter sketches out important implications for therapeutic relevance of Yoga in school counselling and charts out some important policy measures for incorporating Yogic lifestyle in school health education.

Introduction

Yoga has emerged as a major holistic approach popular for promoting health and well-being throughout the world. The significance of Yoga in daily life can be understood from the recent declaration by UNO regarding observance of International Yoga day on 21st June with the support of more than one hundred and forty countries. Recently, in a speech to the U.N. General Assembly, Prime Minister of India observed that Yoga can bring a change in our lifestyle and create awareness in us. In contrast to popular perception of it being identified with a set of postures and breathing practices, Yoga, has been practiced and preached by Indian seers as a part of daily life. *Yoga Sutras* of Patanjali outlined an eightfold path which mentions importance of postures, breath regulation, dietary change, use of sacred sounds etc. for increasing wellness at different levels of being. Several experiential accounts of Yoga practitioners demonstrate that holistic changes in life related to diet, sleep, and daily routine can alleviate multiple physical, emotional and social sufferings (Balkrishna, 2007; *Bhagavad Gita*, 6/17; Ram, 1987; Ramdeo, 2006). In view of plasticity and suitability for change in behaviours, induction of Yogic lifestyle has been favoured during adolescence in many indigenous perspectives in India (Koller, 2006: 97).

In current scenario, while living choices and engagements among adolescents seem to be increasingly and heavily influenced and swayed by plethora of living choices (i.e. fast foods, cold drinks, alcohol, drug, and unhealthy leisure time use etc.) offered by persuasive media and market interfering with mind-body functioning, Yogic lifestyle has become increasingly relevant. It deserves special scrutiny in view of its promising potential to address mental health concerns and social problems such as aggression, violence, suicide, sexual crimes, which are difficult to resolve through mainstream medical model either due to its inability to do so or due to limited availability of expertise and human resources to address the same (Antaramian, Huebner and Valois, 2008; Hans, 1994; Sharma and Misra, 2009; Planning Commission, 2000; Sharma and Sharma, 2008; Singh, 2010; Singh and Misra, 2012; Verma and Saraswathi, 2002; Yarcheski, Mahon, and Yarcheski, 1997). Several scholars have expressed need for inducting such interventions in school setting. Perry and Jessor (1985) have speculated about effectiveness of school-based preventive interventions on differential, but interrelated domains of health: psychological health (subjective sense of well-being), social health (role fulfilment and social effectiveness), personal health (realization of individual potential), and physical health (physical-physiological functioning). Yarcheski, Mahon, and Yarcheski (1997) argued for need of such programme for improving physical health, cognitive ability, academic achievement, social interaction skills, and various indicators of motivational and emotional functioning. Tiwari,

Agarwal, Kumar, and Pandey (2007) expressed their presumptions for relevance of behavioural interventions to get rid of unhealthy behaviours and promotion of wellness. Many practitioners and famous writers have observed that culturally-sensitive and contextually-relevant eastern religious-spiritual practices can be considerably more effective than existing traditional psychological practices in promoting multiple aspects of health (Kakar, 2003; Parashar, 2000; Rao, 2000; Roy, 2000; Sharma and Sharma, 2008).

After considerable neglect, Yogic notions of lifestyle, causes of illness, suffering, mediators of well-being, and wellness practices recently have started getting attention from psychologists (Dalal, 2001; Kapoor, 2002; Misra, 2005; Sinha, 1990). There are studies which have utilized some key elements of Yogic lifestyle for reducing addictions (Kissen and Kissen, 2009; Woolery, Myers, Stemliebm, Zeltzer, 2004), depression (Pilkington, Kirkwood, Rampes, Richardson, 2005), low back pain (Gatantino *et al.*, 2004), symptoms of cancer (Carson *et al.*, 2007; Ragvendra *et al.*, 2007), treatment of arthritis (Kolasinski, Garfinkel, Tsai, Matz, Dyke, Schumacher, 2005), managing stress (Arora and Bhattacharjee, 2008; Granath, Ingvarsson, von Thiele, Lundberg, 2006), cardiovascular disorders (Bharshankar, Bharshankar, Deshpande, Kaore, Gosavi, 2003; Oken *et al.*, 2006), improving sleep quality among cancer patients (Cohen, Warneke, Fouladi, Rodriguez, Chaoul-Reich, 2004) in adults or elderly segment of population.

However, research on the effect of Yogic lifestyle on mental health and well-being among school adolescents is sparse and segmented in conceptual repertoire. Majority of the related studies, which have been conducted among patients or in hospitals, are either rudimentary in their objective or inadequate in their research design to account for relationship between Yogic lifestyle and adolescent well-being. Some previous studies have noted significant changes in some health-related outcomes within a short period of one or two weeks. In one of the prospective controlled study conducted at Integrated Health Clinic, AIIMS, Delhi significant improvement was noted in subjective well-being of normal and diseased sample in age-range of 21-70 years after a brief Yoga based lifestyle intervention only for 10 days (Sharma, Gupta, and Bijlani, 2008). In another study on Yogic lifestyle intervention for a period of two weeks, which included practice of *asanas*, *pranayama*, meditation and consumption of yogic diet, significant reduction was noted in anxiety and depression in persons suffering from gastrointestinal disorder (Mishra and Sinha, 2001). Rani and Rao (2005) noted significant decrease in depression participants of an intervention programme which included some elements of Yoga (including postures, breathing practices, cleansing activities, physical gestures). Broota *et al.* (1995) compared the efficacy of three relaxation techniques: Broota Relaxation Technique, Jacobson's Progressive Muscle Relaxation and a Yogic relaxation practice (*Shavasana*) in reducing symptoms of hypertension and found that Yogic relaxation technique was most effective. The promising possibility of effectiveness of Yoga with behaviour therapy in treating Obsessive Compulsive Disorder has also been subsequently noted (Datta and Broota, 2000). Recent empirical evidences have noted multiple positive effects of postures in reducing anxiety, stress, and psychological disorders (Rani, and Rao, 2005; Rao, 1995; Rao, 2000; Roy, 2000). Hamilton, Nelson, Stevens and Kitzman (2007) reported positive relationship between regular sleep and psychological well-being based on the findings of a study among community residents (N = 502). While, there is abundance of work on risk behaviours (i.e. unprotected sexual activity, drug abuse, alcohol use, violence), there are only few reviews suggesting the possibility about religiosity as an important protective factor for adolescent well-being (Cotton *et. al.*, 2006; Verma and Saraswathi, 2002). The efficacy of many other Yogic lifestyle practices such as dietary habits and regularity in sleep in protecting and promoting health and well-being remain unexplored.

Thus, against the backdrop of lack of studies and potentials of Yogic lifestyle in promoting positive well-being, the present study was aimed at assessing the impact of positive lifestyle changes on adolescent self-reported health. It was assumed that holistic lifestyle changes introduced through YLSIP would promote perception of improvement in all the domains of health. Accordingly, YLSIP was designed to assess the effects of lifestyle changes on adolescent well-being.

Module of Yogic Lifestyle Intervention Programme (YLSIP)

The intervention programme consisted of an integrated module of Yogic lifestyle based on the insights from research literature, personal experiences, and encounters with adolescents in schools. The module was prepared with the following objectives: (a) to create an awareness that health and well-being can be enhanced by changing the lifestyle, (b) to induce adherence for dietary change, (c) to administer Yoga training programme feasible in the setting to reduce health risks and enhance well-being, and (d) to evaluate the efficacy of YLSIP in enhancing health and well-being among adolescents. During planning of YLSIP some of the practical issues related to capability of the participants to adhere with YLSIP, school routine, availability of adolescents for Yoga training programme was taken under consideration. The progression of YLSIP was based on insights derived from theoretical models of behavioural change. It was undertaken in three stages (i.e., preparation, introduction and implementation). Table 4.1 shows the details of strategies, activities, processes and goals during the different stages of YLSIP. The first stage aimed at preparing the adolescents to participate in LSIP. To this end, they were acquainted to the investigator who was providing the intervention. The participants were provided inputs during the second step of stage 1 through an interactive session about the risks of practicing unhealthy habits and benefits of practicing positive lifestyle behaviours.

Table 4.1: Details of Strategies, Activities, Processes and Goals during the Different stages of YLSIP

Stages	*Steps*	*Strategy*	*Activities*	*Process*	*Goal*
Preparation	(i) Rapport Formation				
	(ii) Creating Awareness	Providing information	Interactive session dealing with healthy/unhealthy lifestyle practices	Creating cognitive dissonance	Making the participants to know about the positive effects of lifestyle changes
Introduction	(i) Persuasion	Observational learning	Presentations of role models (i.e. actors, sport persons) through the films, and power point	Modelling	Persuading adolescents to consider imitation
	(ii) Planning	Intentional change	Addressing the pros and cons of the benefits and barriers of changing lifestyle	Reasoning and planning	Inducing the readiness for change in the lifestyle
Implementation	(i) Training	Reward for change and encouragement	Giving positive personal feedback	Reinforce-ment	Compliance for change
	(ii) Persistence	Approval	Video recording of last session, participation of principal and teachers of the school, praise by principal	Recognition	Continue with change in the lifestyle

It was assumed that this would create a cognitive dissonance among them. The second stage aimed at creating readiness among adolescent. Taking cues from social learning theory (Bandura, 1977), fist step of the introduction stage of LSIP included a power point presentation and a film about practicing of some components of LSIP by some of the popular role models (film, sports and public life). Deriving ideas from theory of reasoned action and the observation that people process information thoughtfully only when they perceive it as personally important (Ajzen and Fishbein, 1980), the second step of introduction stage involved addressing the pros and cons of changing lifestyle. The participants were encouraged to talk freely about their individual concerns. In the third stage of intervention, i.e. implementation of a training programme was run for about two weeks. In the first step of implementation, the participants were reinforced by giving personal regards for changing their lifestyle after each Yoga training programme so as to create compliance for lifestyle change.

Each day of YLSIP began with a Yoga session of 45 minutes specially designed for this study on the basis of expert advice, feasibility and relevance to concerns related to academic competence. It included practices related to Yoga, i.e. *Asanas, Pranayama*, *Shavasana* and chanting of *mantras* (i.e. Om, Allahoo, and O Christ) included from different religious traditions. Besides, intervention group participants were engaged in positive change of their dietary habits, avoid unhealthy food items, and follow proper sleep habits and perform Yoga for two weeks.

Subjects and Methods

A sample of 100 school-going adolescents (50 boys and 50 girls) enrolled in junior and senior secondary classes in a residential school participated in the study. The participation in the study was based on two criteria: (1) participants should not have been exposed to the contents of LSIP during the last three months; and (2) they should not be suffering from any disease (*e.g.*, physical disability, chronic diseases, fever etc.) which may impair adherence to the YLSIP. There was equal number of adolescents in intervention and control groups. The mean age of the participants in the intervention group was 14.5 years (SD = 1.89). In the control condition, the mean age was 14.4 yrs (SD = 1.89). The two groups were matched for gender, age and grade. They participated in the study as shown in Fig. 4.1:

For measuring self-reported health, a questionnaire was developed

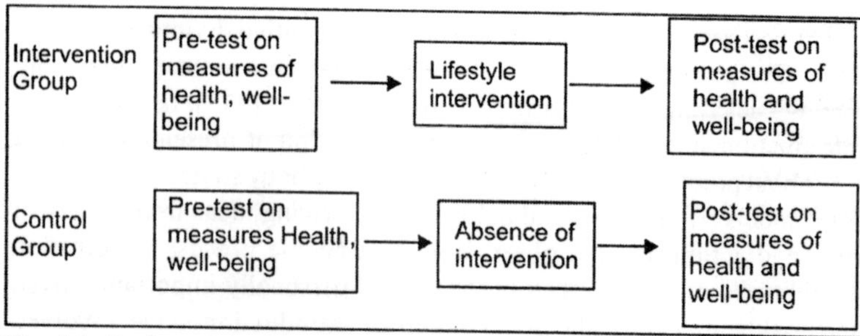

Fig. 4.1: Design of the lifestyle intervention programme (LSIP).

by present researcher using relevant items of existing measures. It consists of 61 items measuring 14 components related to the following domains: bodily illness, insomnia, digestibility, physical fitness, body image, self-esteem, depression, anxiety, goal clarity, adjustment, alienation, and empathy. The items for evaluating *illness* were adapted from the PGI Health Questionnaire (Wig and Verma, 1978). These included common physical complaints such as headache, allergy, constipation, diarrhoea, absence in school due to illness and limitations in performing daily routine activities. The *insomnia* subscale was related to difficulty in sleeping. The items related to *digestion* dealt with the items of hunger and appetite. The *fitness* dimension measured physical stamina, lack of fatigue and freshness after sleep. The items related to *negative body image* were adapted from Body Image Avoidant Questionnaire developed by Riva and Molinari, 1998. It has items related to concerns for appearance and addictiveness for beauty products. The *self-esteem* items dealt with self-confidence and enthusiasm in life. The *anxiety* related items referred to the feelings of embarrassment, irritation and lack of concentration. The *depression* related items dealt with loneliness, guilt and shame. *Clarity of life goal* was assessed by asking about accurate perception of one's life goal. The *adjustment* related items dealt with familial relationships. The *empathy* component dealt with ability for identifying others' concerns and developing trust in the relationships. *Alienation* was measured with the help of anxiety scale of MMPI. It dealt with cohesiveness with social group and ability to share own feelings and thoughts.

The respondents were asked to report their functioning and concerns in different areas of life and rate every item on 5-point scale varying from 'never', 'rarely', 'sometimes', 'usually', to 'always' based on their experiences. The items of illness, insomnia, negative body image, depression, anxiety and alienation were negatively scored so as to denote presence of these negative aspects of health. The items related to digestion, fitness, self-esteem, clarity of life goal, empathy, and adjustment were scored positively. The internal consistency of the scale was found to be satisfactory computed by Cronback Alpha=0.89 (N=100).

Lifestyle Change Inventory: The compliance on multiple components of LSIP during follow-up was assessed through a self-report inventory on 7-point rating scale. The respondents were asked of reporting their adherence to the changes during a usual week in last one year. The researcher for use in the present study developed it.

Table 4.2: Means and SDs of Scores on the Measures of Health and Well-being by Type of Group, Gender and Testing Occasions

Measures	*Intervention Group*				*Control Group*			
	Boys (N= 25)		*Girls (N= 25)*		*Boys (N=25)*		*Girls (N=25)*	
	Pre-test	*Post-test*	*Pre-test*	*Post-test*	*Pre-test*	*Post-test*	*Pre-test*	*Post-test*
Illness	12.80 (3.02)	8.68 (2.60)	11.04 (2.65)	7.96 (2.20)	10.92 (3.17)	11.12 (2.90)	10.32 (2.80)	10.16 (2.71)
Insomnia	4.44 (1.80)	2.88 (1.01)	4.16 (1.77)	3.00 (1.35)	4.04 (1.56)	4.20 (1.77)	4.08 (1.91)	3.84 (1.67)
Digestion	5.96 (2.18)	7.52 (2.02)	7.20 (1.63)	7.36 (1.70)	6.72 (2.11)	7.28 (1.81)	6.88 (1.92)	6.56 (1.82)
Fitness	9.56 (2.98)	12.48 (2.12)	10.52 (2.66)	12.04 (2.73)	10.40 (2.92)	11.36 (1.86)	10.80 (2.25)	10.44 (2.27)
Negative body image	9.72 (3.15)	6.64 (1.86)	8.60 (2.81)	6.44 (2.12)	9.04 (2.85)	8.84 (3.15)	7.64 (2.70)	9.12 (3.05)
Self-esteem	10.56 (2.81)	12.00 (2.08)	10.40 (2.43)	12.52 (1.53)	10.28 (2.42)	10.36 (2.09)	10.80 (2.39)	10.48 (2.70)
Depression	7.68 (2.24)	6.72 (1.54)	7.68 (1.65)	7.60 (1.15)	8.32 (2.15)	7.72 (2.01)	8.16 (1.92)	7.96 (1.61)
Anxiety	9.16 (2.88)	6.56 (2.87)	8.00 (2.53)	6.40 (1.60)	8.00 (2.90)	7.24 (2.81)	8.04 (1.81)	7.64 (1.93)
Goal Clarity	6.32 (2.13)	7.84 (2.26)	6.56 (1.68)	8.00 (1.80)	7.00 (1.97)	6.24 (1.78)	7.40 (1.84)	6.88 (1.56)
Adjustment	11.16 (2.57)	13.24 (1.92)	11.68 (2.17)	13.00 (1.73)	11.76 (2.61)	11.64 (2.53)	12.12 (2.27)	12.00 (2.06)
Alienation	7.64 (2.48)	5.72 (1.94)	7.96 (2.07)	5.76 (1.92)	7.16 (2.73)	7.76 (3.47)	7.20 (1.95)	7.08 (2.21)
Empathy	6.48 (1.89)	8.04 (1.56)	6.20 (1.80)	7.76 (1.61)	6.56 (1.60)	7.00 (1.60)	6.20 (1.44)	6.08 (1.65)

Note: Standard Deviations in parentheses.

Results

Table 4.2 shows performance on the measures of self-reported health. It suggests that 6 negative aspects of health (i.e. illness, insomnia, negative body image, depression, anxiety and alienation) were reduced and 12 positive outcomes of health (i.e. digestion, fitness, self-esteem, goal clarity, adjustment, and empathy) were enhanced in the intervention group. Among control group participants, illness, insomnia and alienation were increased among boys, but reduced among girls, negative body image scores were reduced among control group boys and increased among girls, and depression was reduced among all the control group participants. The scores of digestion, fitness, self-esteem, and empathy were increased among control group boys, but decreased among control group girls. The scores of goal clarity, and adjustment were reduced among all the control group participants.

Subsequently, normality distributions of variables were checked. It was found that variable distributions were somewhat normal, with skewness coefficients ranging from .48 to –.78. After that, separate mixed 2 (type of group) × 2 (kind of gender) × 2 (testing occasions) ANOVAs were conducted on mean scores obtained on various scales. The 2×2×2 analysis partitioned variation due to differences between groups into each pair of independent variables as well as the main effects. All analysis were evaluated at alpha levels of $p < .05$, $p < .01$ and $p < .001$. Table 4.3 displays main effects of the type of group, gender and testing occasions for different scales of self-reported health.

The ANOVA revealed that the intervention group displayed greater mean scores on the measures of self-esteem, and empathy than control group. In regard to gender, it was noted that boys had higher level of illness than girls. The scores for illness, insomnia, negative body image, depression, anxiety and alienation were significantly higher at the pre-test than post-test. The scores for digestion, fitness, self-esteem, goal clarity, adjustment, and empathy were consistently greater at the post-test than pre-test.

The results also indicated interactions that qualified the main effects stated above. The type of group × testing occasions interaction was found significant for illness ($F_{(1,96)} = 39.62, p < .001$), insomnia ($F_{(1,96)} = 13.51, p < .001$), fitness ($F_{(1,96)} = 9.99, p < .01$), negative body image ($F_{(1,96)} = 25.77, p < .001$), self-esteem ($F_{(1,96)} = 13.62, p < .001$), anxiety ($F_{(1,96)} = 8.65, p < .01$), goal clarity ($F_{(1,96)} = 25.73, p < .001$), adjustment ($F_{(1,96)} = 13.6, p < .001$), alienation ($F_{(1,96)} = 22.49, p < .001$), and empathy ($F_{(1,96)} =$

Table 4.3: Summaries of Main Effects of Type of Group, Gender and Testing Occasions Performed for Measures of Self-reported Health (N = 100)

Variables	*Type of Group*				*Gender*				*Testing occasions*			
	INT	*CON*	*MS*	*F (1, 99)*	*B*	*G*	*MS*	*F (1, 99)*	*PRE*	*POST*	*MS*	*F (1, 99)*
Illness	20.24 (4.33)	21.26 (5.25)	13.00	15	21.76 (50)	19.74 (4.43)	51.00	4.52*	11.27 (3.02)	9.48 (2.86)	160.20	38.75***
Insomnia	7.24 (2.39)	8.08 (2.98)	8.82	2.37	7.78 (2.77)	7.54 (2.69)	.72	.19	4.18 (1.74)	3.48 (1.56)	24.50	15.2***
Digestion	14.02 (2.97)	13.72 (3.55)	1.12	.21	13.74 (3.45)	14.00 (3.10)	.84	.15	6.69 (1.99)	7.18 (1.85)	12.00	6.27*
Fitness	22.30 (3.95)	21.50 (3.96)	8.00	1.00	21.90 (3.99)	21.90 (3.96)	.00	.00	10.32 (2.72)	11.58 (2.36)	9.38	17.23***
Negative body image	15.70 (3.93)	17.32 (4.94)	32.80	3.27	17.12 (4.54)	15.90 (4.45)	18.60	1.85	8.75 (2.94)	7.76 (2,85)	49.00	9.509**
Self-esteem	22.74 (3.61)	20.96 (4.13)	39.60	5.17*	21.60 (3.90)	22.10 (4.05)	3.12	.41	10.51 (2.49)	11.34 (2.31)	4.44	10.39**
Depression	4.84 (2.89)	16.08 (3.33)	19.22	3.90	15.22 (3.54)	15.70 (2.74)	2.88	.58	7.96 (1.99)	7.50 (1.65)	10.58	6.17*
Anxiety	5.06 (4.15)	15.46 (4.25)	2.00	.22	15.48 (4.92)	15.04 (3.33)	2.42	.27	8.30 (2.58)	6.96 (2.39)	89.78	26.91***
Goal Clarity	4.36 (3.29)	13.76 (3.01)	4.50	.89	13.70 (3.54)	14.2 (2.70)	6.48	1.29	6.82 (1.93)	7.24 8)	8.82	4.04*
Adjustment	24.54 (3.54)	23.76 (3.94)	7.60	1.06	23.90 (3.97)	24.40 (3.53)	3.12	.43	11.68 (2.40)	2.47 (2.15)	31.20	10.25**
Alienation	13.54 (3.51)	14.60 (4.64)	14.04	1.63	14.14 (4.62)	400 (3.62)	.24	.03	749 (2.32)	6.58 (2.59)	41.40	14.08***
Empathy	14.24 (2.76)	12.92 (2.71)	21.78	5.87*	14.04 (2.72)	13.12 (2.84)	10.58	2.85	6.36 (1.67)	7.22 (1.76)	36.98	20.94***

Note: *SD*s are in parenthesis. **p* <.05, ***p* <.01, ****p* <. 001.

13.87, $p < .001$). Gender × testing occasions interaction was significant for digestion ($F_{(1,96)} = 8.49$, $p < .01$) fitness ($F_{(1,96)} = 5.02$, $p < .05$), and negative body image ($F_{(1,96)} = 4.09$, $p < .05$). Findings show that reduction of illness, insomnia and negative body image was significantly greater in the intervention group than the control group participants. As a result of intervention, there was significant improvement in the intervention group while control group remained at the same level. The scores of negative body image and anxiety were reduced significantly among intervention group participants than their control group counterparts. On the other hand, fitness (c), self-esteem (e), goal clarity (g), and adjustment (h) were enhanced significantly among intervention group participants. Alienation decreased and empathy has enhanced among the intervention group respondents.

Follow-up

A follow-up of the adolescents who participated in the intervention was undertaken after a period of 3 months. To this end, the participants were asked to report the extent to which they were observing the various aspects of lifestyle change which were introduced during the two weeks of LSIP. The compliance was noted for some of the behaviours comparatively more than others after three months of LSIP. Gender was found to be insignificant for compliance of lifestyle behaviours. A majority of lifestyle behaviours were observed in practice by adolescents (72.7% avoiding water during meals, 100% avoiding fast foods, 93.2% avoiding tea, 78.6% getting up before sun rise, 72.7% sleeping before 10 p.m., 72.7% doing *Yoga*, 91.9% reciting *mantras*) for at least once a week. However, a low percentage of adolescents engaged with different other lifestyle behaviours (40.9% avoiding water during meals, for seven days a week, 90.9% avoiding fast foods, 36.4% avoiding fast foods, 72.7% getting up before sun rise, 43.2% sleeping before 10 p.m., 38.6% doing Yoga, 47.7% reciting *mantra*) for five to seven days a week.

Discussion

The purpose of present study was to evaluate effect of Yogic lifestyle on self-reported health among adolescents. The conduct of study included theoretically-oriented and culturally-sensitive Yogic lifestyle intervention among adolescents in which one group was exposed to lifestyle counselling and another group was engaged in a general dialogue for the same duration. The results suggest holistic effects of YLSIP in reducing several health problems and enhancing positive aspects of health and strongly effect on a range of health concerns including illness, insomnia, negative body image, anxiety, depression, and alienation and enhance digestive capacity, physical fitness, and self-esteem, clarity of life goal, adjustment, empathy and academic competence. The effect of intervention was similar among boys and girls. The follow-up results indicated that the effect continued and persisted even after three months. A higher proportion of adolescents reported about compliance with multiple aspects of changes introduced during intervention.

The findings of this study are congruent with results of previous studies on role of Yoga in amelioration of anxiety and depression (Aminabhavi, 1996; Khumar *et al.,* 1993) hyperactivity, attention deficit and improving general health (Abadi, Madgaonkar, and Venkatesam, 2008; Palsane, 1998; Priyadarshini, 2001; Verma, 1997); effectiveness of relaxation training in reducing frequency and intensity of some ailments (i.e. headaches, abdominal pain) (Carr, 2007); impact of breathing exercises, visualization, autosuggestion on controlling arousal, stress, and managing anxiety (Davis *et al.*, 1995; Madders, 1997; Sarafino, 2002).

The present findings have broadened scope of relevance of Yogic lifestyle. It has validated notions of health as a 'reserve stock', to be invested in by adopting health behaviour, or diminished by self-neglect or unhealthy behaviours (Blaxter, 1990; Herzlich, 1973) and sociological proposition that wellness can be increased by improving lifestyle (Antonovosky, 1979). It has affirmed positivistic view of individuals as having resources to solve their own problems in a practical immediate way and wellness as a way of life towards optimization health at physical, mental and spiritual level (Gladding, 2009; Myers, Sweeney and Witmer, 2000). It has further identified role of positive sleep habits as a causal factor, which was previously noted as a correlate by Hamilton, Nelson, Stevens and Kitzman (2007). Regarding to the role of religiosity, it has also provided evidence for religiosity as an important protective factor for adolescent health (Cotton *et al.*, 2006).

There is need to realize about how such holistic change could have taken place among the adolescents and what could have been exact psychological procedures adopted for lifestyle change. In view of success of a range of theoretical elements used in previous intervention studies, the present study utilized techniques of reinforcements, recognition by teachers, self-monitoring, peer support, and perceptions for positive value of lifestyle behaviours (Pandey and Subbakrishna, 2000). During design of effective intervention module, attention was paid to developmental and psychological aspects of adolescent lifestyle. A web of factors such as group participation, plasticity due to age of participants, self-monitoring perception of health needs could have made successful to the programme. A review by Spear and Kulbok (2001) has particularly evinced the relevance of gender, age, peer pressure, attitudes, values and perception of health needs for successful lifestyle interventions. While the content of *LSIP* was decided on the basis of relevance of particular lifestyle components for health; methodological conduct of intervention was based on an eclectic and integrated module designed carefully to create awareness about relevance of lifestyle for health and well-being, introduce positive changes, facilitate voluntary participation and maintain inculcated changes subsequently.

Although, the effects of separate lifestyle practices and role of lifestyle in cure of disease were not examined in the present study, the study has provided an impetus for emergence of new field of lifestyle counselling for curative, preventive and protective roles (Datta and Broota, 2000; Rani and Rao, 2005; Rao, 2000). A group of four case studies provided deeper revelation about holistic contribution of positive lifestyle change. It was interesting to note that one of the participants of the study during introspective observations of participants in video recording session conveyed about improvement in symptoms of a chronic disease, ulcer, created scope for role of lifestyle change in management of several other diseases. Although, currently lifestyle interventions limited to management of cardiovascular diseases and diabetes, this important revelation with other finding of this study is a pointer for immense potential imbued in lifestyle for cure, prevention, protection from illnesses and also improving our wellness.

Although, the findings of present study extend the previous research in many ways; it had some limitations and therefore, the results need to be interpreted with caution. The participation in the study was voluntary and those who were willing to join were recruited in the intervention group. Also, they apparently got special treatment in the school context. This might have raised their motivation for participation. So, it can't be said that random assignment of participants was done. Also, the data were self-report, behavioural, and observational. Despite this limitation the study does point towards the need for school wide lifestyle intervention for adolescents.

It has demonstrated the usefulness of a psycho-social intervention in the lives of adolescents in a residential school setting. It encourages for extension of such intervention on a broader scale with suitable modification as per the requirements of the specific settings. The involvement of peers and teachers in the programme works as a source of motivation and support. Being a collectivistic culture the impact of such intervention increases if the changes take place in group context. However, a close scrutiny of the programme revealed that its goals may be attained more effectively, if the parents and teachers too are addressed and their attitude towards lifestyle and health are changed. The study very clearly brought out the fact that health is a personal as well as a social matter and bringing out any change and sustaining the same would require lifestyle changes with support from the social context in which adolescents live.

Annexure-1

Components of Yoga Training Programme

Phases		*Activities*
Initial Exercises	I	Warming up, rotating the toes, ankle rotation, knees rotation, waist movement, finger movements, arm rotation, elbow movements, wrist movements, neck rolls, shoulder rotation
	II	Quick Relaxation through *Shavasana*
Asanas	I	*Kati Mardanasana*-1 (spinal rotation) *Kati Mardanasana*-2 (spinal rotation)
	II	Quick Relaxation through *Shavasana*
Pranayama	I	*Nadi Shodhana* (Alternate nostril breathing) *Kapalbhati Pranayama* (rapid exhalation)
	II	Quick Relaxation through *Shavasana*

Annexure-2

The Components of LSIP and Mode of Ensuring Compliance

	Components	*Mode of ensuring compliance*
Dietary habits	Proper chewing of food Avoiding water during meals	Self and personal monitoring
Food Intake	Avoiding tea/coffee Avoiding fast foods and cold drinks	Self, peers and Personal monitoring
Sleep Habits	Sleeping before 10 p.m. Waking before sunrise	Self and personal monitoring
Yoga	Physical postures '*Asana*' (10 minutes) *Pranayama* (5 minutes) *Shavasana* (15 minutes)	Self and attendance
Religio-spiritual practice	Chanting *Mantras* (5 minutes)	Self and attendance

References

Ajzen, I. and Fishbein, M. (1980). *Understanding Attitudes and Predicting Social Behaviour*. Englewood Cliffs, NJ: Prentice Hall.

Antaramian, S.P., Huebner, E.S., and Valois, R.F. (2008). Adolescent life satisfaction. *Applied Psychology: An International Review,* 57, 112-126.

Arora, S. and Bhattacharjee, J. (2008). Modulation of immune response in stress by yoga. *International Journal of Yoga*, 1, 45-55.

Bandura, A. (1977). Self-efficacy: Toward a unifying theory of behavioural change. *Psychological Review,* 84, 191-215.

Bharshankar, J.R., Bharshankar, R.N., Deshpande, V.N., Kaore, S.B., and Gosavi, G.B. (2003). Effect of yoga on cardiovascular system in subjects above 40 years. *Indian Journal of Physiological Pharmacology,* 47, 202-206.

Broota, A., Verma, R., and Singh, A. (1995). Role of relaxation in hypertension. *Journal of the Indian Academy of Applied Psychology,* 21, 29-36.

Carson, J.W., Carson, K.M., Porter, L.S., Keefe, F.J., Shaw, H., and Miller, J.M. (2007). Yoga for women with metastatic breast cancer: Results from a pilot study. *Journal of Pain Symptom Management,* 33, 331-41.

Cohen, L., Warneke, C., Fouladi, R.T., Rodriguez, M.A., & Chaoul-Reich, A. (2004) Psychological adjustment and sleep quality in a randomized trial of effects of a Tibetan yoga intervention in patients with lymphoma. *Cancer*, 100, 2253-60.

Cotton, S., Zebracki, K., Rosenthal, S.L., Tsevat, J., and Drotar, D. (2006) Religion/spirituality and adolescent health outcomes: a review. *Journal of Adolescent Health*, 38, 472-480.

Dalal, A.K. (2001). Health Psychology. In J. Pandey (Ed.), *Psychology in India Revisited: Developments in the Discipline.* (Vol. 2, pp. 356-411). New Delhi: Sage.

Datta, J. and Broota, A. (2000). Managing Obsessive Compulsive Disorder (OCD) with yoga and cognitive behavioural therapy. *Journal of Research and Application in Clinical Psychology*, 3, 41-50.

Gatantino, M.L., Bzdewka, T.M., Eissler-Rnsso, J.L., Holbrook, M.L., Mogck, E.P., Geigle, P. *et al.* (2003). The impact of modified hatha yoga on chronic low back pain: A pilot study. *Alternative Therapy Health Medicine*, 10, 56-59.

Granath, J., Ingvarsson, S., von Thiele, U., and Lundberg, U. (2006). Stress management: A randomized study of cognitive behavioural therapy and yoga. *Cognitive Behavioural Therapy*, 35, 3-10.

Hamilton, N.A., Nelson, C.A., Stevens, N., and Kitzman, H. (2007). Sleep and psychological well-being. *Social Indicators Research*, 82(1), 147-163.

Hans, G. (1994). Lifestyle education for student youth: Need and strategy. *The Indian Journal of Social Work, LV* (1), 25-39.

Kaila, H.L. (2003). School based approaches of child guidance and counselling services in Mumbai City. *Journal of Psychological Researches*, 47, 57-60.

Kakar, S. (2003). Psychoanalysis and eastern spiritual traditions. *Journal of Analytical Psychology*, 48, 659-678.

Kapur, M. (2001). Mental health, illness and therapy. In J. Pandey (Ed.), *Psychology in India Revisited: Developments in the Discipline* (Vol. 2): *Personality and Social Psychology* (pp. 412-472). New Delhi: Sage.

Kapoor, R.L. (2002). Can Indian spiritual practices be used in psychotherapy? *Unpublished Manuscript*. Bangalore: National Institute of Advanced Studies.

Kissen, M., and Kissen-Kohn, D.A. (2009). Reducing addictions *via* the self-soothing effects of yoga. *Bull Menninger Clinic*, 73, 34-43.

Kolasinski S.L., Garfinkel M., Tsai A.G., Matz W., Dyke A.V., Schumacher H.R. (2005). Iyengar yoga for treating symptoms of osteoarthritis of the knees: A pilot study. *Journal of Alternative Complementary Medicine*, 11, 689-93.

Koller, J.M. (2006). *The Indian Way: An Introduction of the Philosophies and Religions of India*, Delhi: Pearson Education.

Larson, R.W., Wilson, S., Brown, B.B., Furstenberg, F.F., Jr., and Verma, S. (2002). Changes in adolescent interpersonal experiences: Are they being prepared for adult relationships in the twenty-first century? *Journal of Research on Adolescence*, 12, 31-68.

Misra, G. (2005). From disease to well-being: perspectives from indigenous tradition. In R. Singh; A. Yadav, and N. Sharma (eds.), *Health Psychology* (281-302). New Delhi: Global Vision.

Mishra, M., and Sinha, R.K. (2001). Effects of yogic practices on depression and anxiety. *SIS Journal of Projective Psychology and Mental Health,* 8, 23-27.

Oken, B.S., Zajdel, D., Kishiyama, S., Flegal, K., Dehen, C., Haas, M., *et al.* (2006). Randomized, controlled, six-month trial of yoga in healthy seniors: Effects on cognition and quality of life. *Alternative Therapy Health Medicine,* 12, 40-7.

Parasher, K.P. (2000). Lifestyle for perfect health, *Psychological Studies,* 45(3), 167-172.

Perry, C.L., and Jessor R. (1985). The concept of health promotion and the prevention of adolescent drug abuse. *Health Education Quarterly,* 12, 169-184.

Pilkington, K., Kirkwood, G., Rampes, H., and Richardson, J. (2005). Yoga for depression: The research evidence. *Journal of Affect Disorder,* 89, 13-24.

Ponnuswami, S. (2000). Community care for mental health. *Psychological Studies,* 45, 173-177.

Planning Commission (2000) *Report of the working group on adolescents for the Tenth Five Year Plan.* New Delhi: Government of India.

Raghavendra, R.M., Nagarathna, R., Nagendra, H.R., Gopinath, K.S., Srinath, B.S., Ravi, B.D. *et al.* (2007). Effects of an integrated yoga programme on chemotherapy-induced nausea and emesis in breast cancer patients. *European Cancer Care,* 16, 462-474.

Ram, S. (1987). Dimension of Yoga. In S.N. Mahajan (eds.), *The Science of Yoga and Consciousness* (pp. 11-22). Agra: Y.K. Publishers.

Ramdeo, S. (2006). *Yoga its Philosophy and Practice.* New Delhi: Diamond Pocket Books.

Rani, N.J. and Rao, P.V.K. (2005). Impact of yoga training on body image and depression. *Psychological Studies,* 50 (1), 98-100.

Rao, K. (2000). Stress and its management. In P. Jose (Ed.) *Indian Health—A Reference Document* (pp. 433-435). Kerala: Deepika Publishers.

Riva, G., and Molinari, E. (1998). Replicated factor analysis of the Italian version of body image avoidant questionnaire. *Perceptual Motor Skills,* 86 (3), 1071-1074.

Sharma, R., Gupta, N., and Bijlani, R.L. (2008). Effect of Yoga based lifestyle intervention on subjective well-being. *Indian Journal of Physiological Pharmacology,* 52(2), 123-131.

Sharma, S., and Sharma, M. (2006). Sustaining and enhancing health/well-being of Indian students: The role of certain spiritual and religious interventions. *Psychological Studies,* 51(2-3), 113-118.

Sharma, S. and Sharma, M. (2008). Preventing illness and promoting of health and well-being. *Psychological Studies,* 52 (1), 70-76.

Singh A.R. (2010), Modern medicine: Towards prevention, cure, well-being and longevity. In A.R. Singh and S.A. Singh (eds.), *Psychopharmacology Today: Some Issues, MSM*, (17-29).

Sinha, D. (1990). Concept of Psycho-social well-being. Western and Indian Perspectives. *NIMHANS Journal*, 8, 1-11.

Spear, H.J. and Kulbok, P.A. (2001). Adolescent health behaviours and related factors: A review. *Public Health Nursing*, 18 (2), 82-93.

Tiwari, S.G., Agarwal, G.G., Kumar, A., Pandey, N.M. (2007). Preventing illness: A community based behavioural intervention approach. *Psychological Studies*, 52 (1), 77-84.

Verma, S., and Saraswathi, T.S. (2002). *Adolescence in India: Annotated Bibliography.* New Delhi: Rawat Publications.

Wig and Verma, S.K. (1978). *PGI Health Questionnaire*. Agra: Agra Psychological Research Cell.

Woolery, A., Myers, H., Stemliebm, B., Zeltzer, L. (2004). A yoga intervention for young adults with elevated symptoms of depression. *Alternative Therapy Health Medicine*, 10, 60-63.

Yarcheski, A., Mahon, N.E. and Yarcheski, T.J. (1997). Alternate models of positive health practices in adolescents. *Nursing Research*, 46, 85-92.

5

Therapeutic Application of Music

Indo-Western Perspective

Aradhana Shukla

The relevance of music in our daily life is well accepted as it starts with the cry at birth till death with the chanting up to the cremation place. As the creation of human being appeared, music started till that time and even in every behaviour of human being follow the rhythm which is the essence of behaviour. Any sort of sentiment, hidden inside appears in terms of music so, it is surely fair to say that music is the mediator between the spiritual and the sensual life. It freshens the mood state and inspires him to work well in almost all sorts of behaviour.

Music as a mood state: Music is considered as an important part of human life and behaviour. It is directly related with the affective aspect of human life so, it plays a major and equivalent role in pleasant and unpleasant situations. Although its nature and structure can be different in both places, yet it is quite sure that it will be adequate to consider music as the symbol of human feelings.

The discipline of psychology make the scientific study of all aspects of human behaviour and the affective part that is directly related with music cannot be separated. Music is an attracting art and Psychology is the science of behaviour that comes through the passage of mental processes. Therefore, music and psychology are closely related. It is necessary to analyse interest, attention, imagination, testing, memory, motivation, learning, feeling, thinking, heredity and personality etc. in music which are the basic attributes of Psychology. So, it nurtures the mental power (energy) of human being and has proved itself as a means of mental as well as spiritual development. As Plato has told—"Music is a moral law. It gives a soul to the universe, wings to the minds, flight to the imagination, a charm to sadness, and gaiety and life to everything."

When the *ragas* are played properly and according to their time, not only the human beings but also animals, environment and even vegetation are well controlled. *Deepak* and *Megh ragas* are the examples of it. Thus, it cannot be denied that music has a fascinating power and resulting to which music therapy came in existence.

Many psychologists have defined music therapy according to their own ways—they are listed below: Music therapy is a special type of therapy where forms of a musical interactions and communications are used alongside verbal communication (Gold *et al.*, 2009).

Music therapy can be defined as a systematic process of intervention wherein the therapist helps the client to promote health, using musical experiences and the relationships developing through them as a dynamic force of change (Bruscia, 1998). Music therapy is an established healthcare profession that uses music to address physical, emotional, cognitive and social needs of individuals of all ages (Camasari, 2009).

Music therapy interventions can be designed to promote wellness, manage stress, alleviate pain, express feelings, enhance memory, improve communication and promote physical rehabilitation (American Music Therapy Association, 2009).

Music therapy is directly associated with the music (vocal or instrumental) which lay their apparent effect not as the consequence of change in client-therapist relation, but it enables the client to understand his feelings and problems and organize his behaviour and then life.

Music lays its impact on sympathetic, para-sympathetic and brain nerves through *pancham* (moon) *swar*. *Pancham*, *madhyam*, *gandhar* and *nishad swaras* are more effective in psychological disorders (Joshi, 2011). *Raga* practice of "*ga, re*" (3 minutes), "*ga, re, sa*" (2 minutes) and "*ga, re, saa*" (2 minutes) is found too effective in headache, backache and seasonal diseases of winter. Urinal infection in young boys can be cured or at least minimized by "*re, ga, ma, pa, dha*". Similarly, quick relief for HIV patient is possible through "*ma, re, ga*", and "*pa, ni, dha*". Joshi (2011) also stated that many psychological disorders like hysteria, hypertension, sleeplessness, asthma, depression and constipation are possibly cured through music therapy.

Music therapy has significant effects on clients' mental state. It is a scientific method of effective cures of diseases through therapy of music. It restores, maintains and improves emotional, physical and psychological well-being. The articulation, pitch, tone and specific arrangements of *swaras* (notes) in a particular *raga* stimulates, alleviates and cures various ailments inducing electromagnetic changes in body.

Keeping these views in consideration, a reminiscence regarding treatment through music was started and the advocates of Western music decided to use music in therapeutic conditions. In 1944, first syllabus of music therapy was prepared in Michigan University. Thereafter, in 1944 Cansas University also started the programme. In 1950, an association named as Association for Music Therapy was started. This Association started to give certificates for Music Therapy and registrations were made for clinical practices. This was made clear that Music Therapy increases the "life energy" in the disordered people. As a result, his disorders are cured or at least minimized. Thus, it can be said that Music Therapy is a therapeutic treatment programme which is done by a trained therapist under required circumstances (American Music Therapy Association, 2013). It is an allied therapy in which the therapist uses various musical devices and all its facts like, physical, emotional, mental, social, aesthetic and spiritual assist the client in the attainment of better health by singing, dancing, playing with musical instruments as well as listening and even discussing about the music enhance the affect-cognitive system, socio-motor ability and quality of life. Referrals to music therapy may be suggested by healthcare professionals, but it is also the choice of a client to choose music therapy by his oneself self-referral without any referral. The role of music therapy is very wide and they are found very near to every professional of help and care system. They are very useful for the individuals with special needs. Music Therapy is common in mental hospitals, medical institutions, schools, alcohol and drug recovery programme, psychiatric hospitals and correctional facilities (American Music Therapy Association, 2011).

Historical Perspective and Approaches of Music Therapy

The relative significance of music in everyday human life cannot be denied. Since long back it has been used in terms of healing (Misic *et al.*, 2010). Apollo is considered as the god of music and medicine. Aesculapius advocated the cure of disease through song and music. He told that at first music therapy was used in temples. Plato and Aristotle taught music for the refinement of soul and affect. Music therapy was in existence at Bibical times (Howells and Osborn, 1984). In thirteenth century Arab hospital constructed music room for the patients (Antrim, 2006). But the therapeutic effect of music on soul was discussed by AL. Farabi (872-950) who used it as a healing systems (Haque, 2004). Music therapy with it entitlement started in the aftermath of first and Second World War when it was used for the soliders to get them rid of from the war induced emotions and trauma (Deg Mecic, Dunja and Filakovic, 2005). Models that developed out of music therapy are Neurologic Music Therapy (NMT), Norcloff-Robbins and the Bonny Method of Guided Imagery and Music (Davis, 2008). People suffering from behavioural emotional disorders go in the shelter of music therapist and the music therapists take the help of some current psychological theories like, behavioural therapy, cognitive behavioural therapy and psychodynamic therapy (Deka, 2012; Davis, 2008). NMT studies the function of brains with and without music and then measure the difference, and then uses differences to cause change in the brain through music that will eventually affect the client non-musically. "The brains that engages in music is changed by engaging in music" (Davis, 2008). NMT trains motor responses like tapping first on finger, head movement to see his/her activation during music.

Assessment and Interventions

Similar to any other therapy, music therapy also holds some conduct cares and ethics to understand the client. Formal assessment is crucial for understanding the clients—their background, limitations and needs as well as to create appropriate goal for the process and select the means of achieving them. This serves as the starting step from which to measure the client's progression throughout the therapeutic process and to make adjustments later, if required. The music therapist obtains extensive data on the client including their full medical history, musical (ability to copy a melody or identity changes in rhythm etc.) and non-musical functioning, socio-physical motor, emotional etc. (Crowl 2007). Then the procedure of formal/informal assessment process starts in standardized ways. Crowel (2007) has suggested some most common methods of assessment, they are—

- Interviews with clients and/or family members,
- Structured or unstructured observations,
- Reviewing of clients records, and
- Standardized assessment tests.

After gathering the information, the music therapist decides a treatment which includes specific short-term objectives, long-term goals and an expected time for therapy (Nordoff and Glive, 2008).

When we use music therapy on children we use two types of therapy.

The first, supportive active therapy, is product oriented and it incorporates rhythm activities like clapping, singing or unstructured body movement. The second is might music therapy and it is process oriented like song writing or composing and it is conducted in one-on-one session or a group session (Bunt and Sarab, 2002).

Music therapy intervention programmes can include an average of 18 sessions of treatment. The achievement of a physical rehabilitation goal relies on the child's existing motivation and feeling towards music and their commitment to engage in meaningful rewarding efforts. Session may consist of either active techniques, when the client creates music or receptive techniques. Where the clients listen to, analyze more and respond to music (Hannibal *et al.*, 2012). Both technique are systematic and provide a force on the clients towards rehabilitation (Stanley and Ramsay, 2012).

Indian musicians advocate the direct relation of music to fun in the central attribute of Indian music that it has blended *devatas*, nature, colour *Vedas* time and virtues in are single combination. According to Srivastava (2011) a *raga* solely represents the atmosphere view subject matter nature and in special the affect cognitive status of the composer (our sweetest songs are those that tell of the ruddiest thought). They are depicted in *ragamala* by artists "*Ragamala* pictures being the first instance in the world of presenting music iconographycally should be regarded as a unique Indian achievement" (Srivastava, 2011). The concept of *ragamala* started decline from the beginning of nineteenth century and the attention was paid towards the enlarge public and then new version of music started.

Music Therapy: Indian Scenario

In Indian scenario music was explained as a natural and traditional language through which hidden and unexpressed feelings of human beings are distributed either by throat or by playing any instrument.

There is an important recognition of imagery and creativity in Indian music. It increases our memory, retention, recall, and differentiation. Not only the art of music influences the humans, but also it affects animals and nature. It is the best way of expression, therefore, it reduces many abnormalities and disturbances and provides basic ways of being happy and sprinkle happiness over others.

Sarve bhavantu sukhinah, sarve santu niramayah,
Sarve bhadrani pashyantu, ma kashchit duhkha bhaga bhavet.

> [Every person be happy, every person be out of desease, every person be the perceiver of goodness, wellness and nobody will be the victim (*bhagi*) of sorrow (*duhkha*)].

If we sing *Mahamrityunjaya mantra* according to musical rules we feel happiness, peace. We are healthy in psycho-physical perspective and get a successful and balanced personality.

> *"Om trayambakam yajamahe, sugandhim pushti vardhanam,*
> *Urvarukamiva bandhanat, mrityor mukshiya mamritat.*
> [We worship the three eyed one (Lord Shiva) who is fragrant and who nourishes well to all beings, May He liberate us from death for the sake of immortality even as the cucumber is severed from its bondage (to the creeper)].

It is a life giving *mantra* and it has a great curative effect. Again diseases pronounced incurable by doctors are cured by this *mantra*, when chanted with sincerity, faith and devotion. It is weapon against diseases and a *mantra* to conquer death.

So far as the ground of music therapy in Indian system is concerned it started from Vedic period. In *Samaveda* impact of *raga* as a cure of disease is referred. In Indian music system highest power of *nada* has been elicited through which a therapy emerged. It is the view of science that development of intelligence possible through music. Many nerves call at cortex response on different *swaras*. The waves reach in mid brain. This sense touches nerves and touch the other parts of the nerves and touch the senses. Thus, music is highly gainful in right atmosphere.

There are seven *swaras* in Indian music. They are the ground of music and they are emerged from the seven temperament characteristics of human being. In "*Sangita Parijata*" Pt. Ahobal has said that 22 *Shrutis* of Indian music are directly related with 22 blood vessels. Music lays its direct impact on some human attributes given below:

- It directly and frequently influences the behaviour, temperament feelings and thoughts.
- It augments happiness.
- It develops imagery and creativity.
- It widens moral and intellectual outlook.
- It promotes tolerance, love, social harmony and artistic taste.
- It reduces hynem aggressiveness.

Music not only develops some feeling, but many internal changes are also caused by it. The *sapt swaras* of music come in light by vibrating *shat chakras* and *Bindu vibarga sthana*. They are:

Name of the Ragas	*Name of the Chakras*
Shadaja	Muladhara Chakra
Rishabha	Svadhishthana Chakra
Gandhara	Manipura Chakra
Madhyama	Anahata Chakra
Panchama	Vishuddhi Chakra
Dhaivata	Agya Chakra
Nishada	Bindu Visarga
Tar Shadaja	Sahasrara Chakra

Our Indian Classics have slated seven colours for seven *swaras* of music. They are called *saptaka*. The concept of *raga* has been emerged from here and they are described by seven colours which is as follows:

Name of the Swars	*Name of the Colour*
Shadaja (Sa)	Lotus colour (fluorescent pink)
Rishabha (Re)	Green
Gandhara (Ga)	Orange
Madhyama (Ma)	Yellowish pink
Panchama (Pa)	Red
Dhaivata (Dha)	Yellow
Nishada (Ni)	Black

Therefore, diseases may be cured on the basis of colour deficiency as reported by the client and for this purpose Luscher Colour Test may be applied. So, it is very sure that various *ragas* are able to cure or at least minimize the disease, their description is as follows:

Name of the Raaga	*Its Usage as a Cure of Disease*
Aheer Bhairava	Indigestion, Rheumatic arthritis, hypertension
Aasawari	Confidence building, low Blood Pressure
Bagshri	Insomnia
Basant Bahar	Gallbladder stone, cholecystitis
Bhairavi	Rheumatic arthritis, sinusitis
Bhim Palasi	Anxiety, hypertension
Chandrakauns	Anorexia, heart attack
Darbari	Sedative, easing tension
Darbarikannada	Headache, asthma
Deepak	Indigestion, anorexia, hyperactivity, gallbladder stone, cholecystitis
Gurjaritodi	Cough
Gun kali	Rheumatic arthritis, constipation headache, piles
Hindola	Rheumatic arthritis, backache,
Jaunpuri	Intestinal gas, Diarrhea, Constipation
Kalawati, Kamodini, Multani	Vata related gas
Sohani, Todi, Bhairavi	Pitta related gas
Malkauns	Cough related gas
Dhani, Vihag	Epilepsy
Puria, Darbari, Khamaj	Hysteria
Purvi, Todi, Multani	Blood pressure
Lalit, Kedar	Brain disorder
Aheer Bhairav, Puria	Removing unconsciousness
Sarang Megh	Skin disorder
Shivranjani	Cardiac disorder
Multani	Ophthalmic disorder
Shyam Kalyan	Respiratory system
Bilawal, Tilang	Tuberculosis
Bhairavi	Asthma, cough, tuberculosis
Rag vardhini	Digestive system
Hindol, Malwa, Puria	Typhoid, malaria

As every person has its own differentials intrinsic worth, therefore, this should always be taken into consideration before applying any musical treatment. Moreover, prior to apply music therapy the clinician must have a knowledge of *doshas* (*vata*, *pitta* and *kapha*) because they are important in understanding any disease.

Neuro Scientific Grounds of Music Therapy

Music Therapy may have its impact on psychological health of the individual. Hillecke and associates (2005) presented a heuristic model that works in music therapy. This model has five factors which can be thought as the significant contributors of memory. According to Koelsch (2009), these factors can be named as attention, emotion, cognition, behaviour and communication. They are briefly described below:

1. ***Attention Modulation***: The aim of music therapy is to get relief from pain and provides pleasure. It can very easily catch our attention (Sussman, 2007; Koelsch, 2009). It distorts our attention from the negative stimuli like anxiety, mental pressure, pain, worry etc. and converts them into positive one. This factor states music therapy as pain relieving system during medical process like in tinnitus or attention deficit hypothesis (Nelson and Heart, 2008; Klassen, 2008).

2. ***Emotion Modulation***: The emotion modulation factor is closely related with the treatment of affective disorder like, depression, pathological anxiety and post traumatic stress disease (PTSD). This factor is also associated with peripheral physiological effects and vegetative (or automatic) nervous system. Emotions can also be evoked through music therapy.

3. ***Cognitive Modulation***: This factor includes memory processes that are linked with music. They are encoding, storage and decoding of music information. This factor can also be effective while using the treatment of Alzheimer's patients who need long-term care (Gardener and Swanson, 1993).

4. ***Behaviour Modulation***: This factor deals with the aspects of behavioural conditioning such as movements pattern involved in walking, speaking, grasping etc. with music. A similar action exists between action and emotion.

5. ***Communication Modulation***: Music therapy can be used to train skills of non-verbal communication disorders such as, selective mutism (Findeisen, 2007) and for the training of interpersonal relations.

Some other factors also contribute to the effects of Music Therapy is perceptual modification. It shapes the decoding of acoustic features, like pitch, height and frequency modulation, already at the level of the auditory cortex (Koelsch, 1999). Wong and associates (2007) showed that adults with musical training have more accurate identification of the pitch contour of Chinese tones. This study reveals that Music Therapy has its effects on basic perceptual process during language comprehension.

Types of Music Therapy

1. ***Background Music Therapy***: Background music therapy is transmitted through audio system and it aims to create a normal and calm environment in the hospital (De Sausa, 2005).
2. ***Contemplative Music Therapy***: This is an important therapy and it helps the patients to appreciate the general significance of music and art. It is also termed as reactive musical therapy. This therapy alleviates sadness (De Sausa, 2005).
3. ***Combined Music Therapy***: The combined music therapy may be used in the conjunction with other therapeutic procedure. Sometimes, in the form of music therapy hypnosis is conducted while the subjects listen music. It is the combination of central electro-sleep therapy bad behaviour therapy method (De Sousa, 2005).
4. ***Excutive Music Therapy***: It consists of singing and playing musical instruments. It is done in individual and/or in group setting (De Sausa, 2005).
5. ***Excutive Latro Music Therapy***: This therapy is most frequently used in the treatment of emotionally disabled or mentally retarded dyslexic children (De Sausa, 2005).
6. ***Creative Music Therapy***: In this therapy patients write and compose songs and play on the instruments in terms of catharsis (De Sausa, 2005).

All these musical types are used frequently but according to the qualities and circumstances of the clients. Gold and associates (2009) have stated that "verbal discussion or explanation connected to music is important and they help the client to explore the meaning of experience and relate new experience within therapy to situations in the clients' life".

Tips for Music Therapy

If music is practized by focusing on their *chakras*, vibration will be made in spiral cord (Pandey, 2011). To make Music Therapy more meaningful we should:

- Be in the world of music not by brain but by whole heart.
- Enjoy music not analyze it.
- Listen music three-four times in a day according to our interest.
- In case of hunger, we should not listen music.
- Be with music not only by listening but also singing with.
- Try to play any instrument. It will give us pleasure, peace and relaxation.
- Develop some interest of hearing music in our children.
- Prefer cool and peaceful music for old and ill people.

References

American Music Therapy Association, www.music therapy.org

Bruscia, K.E. (1998). *Defining Music Therapy*. Barcelona Publishers.

Bunt, L. and Sarah, H. (2002). *Music Therapy: Practicalities and Basic Principles of Music Therapy,* Hove and New York: Brunner.

Crowe, B.J. (2007). *Effective clinical practice in music therapy: Music therapy for children, adolescents, and adults with mental disorders*. American Music Therapy Association.

Davis, G.T. (2008). *An introduction to music therapy: theory and practice*. Third edition: *The Music Therapy; Treatment Process*. Silver Spring Maryland, 469-473.

Degmečić, D., Požgain, I., and Filaković, P. (2005). Glazba kao terapija. *International Review of the Aesthetics and Sociology of Music*, 36(2), 287-300.

Deka, (2012). *Inner Power of Music and Music Therapy*. (http://www.efi-news.com/2012/04/inner-power-of-music and music therapy.html).

De Sousa, A. (2005). The role of music therapy in psychiatry. *Alternative Therapies in Health and Medicine*, 11(6), 52.

Findeisen, B. (2007, August). Music therapy in the treatment of young children with selective mutism. In *Workshop at the Conference on Music, Language and Movement,* Herstmonceux Castle, East Sussex, UK.

Gerdner, L.A., and Swanson, E.A. (1993). Effects of individualized music on confused and agitated elderly patients. *Archives of Psychiatric Nursing*, 7(5), 284-291.

Gold, C., Solli, H.P., Krüger, V., and Lie, S.A. (2009). Dose–response relationship in music therapy for people with serious mental disorders: Systematic review and meta-analysis. *Clinical Psychology Review*, 29(3), 193-207.

Gupta, R. (2011). Sangeet: Rogon Ke Upchar Tatha Safal Vyaktitva Ke Nirman Mein Sahyog. In S. Srivastava (ed.) *Sangeet Chikitsa, Vibhinna Vyavaharik Samasyaon Ke Upchara ka Ek Sashakt Madhyam* (Vol. 2). Fazalganj, Kanpur.

Hannibal, N., Pedersen, I.N., Hestbæk, T., Sørensen, T.E., and Munk-Jørgensen, P. (2012). Schizophrenia and personality disorder patients' adherence to music therapy. *Nordic Journal of Psychiatry*, 66(6), 376-379.

Hillecke, T., Nickel, A. and Bolay, H.V. 2005. Scientific perspectives on music therapy. *Annals of New York Academy of Science*, 1060, 271-282.

Joshi, V. (2011). Sangeet Chikitsa evam Anusandhan. In S. Srivastava (ed.) *Sangeet Chikitsa, Vibhina Vyavaharik Samasyaon Ke Upchara ka Ek Sashakt Madhyam* (Vol. 2). Fazalganj, Kanpur.

Klassen, J.A., Liang, Y., Tjosvold, L., Klassen, T.P., and Hartling, L. (2008). Music for pain and anxiety in children undergoing medical procedures: a systematic review of randomized controlled trials. *Ambulatory Pediatrics*, 8(2), 117-128.

Koelsch, S., Schulze, K., Sammler, D., Fritz, T., Müller, K., and Gruber, O. (2009). Functional architecture of verbal and tonal working memory: an FMRI study. *Human Brain Mapping*, 30(3), 859-873.

Koelsch, S. (2005). Neural substrates of processing syntax and semantics in music. *Current Opinion in Neurobiology*, 15(2), 207-212.

Koelsch, S., Schroger, E., and Tervaniemi, M. (1999). Superior pre-attentive auditory processing in musicians. *Neuro Report*, 10, 1309-1313.

Koelsch, S. (2009). Music-syntactic processing and auditory memory: Similarities and differences between ERAN and MMN. *Psychophysiology*, 46(1), 179-190.

Meyer, M., and Jancke, L. (2006). Involvement of the left and right frontal operculum in speech and non-speech perception and production. *Broca's Region*, 218-241.

Nelson, A., Hartl, W., Jauch, K.W., Fricchione, G.L., Benson, H., Warshaw, A.L., and Conrad, C. (2008). The impact of music on hypermetabolism in critical illness. *Current Opinion in Clinical Nutrition and Metabolic Care*, 11(6), 790-794.

Nordoff, P. and Glive, R. Music Therapy in Special Education: Group Instrumental Activities for Physically Disabled Children, New York: The John Day Company.

Paul, S., and Ramsey, D. (2000). Music therapy in physical medicine and rehabilitation. *Australian Occupational Therapy Journal*, 47(3), 111-118.

Roth, E.A. (2014). Music Technology for Neurologic Music Therapy. *Handbook of Neurologic Music Therapy*, 12.

Srivastava, S. (ed.) (2011). *Sangeet Chikitsa, Vibhina Vyavaharik Samasyaon Ke Upchar ka Ek Sashakt Madhyam* (Vol. 2). Fazalganj, Kanpur.

Sussman, E.S. (2007). A new view on the MMN and attention debate: the role of context in processing auditory events. *Journal of Psychophysiology*, 21(3-4), 164-175.

Wong, P.C.E. Skoe, N.M. Russo (2007). Musical experience shapes human brainstem encoding of linguistic pitch pattern, *Nature and Neuroscience*. 10: 420-422.

You tube. web site www.you tube.com.

6

Psychotherapy in India

Past and Present

Anubhuti Dubey and *Radha Maddhessia*

Psychotherapy is a general term referring to therapeutic interaction or treatment contracted between a trained professional and a client, patient, family, couple or group. "Psychotherapy is the treatment by, psychological means, of problems of an emotional nature in which a trained person deliberately establishes a professional relationship with the patient with the object: (1) of removing, modifying or retarding existing symptoms; (2) of mediating disturbed patterns of behaviour; and (3) of promoting positive personality growth and development" (Wolberg, 1967).

Psychotherapy is the utilization of psychological measures in treatment of sick people. It is planned and systematic application of psychological facts and theories to lessen large varieties of human psychogenic dispositions. Psychotherapy is the art of confronting disease and enhancing health by mental influences and the use of psychological methods in the treatment of mental disorder or maladjustment.

Psychotherapy in Past

The core of psychotherapy can be seen as present in all traditional societies all along. In India, it has existed in a submerged form, intertwined with social structures and societal norms. It can be seen in religious practices, in customs, myths and rituals. It has been included in spiritualism, in *yoga*, in Buddhism, in Ayurveda, in the tradition of Unani and in Allopathy as well. From the Hindu mythology, *Mahabharata* is a great textbook of psychopathology and *Gita* a great disquisition in psychotherapy. The Indian tradition includes psychological phenomena like consciousness and joy as core-elements of reality, and it takes 'knowledge of the self' (*adhyatma-vidya*) as the fundamental science.

In a study, Dhairyam (1961) observed the Indian culture and philosophy as being unique in its fostering of spiritual independence and growth in the people. Studies reveal common Indian as under the strong impact of the *Vedas, Upanishads*, *Yoga*, *Bhagavad Gita*, Buddhism and its various schools. Indian philosophy and Indian psychology share a framework and believe that human has tremendous potential hidden in its subsistence in the world. Indian ancient psychology also has an endless array of techniques to raise human consciousness.

Psychotherapy practiced in India is not applicable only to the sick, but was also perceived to be useful in imparting insight in those not stricken by mental illness and thus effecting fulfilment and self-realization. The giver of such remedial and enriching experience assumed a highly exaggerated position in the society. In such a situation, it was neither possible nor considered desirable for the therapist and the client or patient to meet and interact as equals. The relationship was perhaps—akin to the teacher-student disciple relationship. Psychotherapy was, therefore, not a dialectical and argumentative process where truth was reached or approached by a debate between the two or within the heart of the recipient, but was more of a situation where truth was revealed by the therapist and accepted by the client/patient. Not everybody was considered fit for such psychotherapeutic relationship.

Regional concepts and therapies including folk beliefs (Neki, 1977; Choudhry and Mirza, 1983; Hosseini, 1983), *Guru-Chela* relationship (Neki, 1977; Surya and Jayaram, 1964), *Yoga* (Grover *et al.,* 1994; Sethi *et al.,* 1982; Vasudevan *et al.,* 1994; Janakiramaiah *et al.,* 1998) and meditation (Bhaskaran, 1991; Andrade and Andrade, 1991, Chandiramani, 1991) are said to be useful in managing a variety of problems among mentally ill patients. The therapeutic wisdom in the *Bhagavad Gita* (Govindaswamy, 1959; Rao and Parvathidevi, 1974; Rao, 1980; Balodhi and Kesavan, 1986) and in Indian mythology (Shyamsunder, 1993) has important contributions to psychotherapy.

Paradigm of Ramayana

The *Ramayana* imparts knowledge of truths about human nature, norms for living condition and about man's relationship with God. It has much therapeutic wisdom and can be successfully employed in psychotherapy. In the *Ramayana* conceptual themes, similar to those found in traditional psychotherapy can be sanctioned. These themes being well known are easy for patients to accept and analyse with it. The use of examples from the *Ramayana* is especially helpful in patients who are religiously inclined and are under stress (Rajagopalachari, 1993; Narayana, 1987; Acharya, 1998; Varkey, 2000).

The victory of good over evil is the central theme of *Ramayana*. Sri Rama lived as a human being and faced the day-to-day situations and conflicts of life. The *Ramayana* describes many situations where there are moral dilemmas and conflicts between two rights. The other themes with powerful implications for mental health are Sri Rama's tranquility in the face of success and tragedy and the concept of *dharma*. Themes which can be used from a cognitive perspective include: (1) Lakshmana's misinterpretation of Bharata's intent and Sri Rama's counsel; and (2) Hanuman's feelings of inadequacy and Jamvant's focus on potential. The reminiscence and themes can be applied to show the similarity of the issues facing the patient with the aim of increasing insight. They can be used as examples to suggest alternate modes of coping.

The *Ramayana* can be used in contexts where patients have conflicts that require psychological intervention. It can be used in patients with dysthymia, neurotic and stress related disorders and problems, adjustment difficulties, personality problems, maladaptive coping styles, marital discord and relationship difficulties, bereavement, academic, occupational, and phase of life problems. The choice of using such a strategy is not dependent on the diagnostic label but rather on the individual, their religious background, and conflicts. Depending on the similarity to the patient's situation, the therapist would have to match the stories and themes.

Wig (2004) called the story of Hanuman not knowing his true potential, as "Hanuman Complex". It can be used with a patient who has lost confidence and who feels unable to meet life's challenges, as the power to change his life rests with him. He has temporarily lost the knowledge of his own powers due to his illness, or due to this facade of ignorance. Like Hanuman he has to shake off this reluctance and realize his true potential. And as well as it can be used with doctors in training that, when they do psychotherapy, not to assume that power to change the life of the patient lies with them. In fact, the potential to change rests with the patient who has temporarily like Hanuman, lost it. It is the therapist job (like Jamvant) to restore the power back to the patient.

Paradigm of Mahabharata

Experiential anecdotes of therapist in India show the application of Indian concepts in the therapeutic approach. In studies it has been seen how a client in Indian setting could be introduced to psychotherapy using the dialogue of Arjuna and Krishna at the battlefield. The *Bhagavad Gita* is a classical example of crisis intervention psychotherapy.

The *Bhagavad Gita* is one of the greatest contributions of India to the world and is considered to be one of the first revelations from God. The *Bhagavad Gita* is a doctrine of universal truth and is meant for people of every section and age. The *Bhagavad Gita* deals with the most sacred metaphysical science. The *Bhagavad Gita* is also a key authority (Bartley, 2011) dealing with human day-to-day worries, anxieties and inhibitions people facing from time-to-time in everyday life situations. Therefore, it is equally effective for people of any gender, race, religion or culture. The *Bhagavad Gita* is the essence of the *Vedas* and *Upanishads*. It is *brahmavidya* and also a *shastra* of *yoga*.

The *Bhagavad Gita* teaches three things: *Brahma-vidyavam, Yoga-shastre srikrishnaarjuna-samvade.* It means theory, practice and realization. The understanding of theory, practice and realization may lead an individual to cope with day-to-day stresses of life. There is a theoretical physics, practical physics and there is technological implementation of it. The *Bhagavad Gita* draws a temporal sequence of mental events as:

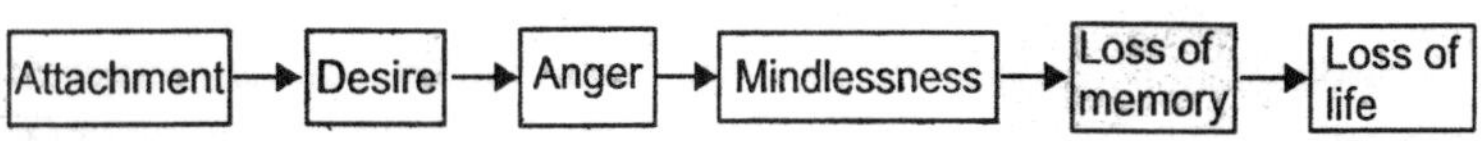

(Bhawuk, 1999)

Theoretical physics is the advanced conceptualization of the fundamental structure of physical reality, and with this insight gained through methodological systematic study of the constituents of matter. Matter becomes more amenable to handle and moves us in the path of self-realization. Human lives are stress-ridden. Stress arising from occupations, career, relationships or finance to name a few. Overall, our morning starts with stresses and end up with stress. It is a vicious cycle of stress which is never ending.

The *Bhagavad Gita* is a key to all worries and anxieties which was spoken by Krishna in the battle of *Kurukshetra—Mahabharata. Bhagavad Gita* has practical and real life application in day-to-day stressors a human faces in his/her life. It can also be proved by the fact that, as the *Bhagavad Gita* was not written in any holy place like temple or *Gurukul* (University) rather it was spoken by Krishna in the field of Battle of *Mahabharata*. Thus, it is quite evident that the *Bhagavad Gita* is the practical application of the stressors, worries one faces in various situations of life. *Gita's* seven hundred concise verses provide a precise guide to the science of self-realization. No other philosophical or religious work reveals in such a lucid and profound way, the nature of consciousness, the self, the universe and the supreme (Bhawuk, 2011).

The *Bhagavad Gita* consists of seven hundred *shlokas* verses in total. These *shlokas* form essence of spirituality. As per the *Bhagavad Gita*, we as a human being are primarily a spirit, a soul/*atman* or a cosmic consciousness that manifested human to work out its *karma* and remove impurities within. The *Bhagavad Gita* meant for reaching stage of enlightenment in one's lifetime.

Since, personality susceptibility are partly conditioned by the dominant inputs contained in the given culture, *anasakti* is analyzed as a multifaceted personality construct consisting of a set of beliefs, attitudes and cognitions consistent with the essence of the ideal. The causal linkage between *anasakti* and health can be argued that the doctrine of *anasakta*, action conveys a message which is central to coping with life stressors. This argument is based on the psychological literature which demonstrates the significance of cognitive and attitudinal systems in determining the manner in which stress inducing situations are encountered (Pearlin, Liberman, Menaghan and Mullan, 1981). One who has been able to relieve himself of the anxieties pertaining to success or failure can apply himself to any task more effectively as compared to others. An *anasakta*, person would perhaps be more effective in pursuing material goals too.

According to Mahatma Gandhi, "I find a solace in the *Bhagavad Gita* that I miss even in the *Sermon on the Mount*. When disappointment stares me in the face of and all alone I see not one ray of light, I go back to the *Bhagavad Gita*. I find a verse here and a verse there and I immediately being to smile in the midst of overwhelming tragedies and my life has been full of external tragedies and if they have left no visible, no indelible scar on me, I owe it all to the teaching of the *Bhagavad Gita* (*Young India*, 1925). Gandhi Ji acknowledged the *Gita* as a proven rich source of mental peace or well-being (happiness). *Gita Nishkama Karma* echoes Abraham Maslow's Meta motivation; the four motives of *Kama, Artha, Dharma* and *Moksha* are like Maslow's hierarchy of needs etc. Swami Brahmavidyananda analyses *Vedanta* and says that in the Indian approach, the process of managing the mind has a spiritual base to it that changes the way you perceive the world. In *Vedanta*, *Ishvara* is the grandiose order, which includes the physical order—harmony, patterns and connections in the movement of our life.

Buddhism Paradigm

Buddhism refers to the stream of consciousness as the basis of subjective feeling of continuity and identity which affects perceptions, thoughts, actions and emotions. In the five modes of knowing (sensory, extra-sensory, holistic, insightful and ethical) in Buddhism, the focus has been on inner transformation, with the ultimate goal being liberation (Premasiri, 2008). According to Buddhism, the knowing should be based on personal experience not on authority, faith, belief or speculation.

Buddhism is an esthetic and it even negates the *atman* or self of Hinduism. Dayal Mirchan, a Mumbai psychiatrist, says "Buddhism has a refined understanding of the mind. The mind, says the Buddha, consists of four processes: Consciousness *(vinnana),* Perception *(sama)*, Sensation *(vedana)* and Reaction *(sankhara)*."

Jainism Paradigm

Jainism is characterized by its typical Soul-psychology. The doctrine of four-fold infinites of the soul: infinite apprehension inflicts power and infinite bless gave rise in Jainism a great deal of interest in Extra Sensory Perception (ESP)—clairvoyance, telepathy and omniscience, subjects now studied under Para-psychology. According to Jainism, the soul is inherently pure and perfect. The soul is clouded by *Karma* as the shining sum is often obscured by either a cloud or mist or a veil of dust.

Ayurveda Paradigm

Ayurveda describes three *gunas* of mind—*Sattva* (balance), *Raja* (arrogance) and *Tama* (indolence). Mind is called '*manas'*. Ayurveda describes that a possibility for disease is due to imbalance of the '*tamas'* or '*rajas*' in the mind. They are the reactive tendencies which vitiate the mind and leads to emotional imbalances, and also results in psychological disturbances. Hence, *Rajas* and *Tamas* are termed as '*Doshas* of mind'. *Tridoshas* are *Vata, Pitta* and *Kapha*. Literally, these terms mean the darkness and brightness of the mind or negative thoughts in the mind or the clearness of the mind. These impurities or imbalances are called '*doshas*'. The reason for any unhealthy condition is the toxins created by the accumulated '*dosha'*. These negative feelings are emotional toxins accumulated in the mind. If they are not driven out by the body in a stipulated period of time, they give rise to neurosis, depression, insomnia etc. If this is further ignored, it turns into permanent disorders like *Unmada*; unreasonable and irrational state of mind like hysteria, *Apasmara* (epilepsy) is also categorized as mental disorder, *Atatvaabhinivesha* and other *Manasroga* under the *Manovaha srotas* or psyche centre. In Ayurveda, there are some different types of sets of behavioural alternation such as *Kama, Krodha, Lobha, Bhrama, Tandra, Murchha, Sannyasa, Maddattaya,* etc.

Mental disorders are treated by the same way in Ayurveda as it follows in treatment of physical illness. It comprises the following:

1. ***Purification***: This traditionally consisted of purges, emetics, enaemas, and bleeding along with instructions for personal hygiene.
2. ***Pacification***: This consisted of outer application of ointments, ingestion of decoctions which are prepared from plants or both.
3. ***Removal of the cause***: This consists of removal of predisposing, maintaining and precipitating factors for the mental illness through changes in lifestyle like regular sleep, dietary changes, abstinence from alcohol, to name a few. It also includes changes in environment such as instructions for family members.

'*Sattvavajaya*' or psychotherapy is one of the three principal categories of the approach to the patients care as described in classics of Ayurveda. In principal, *Sattvavajaya* is applicable in varying forms in all kinds of diseases, but it is essentially applicable in mental diseases. The classical *Sattvavajaya* is based on three principles, viz. (1) Replacement of emotions, (2) Assurances, and (3) Psycho-shock therapy. Ayurveda conceives a set of emotions like *Kama* (lust), *Krodha* (anger), *Lobha* (greed), *Moha, Irshya, Dvesha, Harsha* (happiness), *Vishada* (grief), *Mana* (pride), *Cittodvega* (anxiety) etc. All these are considered to be basic components of psychopathology.

Sattvavajaya considers physician's interference with patient's control on mind. This can be achieved by various ways as: (1) By proper guidance and advice (*sankalpa)* for right decision; (2) By polishing the objectives (*dhyeya)*; (3) By challenging the presumptions (*uhya*); (4) By replacing the ideas (*vicarya*); and (5) By regulating the thought process (*cintya).* *Sattvavajaya* plays a significant role in the maintenance of a harmonious relation among intellect, memory and patience, ultimately leading to a happy healthy state of the individual.

Sattvavajaya is a psychological method of Ayurveda which includes mind control, method of replacement of emotions, mental equanimity, and inhibiting some psychophysical, environmental, psychological, volitional stressors. This can be achieved by adopting some temporal techniques like overmanifestations, undermanifestation, perverted manifestation of five senses of human body, regulation of mind, promotion of intellectual level, by following seasonal regimen and discrimination. *Sattvavajaya* not only prevents the impairment of intellect, dysfunction of memory, but also brings them back to a normal state, whenever they are impaired. Thus, *Sattvavajaya* plays a significant role in the maintenance of a harmonious state among intellect, memory and patience, ultimately leading to a happy healthy state of the individual.

According to *Charaka Samhita*, systematic path of mental diseases includes—*Nidana Parivarjana,* i.e. elimination of basic cause, *Daiva vyapasraya chikitsa*, *Yukti vyapasraya chikitsa*. *Vyapasraya* refers to depending and trusting towards it. *Daivavyapasraya* implies any therapy that depends on the '*Daivya*' (devine) or linked to it and it is concerned to unknown circumstances, which are beyond the purview of reasoning or cannot establish on scientific basis, and therefore, it remain as spiritual therapy. It includes *Mantra* (incantations), *Manidharana* (precious stones), *Oushadam* (amulets), *Mangalam* (propitiatory rites), *Balih* (oblations), *Homah* (sacrifice), *Upavasa* (fasting), *Japa* (prayer), *Vratam* (vows). *Yuktivyapasraya, 'yukti'* means union, connection and it is much rational in its approach to treating disease of psychological and somatic origin. Treatments for mental disorders are given by specific procedures known as *Panchakarma* and presiding suitable palliative measures as drugs (*aushadha*) and diet regimen.

Paradigm of Guru-Chela Relationship and Sahaja

Neki (1974) discussed the '*Guru-chela relationship*' as a therapeutic measure that appears to be particularly tenable where self-discipline rather than self-expression is to be inculcated among the clients and where a creating harmony is sought between the individual and the society. In the Indian tradition, the word '*guru*' has a pair of connotations—being a teacher and a spiritual preceptor. The *guru* acts as a physician of mind and soul with objectivity and competence. The *guru* takes the disciple '*chela*' through an experiential journey of self-exploration with an aim to liberate disciple from all sufferings.

Neki (1975b) proposed '*Sahaja*' as an ideal of mental health which could be merged with '*guru-chela* relationship' for psychotherapy in the

Indian context. *Sahaja* is derived from two words—'*Saha*' (together) and '*Ja*' (born). Thereby, meaning 'born together', i.e. with oneself, hence innate or inborn. *Sahaja* is the state of achieving freedom or liberation and it aims to reaching an ideal state of being by attaining the ultimate human potential.

Paradigm of Meditation and Yoga

The methods of *yoga* and meditation are now-a-days primarily looked as a mean for attaining salvation, as a means to arrive at *samadhi* or *nirvana*. As well as they are seen as means to arrive at physical health and the survival of a corporate lifestyle. In the culture of origin, however, they are part of a coherent knowledge system and they are clearly looked at as a way to arrive at reliable knowledge. This is most clear in the case of *jnanayoga* (the *yoga* of knowledge). One can easily discern elements of the pursuit of truth in *karma*- and *bhaktiyoga* (the paths of work and devotion), which also have methods to reduce the distortions of perception and affect that are part of the ordinary human consciousness.

Deatherage (1975) studied the effectiveness of meditation techniques as a primary or secondary technique with a variety of psychiatric patients. He conceptualized meditation as a self-treatment regimen (highly efficient for the use of the therapists time and therefore, quite cost-effective) that helps patients know their own mental processes and preoccupations, develop the observer self, "and gain the ability to shape or control their mental processes".

Vaughan (1989) listed the following components common to both therapy and meditation—telling the truth, releasing negative emotions, the need for effort and consistency, authenticity and trust-avoiding self-deception, integrity and wholeness—accepting all one's experiences and allowing things to be as they are. Rather than living in a world of illusion and denial, insight and forgiveness directed towards oneself and others, opening the heart and developing and capacity to give and receive love, awareness and non-judgemental attention, liberation from limiting self-concepts, from fear and delusion, and from the past and early conditioning.

Meditation includes *Vipassana* which is to focus attention on the manner in which unconscious conflicts are being processed and recreated in the mind on a moment-to-moment basis. Thus, *Vipassana* offers the possibility of not just understanding such conflicts conceptually, but of actually penetrating and gradually achieving them through meditative insight.

Studies show that for cases of psychoneuroses, *Yoga* is superior to 'pseudo-treatment', i.e. where they were asked to relax and do some postures resembling *Asanas,* and breathing practices resembling '*Pranayama*' and to "write all the thoughts that came to their mind during the treatment (similar to *dharana* and *dhyana*)".

The Electroencephalogram (EEG) records indicate that, meditation can docile amygdale enabling the individual to be less shocked, frustrated, or angry. Transcendental meditation promotes increasing degrees of orderliness, integration, and coherence in the brain leading to a unique style of brain functioning. While a relative excitement is continuously present in the brains of non-enlightened people maintain a low level of excitation, which has a pervasive calming effect on the mind (Travis, 2001). The aspiration for transcendental existence helps overcome the body-centred egoistic strivings and offers a descended view of self. It has implications for work and social relationships. It allows one to be motivated to treat works as a natural duty (*dharma*) to be performed with reference to the demands of the location in one's life space rather than any extrinsic incentive.

Paradigm of Religious and Faith Healers

In India religious and faith healers are widespread all-over the country. A strong faith in the tenets of religion and supernatural phenomena and powers, on part of both the therapists and the clients, is a necessary condition for the success of this kind of therapy. It will perhaps not be incorrect to say that most of the practitioners and patients are Hindus. However, many Muslims are thought to be endowed with great healing properties. The usual method of operation is that the patient seeks the therapist, and comes to him for help. The latter in turn gives him a sympathetic hearing, involves the mercy of God on him. In the process, he may give the patient some sacred ash *(bhabhuti)*, ask him to make certain offerings at the altar, one give him verbal reassurance and suggestion that the problem would be over. Certain other religious rituals, like periodic offerings and worships over long period of time, observation of fasts and other restrictions may be prescribed. Sometimes, the therapist names some offending spirit or the patient's sin or misdeeds (including those ascribed to an earlier birth) and prescribes the remedial measures.

The healer generally enjoys very high reputation in the local area as a holy man; good-intentioned, helpful, compassionate and possessive of extraordinary powers. The vernacular name for faith healer or religious healer varies from one part of the country to another. Some typical examples are *Peer, Sayana, Babajee* and *Ojha*, literally meaning a divine, a learned man, an elder respected man and a Brahmin respectively.

Closed to the roots of Hindu mythology, Najabuddin Unhammad (1222 AD), an Indian physician propagated the Unani system of medicine as he described seven types of mental disorder; *Sauda-a-Tadbee* (Schizophrenia), *Muree Sauda* (Depression), *Ishk* (Delusion of love), *Nisyan* (Organic mental disorder), *Haziyan* (Paranoid state) and *Malikhaloia-a-marak* (Delirium). Psychotherapy was known as *Ilaj-i-Nafsani* in Unani medicine.

During the reigns of King Ashoka, many hospitals were established for patients with mental illness. According to the scribes of *Ashoka Samhita*, hospitals were built with separate enclosures for various practices including keeping the patients and dispensing treatments prevailing during those times.

The Indian tradition has also developed the concept of *ahamkara*, which stands somewhere in between the Western concepts of ego and self-concept. But besides this egoic centre, which belongs to the ordinary waking consciousness, the Indian tradition has also developed a detailed nomenclature for many other, more subtle and non-egoic centre of consciousness; and it has even worked out, especially in certain Buddhist schools, how a consciousness can exist without any centre whatsoever. Varma (1982) used principles from the communication of Buddha in psychotherapy which he viewed as an "interpersonal method of mitigating suffering". He has also conceptualized the use of concepts of *Karma* and *Dharma* in psychotherapy (Varma, 1982). Similarly, the Indian tradition has found below the surface of our waking consciousness not only the dark 'unconscious' that depth psychology has explored, but a whole range of subtle *kosas* or layers of consciousness, that each has their own characteristic nature. It has even worked out many different ways of 'realizing in one's experience (or, perhaps one should rather say, in one's being) a Transcendent beyond all nature. It has found that all these inner layers, types, and centres of conscious existence have their specific influences on the surface personality, and that a direct access to them with sufficient training enables levels of freedom, peace, joy, compassion and understanding much beyond what is possible in the ordinary waking state. Neki (1977) used the concept of '*Sahaja*' and the role of '*Nirvana*' in psychotherapy.

The concept of '*Shaivite*' stemming from the Hindu mythology of God Shiva and representing a phallic symbol can be used in dynamic psychotherapy (Nand, 1961). The legend of *Savitri* has been used as a framework for psychotherapy by Surya and Jayaram (1996).

Present Status of Psychotherapy in India

A historical account of psychotherapy since the second decade of this century has been given by Sinha (1956). Girindrashekhar Bose, the founder of Indian Psychoanalytic Society, can be considered to have brought modern psychotherapy in India. In addition to stimulating other people in psychoanalysis Bose also propounded a theory of 'opposite wishes' and published a book, '*The Concept of Repression*'.

Varma and Ghosh (1975) tried to ascertain the nature and extent of psychotherapy practiced by the Indian psychiatrists. All felt that psychotherapy is a useful mode of treatment. Majority, however, recommended departures from the Western world. Vahia *et al.* (1973) in a study of patients with psychoneurotic and psychosomatic disorders, demonstrated the efficacy of psycho-physiological therapy based on the concepts of Patanjali. The various modifications suggested were that it should be briefer, crisis-oriented, supportive, flexible and comprising different approaches and to be applicable to cultural and social conditions. Greater activity on part of the therapist, greater use of suggestion and reassurance, lesser use of dynamic interpretation, religious blending and entering into a *Guru-chela* relationship were the other departures from the classical model suggested.

In a survey (Sharma *et al.*, 1975), it is reported that approximately eighty per cent of the clinical psychologists practice counselling and guidance, about ¾ of them supportive and eclectic therapies, others are engaged in behaviour therapy, psychodynamic psychotherapy and play therapy. Approximately 1/3rd of their time is taken up by this type of therapy. Sen (1974, 1975a, 1975b) advocates behaviour therapy and therapies based on learning therapy and other psychological approaches also for the clinical psychologists of the 80s. Sharma (1970) mentions that projective tests could be used therapeutically and feels the trend now-a-days is to go from brief to 'briefer' psychotherapies to 'first aid' and 'emergency' and 'crises' therapies. Dhairyam (1975) advocates 'Guru Psychotherapy' and '*Guru-Shishya*' systems. Naug (1975), Majumdar (1975a, 1975b) etc., have also reported case studies where *yoga* and other forms of psychotherapy have been successfully carried out.

A review of the national census data and the National Family Health Survey (NFHS) data suggest that, generally nuclear families are becoming the predominant form of Indian family institution, at least in urban areas. The 1991 census, for the first time reported household growth to be higher than the population growth, suggesting household fragmentation; a trend that gathered further momentum in the 2010 Census. A comparison of the three NFHS data also show that over the years there has been a progressive increase in nuclear families, more in urban areas, with an associated progressive decrease in the number of household members (Bhat *et al.*, 2007; IIPS, 1995).

New and unexpected problems arising out of the rapid changing social scenario also need to be taken into consideration. Family and couple's conflict arising out of factors such as conflicts in families over dowry, or related to intercaste marriages; sexual problems arising out of physical separation of couples due to job timing or placement; disagreement about child rearing practices (both within couples and intergenerational); conflict's related to husband's role in sharing in domestic chores for working couples; problems with unsupervised children, and loss or displacement of role or function of the elderly are only a few of the problems unique to the modern Indian families (Carson, Jain and Ramirez, 2009). In recent times, increased demands on children or adolescents for academic achievements from parents, the culture clash with children going for night-outs, parties, raves and adolescents sexual experimentation have been reported by Indian therapists as common issues while dealing with adolescents (Carson and Chowdhury, 2000). Although most of these problems are the same that troubled the West in the 1960s and the 1970s, our cultural differences make the therapist look and treat these problems.

Kumar and Ram (2001) had discussed the recent trends and status of psychotherapy in a specific therapeutic method and observed that Western psychotherapeutic techniques are being modified to suit the Indian culture. Sengupta and associates (1993) describe the use of psychotherapy in a person with dissociative amnesia following a traumatic incident. Counselling was found to be more effective than moral reasoning as an intervention to increase social competence in girls studying in class five to seven. Social competence was measured in terms of school performance, hard work, appropriate behaviour, learning and happiness (Reddy, 1994). Eight weeks intervention consisting of play therapy and parental counselling was effective in reducing aggressive conduct and improving overall adjustment and family environment in children aged 8 to 12 years (Dogra and Veeraraghavan, 1994). In a much younger age group of pre-school (3-6 years old), Kumari and Chhikara (1997) demonstrated that psychological interventions were effective in enhancing their cognitive development and functioning. Transactional Analysis (TA) was found to increase the emotional maturity of 60 students enrolled in a pre-university course (Srinagar and Rao, 1994a). Sharma and Veeraraghavan (1995) found that 12 to 15 sessions of family behavioural therapy comprising, psycho-education, communication and problem solving skills, resulted in improved social skills and better home environment in 20 patients with schizophrenia.

Modelling techniques were used by Vidyasagar and Mishra (1993) to reduce aggression in ten delinquent males (12 to 24 years). Devi (2002) reported that both differential reinforcement to other behaviour and time out were equally effective in the management of disruptive behaviours among 50 primary school children. Agarwal and Kumari (2000) used a multiple design to treat children with onychophagia (nail biting). Nail biting was associated with anxiety and tension and responded well to the combined application of progressive relaxation and self-monitoring techniques.

India emerging as a major economic power in the world, there is a renewed interest in the Indian thought systems, values and practices as well as in the strength and resilience of Indian society. The Indian culture and its philosophy are now seen behind India's economic success. Indian research acquired greater respectability and is now taken more seriously by the Western psychologists (ironically), and as well as by Indian psychologists themselves.

According to a survey commissioned by the *Yoga Journal*, there were in February 2008, some 15.8 million practitioners of (*Hatha*) yoga in the USA alone, and among the rest of the population, another 8 per cent, 18 million people, were "very or extremely interested in yoga". Effect of yoga and meditation has now been measured almost on variables like blood pressure, anxiety, depression and extroversion.

Torrey (1972a, 1972b) has drawn attention to significant similarities between Western psychotherapy and faith healing and has argued that in spite of apparent differences in the technique in the two cases, the therapeutically active components are remarkably similar. Wittkower and Warnes (1974) have drawn attention to the similarities between psychotherapies practiced all-over the world. In spite of the superficial differences, they feel that such therapies around the world have got the following similarities: (1) There is an intense emotional confiding relationship between the therapist and the patient; and (2) The therapist and the patient share an identical worldview. Neki (1973) quotes Vasavada asserting the parallelism between psychoanalysis and existential analysis on the one hand, and the Yogic and Zen practices on the other.

References

Andrade, C., Andrade, C. (1991). Meditation from an Indian perspective. *Indian Journal of Psychiatry,* 33,82-83.

Balodhi, J.P. and Kesavan, M.S. (1986). *Bhagavad Gita* and Psychotherapy. *NIMHANS Journal,* 4, 139-143.

Bhasakaran, K. (1991). Meditation from a mental health perspective. *Indian Journal of Psychiatry,* 33, 87-94.

Behere, P.B., Das, A., Yadav, R., and Behere, A.P. (2013). Ayurvedic concepts related to psychotherapy. *Indian Journal of Psychiatry,* 55, 311-313.

Bhat *et al.*, (2007). Household Population and Housing Characteristics. *International Institute for Population Sciences (IIPS) and Macro-International.* Vol. 1. Chapter 2. *National Family Health Survey* (NFHS-3), Ministry of Health and Family Welfare, Government of India, 2005-06; Mumbai India, 21-52.

Bhawuk, D.P.S. (1999). Who attains peace: An Indian model of personal harmony? *Indian Psychological Review,* 52 (2 and 3), 40-48.

Bogart, G. (1991). Meditation and psychotherapy: A review of the literature. *The American Journal of Psychiatry,* 45 (3), 383-412.

Carson, D.K., and Chowdhury, A. (2000). Family Therapy in India: A new profession in an Indian land? *Contemporary Family Therapy,* 22, 387-406.

Carson, D.K., Jain, S., and Ramirez, S. (2009). Counselling and Family therapy in India: Evolving Professionals in a rapidly developing nation. *International Journal of Advance Counselling,* 31, 5-46.

Chadda, R.K., and Deb, K.S. (2013). Indian family system, collectivistic society and psychotherapy. *Indian Journal of Psychiatry,* 55, 300-307.

Chandiramani, K. (1991). *Vipassana* meditation: A mirror to the mind. *Indian Journal of Psychiatry,* 33, 293-296.

Choudhry, M.R. and Mirza, L. (1983). Fountain house, Lahore: a unique experiment in cross-cultural collaboration, *Indian Journal of Psychiatry,* 25, 322-327.

Choudhary, S., Vaish, S., Sudarsanan, S., and Bharti, S.P. (2014). Psychotherapy client centred way. *Delhi Psychiatry Journal,* Vol. 17. No. 1, 27-28.

Cornelissen, R.M.M., Misra, G., and Varma, S. (2014). *Introduction to Foundations of Indian Psychology.* Dorling Kindersley (India Pvt. Ltd.) 12-17.

Dalal, A.K., and Misra, G. (2010). *The Core and Context of Indian Psychology, Psychology and Developing Societies,* Sage Publication, 4 (1), 91-92.

Deatherage, G. (1975). The clinical use of mindfulness meditation techniques in short-term psychotherapy. *Journal of Transpersonal Psychology,* 7, 43-133.

Devi, B. (2002). Effectiveness of differential reinforcement of other behaviour and time out in the management of disruptive behaviours among primary school children. *Behavioural Scientists,* 3, 3-6.

Dhairyam, D. (1975). Presidential address to the Vth All Indian Convention of Clinical Psychologists. *Indian Journal of Clinical Psychology,* 2, 1.

Dogra, A., and Veeraraghavan, V. (1994). A study of psychological intervention of children with aggressive conduct disorder. *Indian Journal of Clinical Psychology,* 21, 28-32.

Gandhi, M.K. (1981). *Young India,* 1925. Navjivan Publishing House, Ahmedabad, 1078-1079.

Govindaswamy, M.V. (1959). Surrender-not to self-surrender. *Transaction.* 2, 1-10.

Grover, P., Varma, V.K., Parshad, D. and Varma, S.K. (1994). Role of yoga in treatment of neurotic disorders: current status and future direction. *Indian Journal of Psychiatry,* 36, 153-162.

Hosseini, S.A. (1983). An elementary status of the principles of individual and group psychotherapy and mental health in Islam. *Indian Journal of Psychiatry,* 25, 335-337.

International Institute for Population Studies (IIPS) and ORC Macro. National Family Health Survey (NFHS-1), Ministry of Health and Family Welfare, Government of India 1992-93. India, Mumbai, 1995.

Jacob, A.S., and Krishna, G. (2003). Special article: Spiritualism and psychiatry-II. *Indian Journal of Psychiatry.* 45(IV), 200-201.

Janakiramaiah, *et al.*, (1998). Therapeutic efficacy of Sudarshan Kriya Yoga. *NIMHANS Journal,* 16, 21-28.

Kumar, D. and Ram, N. (2001). Psychotherapy: Current trends. *Eastern Journal of Psychiatry,* 5, 12-18.

Majumdar, S.K. (1975a). A study on pedagophobia psychotherapeutic approach to behaviour modification. *Indian Journal of Clinical Psychology,* 2, 91.

Majumdar, S.K. (1975b). Psychotherapy of Pedagophobia by Reciprocal Inhibition—A Mechanical Technique. *Indian Journal of Clinical Psychology,* 2, 191.

Manickam, L.S. (2013). Integrative change model in psychotherapy: Perspectives from Indian thought. *Indian Journal of Psychiatry*, 55 (Suppl. 2), S322.

Nand, S. (1961). A comparative study of scientific and religious psychotherapy with a special role of the commonest Shaivite model in total psychoanalysis. *Indian Journal of Psychiatry,* 3, 173-261.

Naug, R.N. (1975). Yoga Therapy in neurotic disorders. *Indian Journal of Clinical Psychology,* 2, 87.

Neki, J.S. (1974). A reappraisal of the *Guru-Chela relationship* as a therapeutic paradigm. *International Mental Health Research Newsletter,* 16, 2.

Neki, J.S. (1975b). An Indian ideal of mental health. *Psychiatry,* 36, 1-11.

Neki, J.S. (1977). Psychotherapy in India. *Indian Journal of Psychiatry,* 1, 1-10.

Nizamie, S.H., and Goyal, N. (2010). History of Psychiatry in India. *Indian Journal of Psychiatry,* 52, 7-8.

Pande, N., and Naidu, R.K. (1992). *Anasakti and Health: A Study of Non-Attachment, Psychology and Developing Societies*. Sage Publication, 4, 89, 91-92.

Pearlin, L.T., Liberman, M.A., Menaghan, *E.G. and* Mullan, J.T. (1981). The stress process. *Journal of Health and Social Behaviour,* 22, 337-356.

Premassiri, P.D. (2008). Verities of Cognition in early Buddhism. In K.K. Rao, K.R., A.C. Paranjpe and A.K. Dalal (Eds.). *Handbook of Indian Psychology*, New Delhi: Cambridge University Press, 85-104.

Rao, V.A. (1980). *Gita* and mental sciences. *Indian Journal of Psychiatry,* 22, 19-31.

Rao, V.A. and Parvathidevi, S. (1974). The *Bhagavad Gita* treats body and mind. *Indian Journal of History of Medicine,* 19, 35-44.

Reddy, Y.C., Girimaji, S.C., and Srinath, S. (1997). Clinical profile of mania in children and adolescents from the Indian subcontinent. *Canadian Journal of Psychiatry,* 42, 841-46.

Sen, N.N. (1974). Behaviour therapy in depression: An experimental analysis. *Indian Journal of Clinical Psychology,* 1, 53.

Sen, N.N. (1975a). Behaviour therapy in depression II. Plan and Procedure of case analysis and treatment. *Indian Journal of Clinical Psychology,* 2, 77.

Sen, N.N. (1975b). Clinical Psychology of eighties: Editorial. *Indian Journal of Clinical Psychology,* 2, 1-4.

Sengupta, S.N., Jena, S. and Saxena, S. (1993). Generalized Dissociative Amnesia. *Australian and New Zealand Journal of Psychiatry,* 27, 699-700.

Sethi, B.B., Trivedi, J.K., Srivastava, A. and Yadav, S. (1982). Indigenous therapy in the practice of psychotherapy in India, *Indian Journal of Psychotherapy,* 24, 230-236.

Singh, A., and Modi, R. (2011). Indian Asian thought and well-being (Happiness). *Bilingual Journal of Humanities and Social Sciences,* Vol. 2, 1-2.

Shamasundar, C. (1979). What kind of psychotherapy in the Indian setting. *Indian Journal of Psychiatry,* 21, 36.

Shamasundar, C. (1993). Therapeutic wisdom in Indian mythology. *American Journal of Psychotherapy,* 47, 443-450.

Sharma, V.P. (1970). Psycho-diagnostic tests and psychotherapy. *British Journal of Projective Psychology and Personality Studies,* 15, 13.

Sharma, V.P., Ojha, K.N. and Vagregha, Y.S. (1975). Clinical Psychologist in India II. *Indian Journal of Psychiatry,* 2, 73.

Sinha, T.C. (1956). Development of Psychoanalysis in India. *Indian Journal of Psychoanalysis,* 47, 427.

Srinagar, K. and Rao, T. (1994). An experimental study of the effect of transactional analysis on emotional maturity in PUC students. *Osmania Journal of Psychology,* 17, 18-26.

Sriram, T.G. (1990). Psychotherapy in developing countries: A public health perspective. *Indian Journal of Psychiatry,* 32 (2), 138-142.

Surya, N.C., and Jayaram, S.S. (1964). Some basic considerations in the practice of psychotherapy in the Indian setting. *Indian Journal of Psychiatry,* 6, 153-156.

Surya, N.C., and Jayaram, S.S. (1966). Some basic considerations in the practice of psychotherapy in the Indian setting. *Indian Journal of Psychiatry,* 38, 2-10.

Torrey, E.F. (1972). What Western psychotherapist can learn from witchoctors. *American Journal of Orthopsychiatry,* 42, 69.

Vahia, N.S., Doongaji, D.R., Jeste, D.V., Kapoor, S.N., Ardhapukkar, I. and Nath, S.R. (1973). Further experience in the therapy based upon the concepts based on Patanjali in the treatment of psychiatric disorders. *Indian Journal of Psychiatry,* 15, 32.

Varma, V.K., and Ghosh, A. (1975). Psychotherapy as practiced by the Indian Psychiatrists. Paper presented at the 27th Annual Conference of the Indian Psychiatry Society.

Varma, V.K. (1982). Present state of Psychotherapy in India. *Indian Journal of Psychiatry,* 24 (3), 209-216.

Varma, N., and Singh, A. (2014). Stress management and coping embedded in the *Bhagavad Gita. Indian Journal of Health and Well-being,* 5 (4), 520.

Vasudevan, A., Kumaraiah, V., Mishra, H., and Balodhi, J.P. (1994). Yogic meditation in tension headache. *NIMHANS Journal,* 12, 69-74.

Vaughan, F. (1989). Mapping the territory in search of common ground. *Yoga Journal,* 47.

Veeraraghavan, V. (1995). Violence in families: A biopsychological and naturalistic perspective. *Trends in Social Science Research,* 2, 83-93.

Wig, N.N. (2004). Hanuman complex and its resolution: An illustration of psychology from Indian mythology. *Indian Journal of Psychiatry,* 46 (1), 26.

Wittkower, E.D., and Warnes, H. (1974). Cultural aspects of psychotherapy. *American Journal of Psychotherapy,* 28, 566.

Wolberg, L.R. (1967). *The Technique of Psychotherapy.* New York: Grune & Stratton, p. 3.

7

Early Intervention and Therapy for Autism

Piyali Chakrabarti and *Jessie Holmberg*

In the typical development of infants and children aged 0-6 years old, the normal developmental stages would include development of the body, mind, emotions and social behaviours. Parents may not be able to identify the differences among the various stages unless obvious early symptoms prevail in the child. For children with special needs, their passport to quality life in adulthood begins with provision of quality education in their early years. This gives them a head start towards maximizing their potential in their area of strengths.

Recognizing those children with multiple disabilities could be a challenge as some of the disabilities will manifest during different stages of the child's life. The term 'multiple disabilities' is defined as a child who has more than one type of disability; one would be of a primary nature while the other would be of a secondary nature and it is usually not easily identified by parents. The types of early intervention vary according to the degree of these disabilities. One of the most common disabilities which require early intervention is the Autism Spectrum Disorder (ASD).

Kaplan and Sadock (2003), in their book '*Synopsis of Psychiatry*' discussed that Henry Maudsley was the first psychiatrist known to have worked with children with severe mental disorders. These disorders were heralded by marked deviation, delay, and distortion in the developmental processes and were previously considered as psychoses. They also mentioned that Leo Kanner coined the term 'infantile autism'. Kaplan and Sadock (2003) further discussed the detailed account provided by Kanner for the early childhood syndrome. Children were diagnosed as autistic if they displayed extreme autistic aloneness, failed to assume anticipatory posture, had delayed or deviant language development with echolalia and pronominal reversal (using "you" for "I"), displayed repetitive behaviour verbal or non-verbal, sometimes demonstrated excellent rote memory, had a very limited range of spontaneous activities, were fixated with being in same surrounding and resisting change in any form, obsessive need to complete tasks regardless of priority, difficulty in creating and maintaining relationships with people, and instead having a preference for pictures and inanimate objects. Kaplan and Sadock (2003) pointed out that Kanner suspected that this syndrome was actually underreported and some children with these syndromes were incorrectly diagnosed as schizophrenics or with delayed or stunted mental development. Kaplan and Sadock (2003) also highlight that there has been a dissent in opinion about whether infantile autism is the earliest possible manifestation of schizophrenia or a discrete clinical entity in itself. They also mention that further evidence, however, pointed towards infantile autism and schizophrenia as separate entities.

Early Intervention for Autism

At the onset of ASD signs, parents would seek the professional opinion of a medical doctor to assess and review the developmental normality of the child. A psychologist would be engaged to run a full assessment to determine and affirm if the child has ASD. Parents would need counselling to help them grapple with their own feelings of guilt and to accept that their child would need to be referred to an early intervention centre. At the early intervention centre, the child with ASD would be guided by a set of curriculum pedagogy to help the child in managing his/her behaviour while developing early learning skills. The daily routine in a classroom would be set in a structured manner to enable full participation of the child in a non-threatening environment. Early Interventionist, who is trained in the developmental needs and stages of children with special needs, would apply early learning steps to achieve success in the academic progress. Most times, it would be the goal of the educator to include the child with ASD into the normal school settings. The more this is achieved; the child would benefit higher integration into the real world.

In an early intervention programme, the child with ASD will be provided with adequate curriculum instructions to build his/her strengths in acquiring new skills; in improving behaviours and to remediate areas of weaknesses. Parents will also be supported to understand the behaviour and needs of the child so as to empower them to manage functional situations back home. The early intervention goal for a child with ASD is to give them the best hope for a higher quality life in the future. With the family's active participation, the child will be able to see improvements in his/her core behavioural challenges. With equipped information, resources and training, parents and educators can work towards milestones achievement more effectively. The learning outcome for a child with ASD can be also improved with structured routines and environment which can be challenging when teaching young children with autism. In observing the child, one will find the unique strengths and needs where early intervention can be applied through teaching approaches that are sensitive to these needs. Strategies which are used for typical children would not necessarily be applicable and would like likely to be less effective for the child with autism. Since each individual is unique, the intervention required will not be the same for each child. It would need to some extent of modification to ensure that it is appropriate to the special needs of the individual child.

The goals upon receiving early interventions would be eventually to increase the willingness of the child to engage within different settings of his/her environment. In achieving goals towards independence in the abilities to communicate needs, this would help minimize frustrations being built up in the child. Other goals to achieve would be the cognitive skill development, social competency, play skill development, generalization of skills, and proactive approaches to managing problem behaviour.

Types of Early Intervention

With early prognosis of autism spectrum disorder, the child will be assessed on his/her individual needs in collaboration with the parents. An individual family service programme (IFSP) usually marks the beginning journey of early intervention for the child, in a holistic way. The child's individual educational programme will be written based on the child's current levels of functioning and drafting an agreed anticipated goal for early intervention programme. The type of early intervention services that will be provided to develop the outcome achievements may include either one or all services. These services may include speech and language instruction, occupational therapy, physical therapy, psychological evaluation and specific strategies such as Applied Behaviour Analysis (ABA).

Besides the types of intention methods and strategies, the other aspects of intervention would be the intensity of the programme and age.

Dawson and Osterling (1997) reported that most programmes would involve at least 15 to 20 hours of intervention sessions per week. Harris and Handleman, 2000 and Sheinkopf and Siegal 1998; reported that children who enter early intervention programmes at younger ages make greater progress than those who enter at a later age. These two studies compare children who are older than 4/5 years.

Instructional Strategies and Differentiated Instructions

In supporting teaching and learning process for children with ASD, it must be reminded that no one specific method or intervention can be effective. Integration of various approaches can lead to the development of a curriculum that promotes the best outcomes for an individual child. Early interventionist/teachers can effectively respond to a learner's needs and strengths through the use of differentiated instruction. Through this approach, the specific skills and difficulties of the child with ASD can be addressed by employing a variety of methods that vary according to content, process, learning materials and evaluation.

The content would entail the depth or breadth of the information or skills outlined to be taught while the processes would have the instructional approaches used with the individual child. Teaching materials are important tools used to deliver or illustrate the content. The teaching materials or end product would depend on the learning situation and could be in the form of a worksheet, project, craft work etc. The skills taught in achieving the outcome would have ended up with acquired skills and knowledge for the child. Through specific lesson plans, early interventionist/teacher would be able to determine the most effective strategies for the child with ASD in a learning situation. It is necessary for him/her to consider the learning goals for the child in these areas, such as: what do we want the child to learn; skills or knowledge to be acquired; why is the learning important for him/her in achieving what type of learning goals aligned to the Individual Educational Plan for the child; how best can the activities and materials be delivered and evaluation of its effectives to view if the child has demonstrated learning.

In order to differentiate instruction, the early interventionist/teacher would have to consider adaptations to the curriculum, instruction and manage his/her own expectations. This should take lead from the child's readiness to learn, interests and learning abilities/profile. The types of differentiated instructions which should be considered are groupings, activities, level of support needed, task expectations, materials and resources as well as assessments and evaluation.

Structured Learning Environment

Being in a predictable environment is most effective for a child with ASD to learn. They need to know what is expected of them and what comes next in order for them to learn and generalize skills. Classroom rules and activities need to be clear, consistent and expectations of appropriate behaviour must be an ongoing process. Visual support can be very helpful in this instance. Using of assistive technology can help to increase, maintain and improve functional learning. Resources such as an IPad can be used by the early interventionist/teacher to provide alternative methods to access information and reinforce learning. The visual and auditory output can help to sustain and capture learning moments. Since the learning needs of a child with ASD are diverse, specific technological needs should be evaluated by the respective therapists and the use of these technologies must be carefully planned for effectiveness. For example, children with ASD vary in their sensitivity and tolerance to sensory stimulation in the environment. In choosing the technological software or equipment, one must be aware of the sensory preferences or sensitivities of the child and consider the possibilities that might impact his/her learning due to anxiety level.

Effective Early Intervention for ASD

Generally, the contributing factors to measuring an effective programme are by a "one size fits all" concept. The programme must be individualized and implemented in a flexible manner depending on the individual diagnosis and the spectrum of the autistic nature of the child. The type of intervention is based on current research and effective practices which can involve the use of a variety of methodologies and approaches, based on the comprehensive assessment results. As such, it should be reflective of the individual needs and outcome based. Most of these programmes which are effective would witness the fact that with family involvement, there would be progress in child development. The most important factor according to "Best Practice Guidelines" would be the intensity of intervention time which should happen between 25 and 40 hours a week. Other factors taken into consideration would be the individualization of the curriculum and the level of structure in the learning environment. In a classroom setting, the student to teacher ratio should be low at a preferred two to one. The curriculum should be developmentally appropriate and sequenced, as well as behaviourally based to support learning. Empirical evidence has proven that using applied behaviour analysis techniques such as discrete trail training, pivotal response training, and verbal behaviour, do play an integral part in the process of learning and development.

Early Interventionists may also include other techniques to assist in effectiveness of his/her intervention methods. These could be in the form of incidental teaching techniques which can take place in various settings. The effectiveness of learning can also be measured when learning is brought into different environment particularly in functional and meaningful ways. This is to ensure that generalization and maintenance of new skills can be evaluated. Besides having a set of routines to encourage a systematic method to support learning, consistency across environments should be set. Learning must be designed to allow transition from an interdependent stage to independence.

In monitoring the intervention system to arrive at the desired outcome for the individual, data recording in all aspects of learning is an integral factor. The environment set for a structured and organized space, the teaching areas should also be distraction free. Children with autism tend to learn well with visual schedules of the daily routine which are assisted through the use of photographs or Picture Exchange Communication icons. These visual pictures should be generalized and used in different settings. They can be incorporated into the interventions involving motor skills development, occupational therapy, sensory integration therapy or even used as part of the social skills instruction. In engaging children with autism in the various intervention sessions, learning to communicate in a language enriched environment would be useful. Methods of using the Picture Exchange Communication System, Whole Language Approach, Hannon (More than Words), knowledge of which should be imparted to parents and caregivers to allow functional use of communication with family members at home and in other environment.

Evaluate if the Intervention is Effective

The only way to evaluate if an intervention method is effective is to see the data. These data should be collected and reported on a frequent basis. Parents have the right to ask for the report if it is not made available to them. If there is no data to support the efficacy of the intervention, then the parents and educators should note that the intervention sessions would be of no relevance to the goals set when they are not measured. The data collected at intervals would provide parents and teachers the capability to make timely decisions about interventions. In any case, if the data show the child is not making significant improvements in the expected time frame, considerations could be made to find other intervention options or modification of the methods could be suggested. On the other hand, should the data show that the child is making good progress, one should be able to affirm that the intervention method is right on track. If interventionists are not collecting data, there is no way to quantify the need for change hence, there is no way to make informed decisions about the efficacy of the interventions being used.

Be Involved in Child's Intervention

The family's participation is vital to the child's success. The fact remains that parents are the child's first educator/s therefore, getting involved in the intervention process and in the child's therapy programmes, should, to a large extent, achieve successful outcomes. When parents are involved in the development and implementation of interventions, the intervention procedures are more likely to be used within functional settings in the home and other environment. The child will be able to learn and use skills more quickly and effectively. As parents and family members are the people who spend the most amount of time with the special needs child, they should be further involved in the development of intervention strategies. They should receive extensive training from the professionals who work with their child so as to allow them to implement the interventions well, at all times. In giving the right support to the therapists working with the special needs child, parents could help the child generalize the skills learnt through the intervention sessions.

***Power to Parents*!**

Please know that parents have a very important role in this assessment, because they have information about their child that no one else has. When they understand the process, they can work effectively with the rest of the team. What parents know about their child will be used to help develop effective instruction (Fig. 7.1).

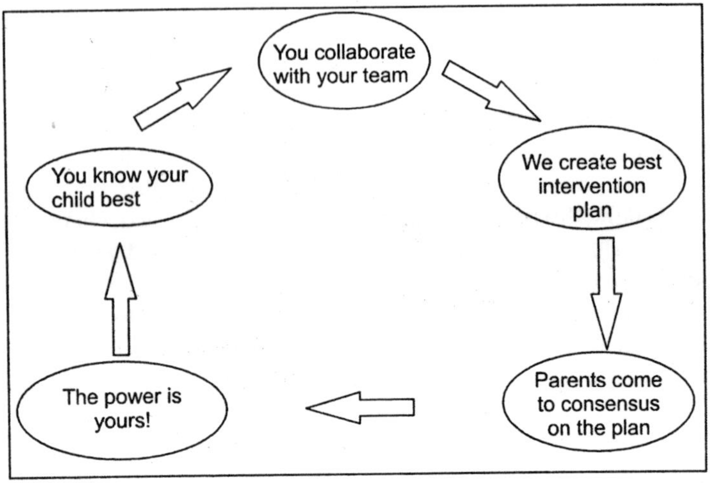

Fig. 7.1: Flow chart of power of parents

Conclusion

No intervention is effective without family support and parents' involvement. Our *mantra* as always remains power 'power to parents'! Together we can help a child attain his/her potential to his/her fullest.

References

Dawson, G. and Osterling, J. (1997). Early intervention in autism: Effectiveness and common elements of current approaches. In M.J. Guralnick (Ed.), *The Effectiveness of Early Intervention: Second Generation Research* (pp. 307-326). Baltimore, MD: Paul H. Brookes.

Harris, S.L. and Handleman, J.S. (2000). Age and IQ at intake as predictors of placement for young children with autism: A four-to six-year follow-up. *Journal of Autism and Developmental Disorders*, 30(2), 137-142.

Kaplan, H.I. and Sadock, B.J. (2003). *Synopsis of Psychiatry: Behavioural Sciences/Clinical Psychiatry*, Williams & Wilkins Co.

Sheinkopf, S.J. and Siegel, B. (1998). Home-based behavioural treatment of young children with autism. *Journal of Autism and Developmental Disorders*, 28(1), 15-23.

8

Depression and Its Correlates

Evaluating the Imagery Re-scripting Treatment Approach

E.T.T.M. Pasipanodya, Yogesh Kumar Arya and *Tushar Singh*

Introduction

According to the World Health Organization (W.H.O., 2002), there is an alarming increase in the number of mental health cases as they account for almost half of the total burden for disease. Among these mental health cases depression is one, which contributes significantly to the increasing mental health problems. A large number of documented research works have labelled depression as both a common illness and experience that is estimated to be the leading burdensome disease by 2030. Seligman (1975) has termed it as the 'common cold' of psychiatric disorders. The W.H.O. (2004) data on depression, estimated that nearly 350 million people suffer from depression and 1 out of every 20 people experience an episode of depression at least once a year throughout their lifetime. Recent estimates indicate that almost 20 per cent of the American population experiences a significant episode of depression at a decisive point in their lives making depression the most prevalent of all psychological disorders (Kessler and Wang, 2009). In many developing countries, depression is a common mental disorder that has less than 1 per cent of the total health expenditure allocated to it. Due to high population rates, pervasive poverty, violence and political instability, the prevalence and rates of depression are high in these countries. In India, the prevalence of severe mental disorders is about 10-20 per 1,00,000 individuals. Globally, the lifetime prevalence of depression is 12.1 per cent, which accounts for 5 per cent of the total burden of diseases and suicide mortality of 16/1,00,000 individuals (W.H.O., 2004). With respect to overall disability, the World Health

Organization has listed depression as the sole troublesome disorder (Murray and Lopez, 1996).

Diagnostic Classification of Depression

Depression is characterized by a mixture of behavioural, emotional, and cognitive symptoms. These include psychomotor agitation, insomnia or hypersomnia, decreased appetite, fatigue, extreme feelings of guilt or worthlessness, marked weight loss and loss of interest in activities that were once pleasurable. W.H.O. defines depression as a common mental disorder characterized by sustained negative affect and emotion dysregulation as its hallmark features. To meet diagnostic criteria, a set of these symptoms has to be present for at least a two week period at a time. Therefore, for a diagnosis to be given, persistent negative affect, emotion dysregulation or loss of pleasure should be one of the persistent symptoms. Therefore, depression can be defined as a disorder of impaired mood regulation that has continuous pessimistic mood and a persistent reduction in positive affect being its hallmark features. It is, therefore, important to have treatment techniques that will bridge the gap between treatment regimens and reality.

There exists a vast array of theoretical and experimental literature to show that depression casts a wide and deep net that cuts across multiple dimensions in psychological as well as in the cognitive functioning of an individual.

Cognitive Theories of Depression

The cognitive theories of depression provide an impetus for extraordinary and productive programmes for research that can be advanced to best suit treatment techniques. However, both basic methods and theory have progressed at a very slow pace. Much of the hallmark foundation of what is known about depression originated from the work of Beck (1976). The underlying assumptions of these theories highlight the importance of cognitions in maintaining dysfunctional emotion, behaviour, and physiological symptoms. Over the past few decades, mood-congruent memory has led to the diversification of interest in depression to other facets of human functioning such as cognitive inhibition, emotion regulation/ dysregulation, autobiographical memory etc. Cognitive theories of depression can be summed up as either being representative of information processing biases or preferential attentional biases that render the individual more apt to favour schema-congruent information while ignoring all other cues from the environment.

However, newer trends in research have advanced cognitive theories as being represented by affect (emotion valence), which can structured into the cognitive models of emotional disorders. The sole aim of this ideology is to use experimentally testable concepts and theories derived from literature that will be employed in treatment techniques. Affect based research postulates that affective memories may also represent stable vulnerability factors for depression onset, relapse, and recurrence. If they are left unaddressed, they can lead to an onset of vicious depressive episodes as well as recurrent episodes. Therefore, there is a continuous retrieval of dysfunctional respondent-functional-appraisal memories as compared to the inhibition of respondent-functional memories.

Cognitive theories of depression posit depressive episodes as being the ubiquitous activation of conglomerate and contiguous dysfunctional beliefs, meanings, and memories that operate in coordination with emotions. The end result may lead to motivational behaviour and physiological response culminating into distinct biases that influence how an individual incorporates and responds to new information.

Emerging evidences from earlier studies seems to identify negative mood as generally being associated with or consists in part of the activation of mood-congruent representations in working memory (Isen, 1984; Siemer, 2005). It is assumed that this association may lead to the onset or maintenance of a depressive episode. There is, therefore, an urgent need to structure emotion based treatment etiologies that will foster psycho-social well-being of those suffering from depression.

Factors Affecting Depression

Depression is beset by sustained negative affect and the dysregulation of emotion. Although there are many causal factors for the (onset), maintenance or triggering elements in depression, a number of them have been studied independently of each other. A variety of studies (Blaney, 1986; Isen, 1984; Matthews and Macleod, 2005; Rusting, 1998; Siemer, 2005) seem to have vehemently exhausted the importance of unitary factors in depression. However, there exists the need to adjoin their findings so as to establish a bridging relationship between all the significant variables in depression.

***(a) Cognitive inhibition and emotion regulation*:** Human are social beings who are thought to be a blend of feelings and emotions. What seems real and valid to most people are their feelings and emotions. In this regard, researchers have identified deficits in the regulation of emotion and cognitive inhibition in depression to be related. An individual's ability to resonate with positive feelings is reduced due to their failure to inhibit negative mood-congruent material. Ultimately, this may lead to extreme vibrations of unpleasant emotions (the conduits of melancholy, dispiritedness and despondency). Based on the importance of emotions in depression, empirical work suggests that there should be a systematic desensitization moderated by a remodelling of the individual's mental set (Berger and McGaugh, 1965).

Depression is a disorder of impaired mood regulation. Research suggests that dysfunctional emotion regulation is the hallmark feature of this negative mood state. Identifying the cognitive processes associated with the use of emotion regulation strategies and individual differences will help in treating depression. Research on mood disorders has shown that there are two important related aspects to healthy emotional well-being namely emotion regulation and cognitive inhibition. Emotion regulation is dependent on inhibitory processes which in turn constitutes a variety of domains in affective disorders (Matthews and MacLeod, 2005). Emerging evidence posits that depression is marked by deficits in the inhibition of mood-congruent material that may result in the prolonged processing of negative, goal irrelevant material thereby hindering recovery from negative mood (e.g., Holmes and Matthews, 2010). Theoretical as well as empirical evidence in the study of depression seems to highlight the importance of cognitive inhibition.

Mathews and MacLeod (2005) have theoretically prioritized that cognitive inhibition is the major factor leading to memory and attention biases in depression, which consequently sets the stage for ruminative responses to stressful events and mood states. Therefore, the best way to cope with such an imminent outcome is to control for the prolonged processing of dysfunctional mood-congruent negative and goal irrelevant material in memory.

To sum up, the relationship between emotion regulation and depression is mediated by cognitive inhibition which is selective to the prolonged processing of negative material in memory. A bias in the processing of emotional material seems to suggest that there is an inability to regulate negative mood signifying cognitive biases in the inhibition of negative schema relevant material (Joormann & Gotlib, 2010).

***(b) Depressive Rumination*:** Nolen-Hoeksema (1991), in her Response Styles theory, highlights the importance of compulsory and yet unintentional focusing of attention on the distress symptoms that characterize negative mood and depression. Ruminative tendencies in depression tend to focus on the causal factors and ultimate consequences of these factors rather than planful problem solving (e.g. Clark, Beck and Alford, 1999; Nolen-Hoeksema, 1991). Depressive rumination represents the recycling of the contents of thoughts and not their associated meanings. Prolonging this process is detrimental to an individual as it resonate feelings centred on negativity of the self, the world and the future setting the tone for other factors of depression. Rumination consists of multiple maladaptive processes that may lead to a sequel of depressed mood. These processes facilitate the recalling of negative events about the individual's past as well as the precipitating experiences that have led to the current circumstances.

Furthermore, ruminative tendencies may lead to the maintenance of negative material in working memory as well as the retrieval of mood-congruent material from memory. The prolonging of this negative mood state may lead to the development of negative cognitions that play a role in the onset and preservation of affective disorders. It is noteworthy to mention that rumination is not an automatic response to stressful life events or the experience of negative mood. Rather, it is about thinking of one's self in relation to the social environment in a prolonged and repetitive manner upon encountering stressful events or emotional states that may set the stage for ruminative response styles. Beck (1979) suggested that rumination was consistent with negative schemas that are characteristic of depression, as well as mental representations regarding past events and experiences containing dysfunctional attitudes about the self. Furthermore, rumination enhances negative thought styles that are associated with depression, forcing the individuals to make use of negative memories and thoughts to understand their distressing condition. Rumination compels the depressed individuals to focus on why they feel the way they do as opposed to coming up with constructive problem-solving strategies. The negative connotations represented by ruminative thinking styles should be viewed as learned behaviours that may lead depressed individuals to respond in a predetermined manner.

(c) Self-Complexity: Research in depression is drawing from social psychology to try and explain the phenomenon that underlies the tragic vicious self-defeating aspect of depression (Linville, 1985; 1987). Self-complexity is a term that is used to describe a person's perceived knowledge of oneself. Linville (1985) denotes that self-complexity is representative of the number of distinct cognitive structures or self-aspects that an individual believes they possess. Although these known self-aspects are multiple and infinite, they can include context-dependent social roles, activities superordinate traits, goals of the individual etc., which combine to form the larger associative network of the self-concept. Self-complexity is structured on the premise that the self is cognitively represented as a multifaceted arrangement of self-relevant knowledge invoked to process information about the individual (Gergen, 1991). Research in this area has focused on relating the self-complexity representations to affective and evaluative responses.

The self-complexity model concludes that, there are marginal difference between individuals who have high self-complexity (independent self-aspects, i.e. cognitive representations) and those who have low self-complexity (Montemayor and Eisen, 1977; Mullener and Laird, 1971). The observed differences in integration are not only measurable *via* the number of cognitive representations of the self, but also differences in affective valence. Therefore, self-relevant cognitions are important constructs to study in order to understand thinking patterns in depression (Beck, 1976; Deci and Ryan, 2003; Muraven and Baumister, 2000).

***(d) Autobiographical Memory*:** Autobiographical memory is the aspect of memory that is directly responsible for the recollection of personally experienced past events. Autobiographical memory is pivotal in individual functioning as it gives understanding and relevance to "sense of self". A clear understanding of one's "sense of self" is vital in pursuing current goals in the light of past problem-solving (Conway and Pleydell-Pearce, 2000; Nelson and Fivush, 2004). Autobiographical memory is a tractable phenomenon to study in emotional disorders as it is the memory store for personally experienced events (Castel and Craik, 2003; Hertel and Gerstle, 2003; Tulving, 2002; Tulving *et al.*, 1994). Furthermore, other cognitive aspects pivotal in depression e.g., self-complexity, rumination, cognitive inhibition, emotion-regulation etc. are directly affected in how one organizes and understands "the self" with reference to autobiographical memory.

Conway and Pleydell-Pearce (2000) have built their hierarchical search model of personal event retrieval on the idea that autobiographical memory is a self-memory system (SMS). Their model highlights the importance of accessing self-relevant memories using categorical versus specific methods. In this system, there is a likelihood that the recollections might be biased by existing mood states, which may relay into the commencement and preservation of mood disorders. The effect that over general memory has on mood disorders has started to gain ground in depression. Research states that those individuals who suffer from depression or prone to have an onset of a depressive episode use over general access of memory in order to limit their impact. The Galton cue-word paradigm has demonstrated that there are mood-congruent biases in response to experimental manipulation (Teasdale and Fogarty, 1979). Findings from similar studies suggest that autobiographical memory is a tractable phenomenon to study in relation to mood (e.g. Lloyd and Lishman, 1975; Clark and Teasdale, 1982; Teasdale and Fogarty, 1979).

(e) ***Mental Imagery***: Mental imagery is the experience of accessing perceptual information from memory. Mental imagery allows an individual to relive past events by drawing on autobiographical memories through imagination etc. (Schacter and Addis, 2007). Until recently it had been assumed that human cognition was more verbal than it was visual. However, it has now been conceptualized as much of what we remember as memories or recall is in the form of visual images. Findings from mental imagery research have led researchers to postulate that human cognitions in the form of mental images have a profound impact on affect than their verbal counterparts (Singh and Pande, 2007). This line of thinking is in consonant with some of the published data that highlights the presence of emotion based mental imagery to be prevalent in depression, as well as in other mood disorders (Holmes and Matthews, 2010).

A mental image is an experience that on most occasions significantly resembles the experience of perceiving some object, event or scene as it is happening *"here and now"*. Mental imagery allows an individual to relieve experiences as well as to create new novel combinations of imagery of never experienced images. These novel combinations allow us to "time travel" mentally, to what might happen in the future (Schater and Addis, 2007). Thus, we are more likely to be influenced by the events stimulated by imagery than those events that are stimulated by verbal thought only. This line of thinking is supported by the work of Libby, Shaeffer, Eiback and Slemmer (2007).

Mental imagery is critical in exacerbating states of normal and abnormal mood. Emerging evidence suggests that mental imagery acts as an emotional amplifier of affect and may be highly elevated in depression. Holmes and Matthews (2005) suggest that emotional processing in the brain is particularly sensitive to visual imagery rather than verbal thought. Data suggests that depressed individuals seem to employ the over general use of mental imagery that is responsible for the high levels of intrusive imagery. In depressive states, these intrusive images are likely to initiate the action leading to further deterioration of the condition as depressed individuals are highly susceptible to use mental imagery (think in images rather than words). The tendency to rapidly respond to imagery will also affect similar processes involved in mental imagery that overlap with those in perception (Kosslyn *et al.*, 2001).

Modern clinical psychologists argue that mental representations are the stimulation or recreation of experienced as well as never experienced perceptual events (Kosslyn, Ganis & Thompson, 2001). This presents a new arena of study in clinical and cognitive psychology. Since the published research in this area of depression concerning mental imagery is limited, there is need to establish primary domains of interest to clinical and cognitive psychology. The establishment of these primary fields should highlight cognitive bias modification while at the same time addressing treatments that are schema-focused such as cognitive restructuring, imagery re-scripting, stage-wise processing of mental representations etc.

Coping with Depression: The Imagery Re-scripting Method

It is clearly evident from the literature reviewed above that mental imagery has a special relationship with emotion to the extent that images may invoke emotion and *vice versa* (Holmes, 2007). Thus, mental imagery is identified as being a dominant, persistent, and distressing feature reported in a variety of mood disorders (Smucker, 1997). The dysfunctional factors that aide the onset, maintenance, recurrence, and relapse of depression (i.e. cognitive inhibition and emotion regulation, autobiographical memory, rumination, and self-complexity), have been found to be influenced greatly by mental imagery. The duration, course, and intensity in which depressive episodes are experienced, are influenced by mental imagery (Clark, 1992; Gold and Wegner, 1985). Thus, researchers (e.g. Beck, Emery, and Greenberg, 1995) are of the view that an effective treatment technique for depression must be imagery based, which is aimed at directly challenging the associated contents and meanings.

The presence of faulty distressing intrusive sensory images in depressive episodes have been suggested as being generated and maintained by the same mechanisms responsible for visual perception (Burgess, Becker, King, and O'Keefe, 2001; Byrne, Becker, and Burgess, 2007). Therefore, the effective treatment of depression requires a technique that changes faulty images to positive images. Imagery rescripting is proposed as the technique for effective treatment for depression. This technique has been used in a number of psychopathological disorders that possess distressing sensory images and have been reported to be very successful (e.g. Ehlers and Clark, 2000; Grey, Young, and Holmes, 2002).

Although there are a variety of imagery based techniques in cognitive behaviour therapy, imagery rescripting is differentiated from them due to its ability to integrate the use of visual, verbal, and schema modifications with the aim to eliminate intrusive thoughts. Imagery rescripting accesses the entire memory network representing the distressing sensory images to modify dysfunctional beliefs and promotes positive prospective views about the self, the world, and the future.

Ehlers and Clark (2000) argue that mental imagery influences emotional processing and balance in mood disorders. Therefore, directly modifying negative imagery by promoting positive alternatives *via* imagery rescripting will be a better treatment modality in depression. Imagery rescripting directly changes the meanings and emotions associated with distressing images and their memory representations. Grey (2002), have demonstrated the efficacy of imagery re-structuring with flashbacks in PTSD (Grey, Young, and Holmes, 2002). Their research demonstrated that pre-existing distressing negative mental images (IR "Type A") are re-scripted into newer more benign positive images (IR "Type B"). Similarly, in a study of PTSD patients, Arntz, Kintdt, and Tiesema (2007) contrasted different imagery based techniques (imaginal exposure *vs.* imaginal exposure enhanced with imagery rescripting) and found that imaginal exposure enhanced with imagery rescripting not only changed the outlook of the patient, but also made the treatment more acceptable by the patients and therapists. The results of this study show that imagery rescripting can be used in conjunction with other treatment efficacies or as a stand-alone treatment technique. Wheatley *et al.* (2009) also conducted a study on 10 depressed participants with a long history of depression. The mean length of the depressive episodes was 2.3 years. The results of this study showed that while half of the participants scored in the severe range of the Beck depression inventory scores, there was a considerable average reduction of 16.60 (SD13.47) after an average of 8.1 sessions. The observed reduction is symptoms were also reported to be well maintained after a 1-year period.

Therefore, it is evident that imagery re-scripting is a technique that directly challenges depressive cognitions and may prove efficient in alleviating negative cognitions observed in depression. More research is needed in this area in order to understand the underlying mechanisms of how imagery rescripting changes the meanings and cognitions associated with faulty sensory images in depression.

Conclusion

To conclude, there are strong evidences that a majority of the factors that either influence or predispose individuals to depression are primarily emotion based and influenced by mood-congruent images (Joormann and Gotlib, 2010). While there are various treatment techniques to this crisis, the shortage of transportable (efficacious and universal treatments) models is widely recognized as the major problem. Therapeutic techniques should contain education and training about the modification of negative cognitions and behavioural coping strategies in response to social stimuli. The goal of these techniques should be enhancing and developing psychosocial competence.

There is also a general agreement among researchers (e.g. Matthews and MacLeod, 2005) that there is something special about reasoning by using mental images. Higher executive cognitive processes are not simply embedded in the brain which is entrenched in the body. They are representative of ideas and mental experiences. Therefore, modern research and techniques should focus on deriving and analyzing the intentions of emotions and their goal-directedness in developing treatment techniques for cognitive-affective disorders like depression. Techniques based on mental imagery are of paramount value in these affective-cognitive disorders because of its powerful impact on emotion. However, despite a vast array of literature on depression, there exists a huge gap of researches documenting the efficacy of mental imagery and its techniques such as imagery re-scripting on restoring emotional well-being in depression.

Thus, there is a need to conduct researches on mental imagery techniques that have correctness conditions for correcting faulty imagery and emotions in affective disorders. Such methodologies should focus on promoting the intentional evaluation of emotion. Imagery re-scripting technique has emerged as an effective technique that directly challenges depressive cognitions and may prove efficient in alleviating negative cognitions observed in depression.

It has been the case with many researchers to advocate for one theory, model or treatment regime than the other, doing little to bridge the gap between reality and the epidemiology of depression. However, the goal of therapeutic techniques should be full recovery that encompasses total remission of symptoms and a return to premorbid psycho-social functioning. Therefore, we suggest that future research should concentrate on therapeutic coalitions of various treatment techniques keeping imagery rescripting in a central position.

References

Arntz, A., de Groot, C., and Kindt, M. (2005). Emotional memory is perceptual. *Journal of Behaviour Therapy and Experimental Psychiatry*, 36(1), 19-34.

Arntz, A., Kindt, M., and Tiesema, M. (2007). Treatment of PTSD: A comparison of imaginal exposure with and without imagery rescripting. *Journal of Behaviour Therapy and Experimental Psychiatry*, 38(4), 345-370. http://www.sciencedirect.com/science/articlc/pii/S0005791607000651

Beck A.T. (1976). *Cognitive therapy and the emotional disorders*. New York: International Universities Press.

Beck, A.T., Emery, G. and Greenberg, R.L. (1985). *Anxiety Disorders and Phobias: A Cognitive Perspective*. New York, NY: Basic Books.

Beck, A.T., Rush, J.A., Shaw, B.F., and Emery, G. (1979). *Cognitive Therapy of Depression*. New York: The Guilford Press, 12-13.

Berger, L., and McGaugh, J.L. (1965). Critique and reformulation of "learning theory" approaches to psychotherapy and neuroses. *Psychological Bulletin*, 63, 338-358.

Blaney, P.H. (1986). Affect and memory: A review. *Psychological Bulletin*, 99(2), 229-246.

Burgess, N., Becker, S., King, J.A., and O'Keefe, J. (2001). Memory for events and their spatial context: Models and experiments. *Philosophical Transactions of the Royal Society of London B: Biological Sciences*, 356 (1413), 1493-1503.

Byrne, P., Becker, S., and Burgess, N. (2007). Remembering the past and imagining the future: A neural model of spatial memory and imagery. *Psychological Review*, 114, 340-375.

Castel, A.D. and Craik, F.I.M. (2003). The effects of ageing and divided attention of memory for item and associative information. *Psychology and Ageing*, 18, 873-885.

Clark, D.A. (1992). Depressive, anxious and intrusive thoughts in psychiatric inpatients and outpatients. *Behaviour Research and Therapy*, 256, 93-102.

Clark, D.A., Beck, A.T. and Alford, B.A. (1999). *Scientific Foundations of Cognitive Theory and Therapy of Depression*. New York: Wiley.

Clark, D.M., and Teasdale, J.D. (1982). Diurnal variations in clinical depression and accessibility of memories of positive and negative experiences. *Journal of Abnormal Psychology*, 91, 87-95.

Conway, M.A., Plcydell-Pearce, C.W., Whitecross, S.E., and Sharpe, H. (2003). Cultural and historical context. *Journal of Adolescence*, 19, 405-416.

Deci, E.L., and Ryan, R.M. (2010). *Self-determination.* John Wiley & Sons, Inc.

Ehlers, A., and Clark, D.M. (2000). A Cognitive Model of Post-traumatic stress disorder. *Behaviour Research and Therapy,* 38(4), 319-345.

Gergen, K.J. (1991). *The Saturated Self: Dilemmas of Identity in Comparative Life.* New York: Basic Books.

Gold, D.B. and Wegner, D.M. (1995). Origins of Ruminative thought: Trauma, incompleteness, non-disclosure, and suppression. *Journal of Applied Social Psychiatry,* 256, 1245-1261.

Grey, N., Young, K., and Holmes, E. (2002). Cognitive restructuring within reliving: A treatment for peri-traumatice motional hotspots in PTSD. *Behavioural and Cognitive Psychotherapy,* 30, 37-56.

Hertel, P.T., and Gerstle, M. (2003). Depressive Deficits in Forgetting. *Psychological Science,* 14(6), 573-578.

Holmes, E.A., and Mathews, A. (2005). Mental Imagery and Emotion: A special relationship? *Emotion* (Washington, DC.), 5, 489-497.

Holmes, E.A., and Mathews, A. (2010). Mental imagery in emotion and emotional disorders. *Clinical Psychology Review,* 30, 349-362.

Holmes, E.A., Mathews, A., Dalgleish, T., and Mackintosh, B. (2006). Positive interpretation training: Effects of mental imagery *versus* verbal training on positive mood. *Behaviour Therapy,* 37(3), 237-247.

Holmes, E.A., Arntz, A., and Smucker, M.R. (2007). Imagery rescripting in cognitive behaviour therapy: Images, treatment techniques and outcomes. *Journal of Behaviour Therapy and Experimental Psychiatry,* 38, 297-305.

Isen, A.M. (1984). Toward understanding the role of affect in cognition. In R.S. Wyer and T.S. Srull (Eds.), *Handbook of Social Cognition* (pp. 179-236). Hillsdale, NJ: Erlbaum.

Joormann, J., and Gotlib, I.H. (2010). Emotion regulation in depression: Relation to cognitive inhibition. *Cognition and Emotion,* 24(2), 281-298.

Kessler, R.C., and Wang, P.S. (2009). Epidemiology of depression. In Gotlib, I.H., and Hammen, C.L. (Eds.). *Handbook of Depression,* 2nd ed., pp. 5-22. New York: Guilford.

Kosslyn, S.M., Ganis, G., and Thompson, W. (2001). Neural foundations of imagery. *Nature Reviews Neuroscience,* 2, 635-642.

Libby, L.K., Shaeffer, E.M., and Eibach, R.P. (2009). Seeing meaning in action: A bidirectional link between visual perspective and action identification level. *Journal of Experimental Psychology: General,* 138(4), 503-516.

Linville, P.W. (1985). Self-complexity and affective extremity: Don't put all of your eggs in one cognitive basket. *Social Cognition,* 3(1), 94-120.

Linville, P.W. (1987). Self-complexity as a cognitive buffer against stress-related illness and depression. *Journal of Personality and Social Psychology,* 52(4), 663-676.

Lloyd, G.G., and Lishman, W.A. (1975). Effects of depression on the speed of recall of pleasant and unpleasant experiences. *Psychological Medicine,* 5, 173-180.

Mathews, A., and MacLeod, C. (2005). Cognitive vulnerability to emotional disorders. *Annual Review of Clinical Psychology*, 1, 167-195.

Montemayor, R., and Eisen, M. (1977). The development of self-conceptions from childhood to adolescence. *Developmental Psychology*, 13(4), 314-319.

Mullener, N. and Laird, J.D. (1971). Some developmental changes in the organization of self-evaluations. *Developmental Psychology*, 5(2), 233-236.

Muraven, M., and Baumeister, R.F. (2000). Self-regulation and depletion of limited resources: Does self-control resemble a muscle? *Psychological Bulletin*, 126(2), 247-259.

Murray, C.J.L., Lopez, A.D. (1997). Global mortality, disability and the contribution of risk factors: Global burden of disease study. *Lancet,* 394: 1436-1442.

Nelson, K., and Fivush, R. (2004). The Emergence of Autobiographical Memory: A Social Cultural Developmental Theory. *Psychological Review*, 111(2), 486-511.

Nolen-Hoeksema, S. (1991). Responses to depression and their effects on the duration of depressive episodes. *Journal of Abnormal Psychology*, 100(4), 569-582.

Rusting, C.L. (1998). Personality, mood, and cognitive processing of emotional information: Three conceptual frameworks. *Psychological Bulletin*, 124(2), 165-196.

Schacter, D.L. and Addis, D.R. (2007). The cognitive neuroscience of constructive memory: Remembering the past and imagining the future. *Philosophical Transactions of the Royal Society B: Biological Sciences*, 362(1481), 773-786.

Siemer, M. (2005). Mood congruent cognitions constitute mood experience. *Emotion,* 59(3), 296-300.

Singh, T. and Pande, (2007). Visual imagery, Affect and Problem Solving. *Psychological Studies,* 52 (3), 244-247.

Smucker, M.R. (1997). Post-traumatic stress disorder. In R.L. Leahy (Ed.), *Practicing Cognitive Therapy* (pp. 193-220). Northvale, NJ: Jason Aronson.

Teasdale, J.D. and Fogarty, S.J. (1979). Differential effects of induced mood on retrieval of pleasant and unpleasant events from episodic memory. *Journal of Abnormal Psychology*, 88(3), 248-257.

Tulving, E. (2002). Episodic memory: from mind to brain. *Annual Review of Psychology*, 53(1), 1-25.

Tulving, E., Kapur, S., Craik F.I.M., Moscovitch M., Houle, S. (1994). Hemispheric encoding/retrieval. Asymmetry in episodic memory: Positron emission tomography findings. *Proceedings of the National Academy of Sciences of the USA*, 91:2016-2020.

Wheatley, J., Brewin, C.R., Patel, T., Hackmann, A., Wells, A., Fisher, P., *et al.* (2007). 'I'll believe it when I see it': Imagery rescripting of intrusive sensory memories in depression. *Journal of Behaviour Therapy and Experimental Psychiatry,* 38(4), 371-385.

World Health Organization, (2002). *The Global Burden of Disease.* Retrieved from http://www.who.int/evidence

9

Multicultural Counselling

Perspectives and Guidelines

Dhananjay Kumar

Introduction

Multicultural counselling has different meanings depending on the context of use. Multicultural counselling refers to supporting and helping activities where the counsellors and counsellees are different from each other in terms of ethnicity, race, culture etc. Becoming a multicultural counsellor is not only mean gaining more knowledge of other cultures, but it includes also understanding the complex processes through which people become members of communities and societies and construct their worldviews, basic attitudes, values, norms (Geertz, 1973; Maruyama, 1992; Seeley, 2000). "Multicultural" refers to interactions between individuals from minority racial and ethnic groups, including biracial and multiracial individuals in different groups and countries. Minority population are frequently identified as people of colour. Nonetheless, various Multicultural guidelines recognize that there is great heterogeneity within each of these groups. The definition of multicultural has to be contextualized. For instance, individuals of Indian subcontinent and of Arab descent will identify as peoples of colour in some areas of the United States. Additionally, the Multicultural counselling applies to practitioners' work with people from other countries, international students, immigrants and seasonal or temporary workers.

Counsellors and other professionals need multicultural competencies in order to develop better understanding of cultural diversity of their clients. The most well-known way in conceptualizing multicultural counselling competencies is the one developed by Sue *et al.* (1992; 1996). They divide the multicultural competencies into three characteristics related with three dimensions: awareness of counsellors' own assumptions, values and biases; understanding of the worldview of a culturally different clients and an ability to develop appropriate intervention strategies and techniques. Each of these characteristics include the following three dimensions: beliefs and attitudes, knowledge, and skills.

Culture and its Dimensions

The classic definition by Herkovits (1948), sees culture as that part of the environment that is created or shaped by human beings. Other definitions place the main stress on those elements in culture which cannot be observed as clearly as the visible elements in our environment. Among the more comprehensive definitions of culture as it relates to multiculturalism is that of Pedersen (1991), in which he described the following elements: Demographic variables (age, sex, place of residence), Status variables (social, educational, economic), Affiliations (formal and informal), and Ethnographic variables (nationality, ethnicity, language, and religion).

Culture is also defined as the belief systems and value orientations that influence norms, customs, practices, and social institutions, psychological processes including language, cognition, perception, and organizations (Fiske, Kitayama, Markus, and Nisbett, 1998). Culture is not a static concept but one that changes as it is transferred by one generation to the next (Leighton, 1967), and by the interaction of different groups.

This and other broad definitions of culture suggest that we are dealing with a complex phenomenon which is present in all counselling situations. Cultural difference, here, can have different meanings depending on the way it is interpreted. The trend that emphasizes cultural differences, particularly based on ethnicity or race, is often called as culture-specific (emic), whereas the trend that puts more stress on similarities is called universalistic trend (etic). Culture-specific perspective conceptualizes cultural differences in a way that people from other cultures can feel that they are noted and respected as people of their own culture of origin. Universalistic perspective holds that people from different cultures share similarities and that all counselling is multicultural in the sense that each individual has his or her own unique personal history and belongs to various cultures characterized by gender, social class, sexual orientation, political background, religion etc. Both of them provide important perspectives, but a balance between them is needed. Further, multicultural counselling represents systematic attempts to deal with cultural diversity in counselling. In addition, multicultural counselling also refers to a theoretical force or theoretical trend, which can be seen as the most recent addition to the theoretical forces of counselling (Hackney and Cormier 1996; Pedersen, 1991; Sue, Ivey and Pedersen 1996). Multicultural counselling implies the recognition of the major impact the culture has on us as human beings. Human existence as expressed in thoughts, values, behaviours, attitudes, cannot be understood without considering us as members of larger communities, societies, and civilizations. Meanings and perceptions are constructed together with other people. Culture affects us and we affect the development of the culture together with other people to take into account the challenges posed by these cultural factors.

To describe cultural differences in a rational and comprehensive way, researchers have identified a number of cultural dimensions. Hofstede (1980) carried out one of the earliest studies of this type. He initially identified four main cultural dimensions, and later added fifth one (Hofstede and Bond, 1988) that appeared to be common to all cultures, (Hofstede, 1991, 2001). These dimensions include different cultural values: power distance, uncertainty avoidance, individualism *versus* collectivism, masculinity *versus* femininity, and Confucian dynamism. Power distance is the distance between individuals at different levels of a hierarchy. This dimension does not only relate to the workplace, but any social, political and economic relationship. Uncertainty avoidance is the extent to which people organize themselves and their activities in order to avoid uncertain or unexpected situations. The degree of tolerance of the unknown also varies among different cultures. Individualism *versus* collectivism is related with the relations between an individual and his or her community. In individualistic societies, individuals generally tend to look after themselves and their immediate family. Collectivistic societies show social ties and form strong, cohesive in-group feelings. Their members care each other with unquestioning loyalty to their in-group. Masculinity *versus* femininity refers to the gender division of roles and values in societies. In masculinity-oriented cultures, men are supposed to be assertive, tough, and focused on material success; women are expected to be more modest, tender, and concerned with quality of life. On the other hand, in femininity inclined cultures, no such marked distinction in social gender roles found. Confucian dynamism is a cultural dimension that became evident when Hofstede worked in the Far East, where Confucius' teachings are common. The Hofstede's Model has shaped much of the successive research in intercultural relations.

Trompenaars (1994) revised Hofstede's Model, emphasizing different theoretical hypotheses and methodological practices. While Hofstede based his premises on theories stemming from individual psychology and A. Maslow's hierarchy of human needs, Trompenaars focused his perspective on social behaviours and relational orientations. Trompenaars recognized three main cultural variables, one of them with five sub-categories, thus a total of seven dimensions were described.

The first one is relationships with people, which includes universalism *versus* particularism, individualism *versus* collectivism, affective *versus* neutral, specific *versus* diffuse, and achievement *versus* ascription. The other two cultural variables are attitudes to time and attitudes to the environment. According to Trompenaars, universalism refers to the need to respect certain standards that are universally accepted and to treat all people in the same way, whereas particularism is based on the evaluation of precise circumstances. In some cultures, professional relationships are usually limited to the specific circumstance of the time and the place dedicated to the working environment; in others, they tend to be diffuse, that is, they involve colleagues' personal and private life. The dimension of achievement *versus* ascription distinguishes between cultures where people are evaluated on the basis of the achievements they achieve and those who considered according to their status and prestige ascribed to them.

The second main cultural dimension suggested by Trompenaars is attitudes to time, that implies the consideration people have of past, present, and future time. A further distinction regards time management. Some people are used to doing one thing after another, and do not begin doing something else until they have completed the previous activity. These people are known as sequential. On the other hand, there are others who tend to do many things at the same time and have a synchronic attitude to the management of their time.

The third dimension values attitudes towards the environment. Some societies believe that they should control nature by developing a specific technology; others prefer to accept natural laws and forces, without trying to change them.

As a theoretical and practical approach in modern counselling systems, multicultural counselling is still a new development, but growing rapidly. The current phase in the development of multicultural counselling often referred to as a "fourth force in counselling".

Approaches of Multicultural Counselling

The roots of multicultural counselling lie mainly in changes of psychology, where a more critical understanding of the limitations of traditional Western psychology with its culture-bounded history emerged (Robinson and Morris, 2000). While the term minority counselling was frequently used during the 1960s, today cross-cultural and multicultural counselling are more in use (Jackson, 1995). These changes in terminology later reflected in the names of professional organizations as well. Such as the Association for Non-White Concerns in Personnel and Guidance (ANWC), established during the 1970s, later changed its name to the Association for Multicultural Counselling and Development (AMCD).

The special issue of *Journal of Counselling and Development* focusing on multiculturalism as a fourth force in counselling was among the first publications which explicitly opened the discussion around this particular perspective. The traditional theories of counselling have evolved in a Western cultural environment. Each of these theories is important, but in some respect they are narrow. Aspects of human nature and all of them almost completely lack the dimension of cultural diversity. Therefore, a more holistic theoretical approach to counselling and therapy was required to meet the needs of culturally and ethnically diverse populations. And, thus two distinct trends emerged in the field of multicultural counselling.

The universal trend emphasizes that all counselling is multicultural in the sense that, all individuals belong to many cultures that have different values (Fukuyama, 1990; Gladding, 1996; Patterson, 1996). Pedersen (1991) discusses multicultural counselling as a generic approach in counselling. In multicultural counselling, a counsellor and a client have some similarities and differences. The differences are generated by a certain culture *via* the effects of socialization or child-rearing (Locke 1990, 18). Given that people have unique personal histories that make them different, all counselling relationships can therefore be considered multicultural. Some authors supporting the universal trend have also analyzed the applicability of some conventional theories in multicultural counselling. For instance, Patterson (1996) claims that Carl Rogers' theory of person-centred counselling is neither culture, nor time specific.

Others, such as Courtland (1996), have adopted an opposing, culture-specific view, and emphasize specific national cultural traits. The culture-specific trend emphasizes the importance of understanding and responding to the special nature of certain cultural groups in counselling and at the same time of keeping in mind that clients should be seen both as individuals and as members of a culturally different group (Locke, 1990, 1992; Nwachuku and Ivey, 1991). According to this trend, a cultural group is defined mainly by race and ethnic background. Culture-specific counselling first tries to form an understanding of the culture and then moves on to action where the theory is applied. Nwachuku and Ivey (1991), who focus on counselling skills in their model of culture-specific counselling, point out that without paying proper attention to specific cultural groups we may apply generalizations and stereotypes based on our dominant Western thinking. Sue *et al.* (1992) point out that the universal and focused multicultural trends are not necessarily contradictory. Both offer legitimate issues and views that can enrich our understanding of multicultural counselling.

Correa (1990) describes that "it is of utmost importance to understand that ignoring differences among people is just as dangerous as stereotyping groups of people from different cultures." Wrenn's (1962) concept of cultural encapsulation is related to an extreme form of the universalistic ("etic") approach to cultural differences. The extreme "etic" approach disregards cultural diversity and overemphasizes universal elements. In contrast, the extreme culture-specific ("emic") approach overemphasizes cultural differences and disregards similarities. For practitioners, it is important to seek a balance between these extremes (Draguns, 1981; Pederson, 1996).

Four major theoretical approaches or systems can be identified in counselling and psychotherapy: psychodynamic, cognitive-behavioural, existential-humanistic and multicultural counselling.

The first theoretical force covers psychodynamic theories, which include psychoanalytic therapy (Sigmund Freud) which is based on psychoanalysis and Jungian therapy (Carl Jung), the theoretical base of which is analytical. The cognitive-behavioural theories form the second theoretical force. According to the cognitive-behavioural approach, the behaviour and feelings of people are affected by consequences, rewards and punishments, and by the way that we perceive and think about our lives. The existential-humanistic theories belong to the third theoretical force.

The counselling models are usually divided into certain logical phases. The emphasis on logical thinking contrasts markedly with the philosophy of some other cultures, which perceive the world from a more holistic perspective and emphasize the harmonic aspect of the world. Many non-Western cultures emphasize intuition and non-linear thinking, which differ considerably from an analytical reductionist demand for cause and effect often implied or explicitly expressed in Western thinking. As a response to these and other related challenges, multicultural counselling as a theoretical approach is seeking ways to recognize the limitations of Western theories and narrowing the gap between the West and the other cultural experiences.

Models and Guidelines

Multicultural Counselling and Therapy (MCT) was developed by a number of authors, especially by Ivey, Sue and Pedersen (1996). MCT has contributed to changing the thinking in psychology from a Eurocentric deductive theoretical approach to a perspective-centred, inductive approach to the study of human behaviour. MCT can be seen as a meta-theoretical approach, because it acknowledges that all modes and theories of helping arise from a particular cultural context and those cultural views of reality are social agreements developed in relation to interpersonal exchange. It rests on the assumptions that all theories of counselling are culture-bound and that their values, assumptions and philosophical bases must be made explicit. It is important to notice that as a meta-theory, MCT does not intend to replace the other existing theoretical approaches and methods, but it calls for a proper cultural analysis of them and encourages counsellors to widen their repertoire of theories and methods to be able to flexibly respond to the needs of diverse clients in counselling (Sue *et al.*, 1996).

First Proposition of MCT theory offers an organizational framework for understanding the numerous helping approaches. It recognizes that theories of counselling developed in the Western world and those indigenous to non-Western cultures are neither right nor wrong or good or bad. Each theory represents a different worldview.

Second Proposition stresses that both counsellor and client's identities are formed and embedded in multiple levels of experiences and contexts. The totality and interrelationships of experiences and contexts must be the focus of treatment.

Third Proposition states that development of cultural identity is a major determinant of counsellor and client attitudes toward the self, others of the same group, others of a different group, and the dominant group.

Fourth Proposition emphasizes that the effectiveness of MCT theory is most likely to enhance when the counsellor uses modalities and defines goals consistent with the life experience or cultural values of the client.

Fifth Proposition stresses the importance of multiple helping roles developed by many culturally different groups and societies.

The liberation of consciousness is a basic goal of MCT theory according to *Proposition Six*. MCT emphasizes the importance of expanding personal, family, group, and organizational consciousness of the place of self-in-relation, family-in-relation, and organization-in-relation.

The American Psychological Association have given its Guidelines on Multicultural Education Training, Research, Practice and Organizational Change for Psychologists as APA official policy in 2002. The Multicultural Guidelines outline the respect and inclusiveness for the heritage of all cultural groups, the recognition of cultural contexts of individuals and group experiences. The role of external forces such as history, economics, sociology, politics, geography, and ecology in people's lives are also emphasized.

The APA Multicultural Guidelines provide psychologists with Rationale for addressing multiculturalism and diversity in education, training, research, practice, and organizational change; the Basic information, terminology, and empirical research from psychology and other fields; References to enhance continuing education, training, research, practice and organizational change methodologies; and Paradigms that expand the purview of psychology as a profession.

These Guidelines are aspirational in nature; they are not mandatory or exhaustive and may not be applicable to every practice-oriented situation. They should neither be applied rigidly nor without regard for individual differences, subgroup variations, clients' specific life circumstances, socio-political, and ecological influences. The Multicultural Guidelines are continuously evolving.

Multicultural Guideline 1: "Psychologists are encouraged to recognize that, they may hold attitudes and beliefs that can detrimental influence on their perceptions of and interactions with individuals who are ethnically and racially different from themselves."

Multicultural Guideline 2: "Psychologists are encouraged to recognize the importance of multicultural sensitivity/responsiveness, knowledge and understanding about ethnically and racially different individuals."

Multicultural Guideline 3: "Psychologists are encouraged to employ the constructs of multiculturalism and diversity in psychological education."

Multicultural Guideline 4: "Psychological researchers are encouraged to recognize the importance of conducting culture-centred and ethical psychological research among persons from ethnic, linguistic and racial minority backgrounds."

***Multicultural Guideline 5*:** "Psychologists needed to apply culturally appropriate skills in clinical and other applied psychological practices."

***Multicultural Guideline 6*:** "Psychologists are encouraged to use organizational change processes to support culturally informed organizational development and practices."

References

Betancourt, J.R.; Green, A.R.; Carrillo, J.E.; and Ananch-Firempong, O. (2003 July-August). Defining cultural competence: A practical framework for addressing racial/ethnic disparities in health and healthcare. *Public Health Reports*, 118; 293-302.

Correa, V.I. (1990). Involving culturally diverse families in the education process. In S.H. Fradd and M.J. Weismantel (Eds.) *Meeting the needs of culturally and linguistically different students: A handbook for educators*. Austin, TX: Pro-Ed, 130-144.

Courtland, C. (1996). *Multicultural Issues in Counselling*. Alexandria, VA: American Counselling Association.

Cross, T., Bazron, B., Dennis, K. and Issacs, M. (1989). *Towards a culturally competent system of care: A monograph on effective services for minority children who are severely emotionally disturbed*. (pp. 13-17). Washington, DC: CASPP Technical Assistance Center, Georgetown University Child Development Center.

Draguns, J.G. (1981). Cross-cultural counselling and psychotherapy: History, issues, current status. In A.J. Marsella and P.B. Pedersen (eds.) *Cross-cultural Counselling and Psychotherapy*. New York: Pergamon, 3-27.

Dumont, L. (1986). *Essays on Individualism*. Chicago: University of Chicago Press.

Evans, K.M., Rotter, J.C. and Gold, J.M. (eds.) (2002). *Synthesizing family, career, and culture: A model for counselling in the twenty-first century*. ERIC, ED 461816.

Fiske, A.P., Kitayama, S., Markus, H.R., and Nisbett, R.E. (1998). The cultural matrix of social psychology. In D.T. Gilbert and S.T. Fiske (eds.). *The Handbook of Social Psychology*. Vol. 2 (4th ed.), (pp. 915-918). New York: McGraw-Hill.

Fukuyama, M.A. (1990). Taking a universal approach to multicultural counselling. *Counselor Education and Supervision*, 30, 6-17.

Gaw, A.C. (ed.) (1993). *Culture, Ethnicity, and Mental Illness*. Washington, DC: American Psychiatric Press.

Geertz, C. (1983). *Local knowledge: Further Essays in Interpretive Anthropology*. New York: Basic Books.

Gladding, S.T. (1996). *Counselling: A Comprehensive Profession*. 3rd edition. Englewood Cliffs, New Jersey: Prentice Hall.

Guidelines. (1993). Guidelines for providers of psychological services to ethnic, linguistic, and culturally diverse populations. *American Psychologists,* 48 (1), 45-48.

Guidelines on Multicultural Education, Training, Research, Practice, and Organizational Change for Psychologists. American Psychological Association. *Approved as APA Policy by the APA Council of Representatives,* 2002.

Hackney, L.H. and Cormier, L.S. (1996). *The Professional Counsellor: A Process Guide to Helping*. 3rd ed. London: Allyn and Bacon.

Hansen, N.D., Pepitone-Arreola-Rockwell, F. and Greene, A.F. (2000). Multicultural competence: Criteria and case examples. *Professional Psychology: Research and Practice*, 31, 652-660.

Helms, J.E. (1992). Why is there no study of cultural equivalence in standardized cognitive ability testing? *American Psychologist*, 47, 1083-1101.

Herkovits, M.J. (1948). Man and his works: *The Science Cultural Anthropology*. New York: Knopf.

Herring. R.G. (1997). *Multicultural Counselling in Schools. A Synergetic approach*. Alexandria, VA: American Counselling Association.

Hofstede, G. and Bond, M.H. (1988). Confucius and economic growth: New trends in culture's consequences. *Organizational Dynamics*, 16 (4), 4-21.

Hofstede, G. (1991). *Cultures and organisations: Software of the mind: Intercultural cooperation and its importance for survival*. London: McGraw Hill.

Hofstede, G. (2001). *Culture's consequences: Comparing Values, Behaviours, Institutions, and Organizations Across Nations*. Thousand Oaks: Sage.

In D.W. Sue, A.E. Ivey and P.B. Pedersen (1996). *A Theory of Multicultural Counselling and Therapy*. Pacific Grove: Brooks/Cole, 155-176.

Ivey, A. (1987). The multicultural practice of therapy: Ethics, empathy, and dialectics. *Journal of Social and Clinical Psychology*, 5, 195-204.

Ivey, A.E. (1994). *Intentional Interviewing and Counselling*. California: Brooks/ Cole Publishing Company.

Ivey, A.E. (2003). Hans Zacharias Hoxter: Building counselling internationally. *International Journal for the Advancement of Counselling,* 25 (2-3), 95-108.

Jackson, M.L. (1995). Multicultural counselling. Historical perspectives. In J.G. Ponterotto, J.M. Casas, L.A. Suzuki, and C.M. Alexander (eds.) *Handbook of Multicultural Counselling*. Thousand Oaks, CA: Sage, 3-16.

Lee, E. (1989). Assessment and treatment of Chinese-American immigrant families. *Journal of Psychotherapy and the Family*, 6 (1-2), 99-122.

Leighton, A. (1967). Is social environment a cause of psychiatric disorder? In R.R. Monroe, G.D. Klee, and E.B. Brody (eds.) *Psychiatric Research Report*. No. 22, Washington, DC: National Institute of Mental Health.

Locke, D.C. (1990). A not so provincial view on multicultural counselling. *Counsellor Education and Supervision*, 30, 18-25.

Locke, D.C. (1992). *Increasing Multicultural Understanding: A Comprehensive Model*. Newbury Park, CA: Sage.

Locust, C. (1990). Wounding the spirit: Discrimination of traditional American Indian beliefs systems. In G.E. Thomas (ed.) *U.S. Race Relations*. New York: Hemisphere Publishing, 219-232.

Lovén, A. (2000). Kvalet infôr Valet [The Trouble of Choosing]. Malmö: Lärarhögskolan. Institutionen för Pedagogik.

Marin, G. (1994). The experience of being a Hispanic in the United States. In W.J. Lonner and R. Malpass (eds.) *Psychology and Culture*. Boston, MA: Allyn & Bacon, 23-27.

Marin, G. and Marin, B.V. (1991). *Research with Hispanic Populations*. Newbury Park, CA: Sage.

Maruyama, M. (1992). *Context and Complexity: Cultivating Contextual Understanding*. New York: Springer-Verlag.

Merali, N. (1999). Resolution of value conflicts in multicultural counselling. *Canadian Journal of Counselling*, 33 (1), 28-36.

Mio, J.S., Trimble, J.E., Arredondo, P., Cheatham, H.E. and Sue, D. (eds.) (1999). *Key words in Multicultural Interventions: A Dictionary*. Westport, CT: Greenwood Press.

Nwachuku, U.T. and Ivey, A.E. (1991). Culture specific counselling: An alternative training model. *Journal of Counselling and Development*, 70, 106-111.

Patterson, C.H. (1996). Multicultural counselling: From diversity to universality. *Journal of Counselling and Development*, 74 (3), 227-231.

Pedersen, P.B. (1991). Multiculturalism as a fourth force in counselling [special issue]. *Journal of Counselling and Development*, 70 (1).

Pederson, P. (1996). The importance of both similarities and differences in multicultural counselling: Reaction to C.H. Patterson. *Journal of Counselling and Development*, 74 (3), 236-237.

Robinson, D.T. and Morris, J.R. (2000). Multicultural counselling: Historical context and current training considerations. *Western Journal of Black Studies*, 24 (4), 239-53.

Sauli Puukari and Mika Launikari Sue, D.W. (1981). *Counselling the Culturally Different*. New York: John Wiley.

Sue, S. and Sue, D.W. (1971). Chinese-American Personality and Mental Health. *Amerasia Journal*, 2, 39-49.

Trompenaars, F. (1994). *Riding the Waves of Culture: Understanding Diversity in Global Business*. London: The Economist Books.

Vontress, C.E. (1969). Counselling the culturally different in our society. *Journal of Employment Counselling*, 6 (1), 9-16.

Vontress, C.E. (1971). *Counselling Negroes: Series 6. Minority groups and guidance*. Boston: Houghton Mifflin.

Wrenn, C.G. (1962). The culturally encapsulated counsellor. *Harvard Educational Review*, 32, 444-449.

10

Cognitive-Behavioural Paradigm

Efficacy and Applications

Anita Sharma

People are disturbed not so much by events, but by the views which take of them. —**Epictetus**, Greek Philosopher

Introduction

Cognitive-behavioural Therapy (CBT) pioneered by Beck (1970) and Ellis (1962) refers to a family of interventions that share the basic fact that psychological disorders and mental distress are triggered by cognitive factors. The therapy proposes that distorted cognitions contribute to development of psychological distress and maladaptive behaviour. According to Beck's model, the maladaptive cognitions include general beliefs, or schemas, about the world, the self, and the future lead to specific and automatic thoughts in particular situations. The model assumes to relieve emotional disturbances by helping people changing their maladaptive beliefs and undesirable behaviour. This therapy is also termed as change-oriented therapy. The thrust of cognitive therapy is on making their clients active, practical and rational beings. In cognitive therapy, the therapist and client work collaboratively and actively as a team. Clients are motivated to try out various "experiments" in their lives, in order to spark change and growth. Cognitive therapy is relatively briefer to other forms of therapy. The emphasis is more on improving the present than on discussing the past.

Cognitive-Behaviour Therapy (CBT) is a relatively short-term, focused approach in treating several types of emotional, behavioural and clinical problems. It is a collaborative and individualized programme that helps clients to identify and locate helpless and irrational thoughts and behaviours and learn or relearn sound coping skills and habits.

It is developing continuously, and includes alternate therapies, like Mindfulness Based Cognitive Therapy (MBCT), Acceptance and Commitment Therapy (ACT), Dialectical Behaviour Therapy (DBT), Schema Therapy. In line with the medical model of psychiatry, the ultimate goal of treatment programme is symptom reduction, improvement in functioning, and controlling the disorder. In order to achieve this goal, the client becomes an active participant in a collaborative problem-solving process to test and challenge the validity of maladaptive cognitions and to modify maladaptive behavioural patterns. Thus, modern CBT refers to a class of interventions that combine a variety of cognitive, behavioural, and emotion-focused techniques (Hofmann, 2011) although these strategies greatly emphasize cognitive factors, physiological, emotional, and behavioural components are also recognized for the role that they play in the maintenance of the disorder.

CBT stems from both 'cognitive psychology' with its emphasis on the effects of thoughts on behaviour, i.e. on cognitive processes as mediators which refer to the individual's feelings, thoughts, attributions, self-statements and other cognitive variables while behaviour therapy looks at associated, i.e. it typically focuses on the directly observable behaviour in the individual's immediate environmental setting that may be modified. When combined skilfully, these two approaches provide a very powerful method to help overcome a wide range of emotional and behavioural problems.

Depending on the problem, CBT may involve a mix of both therapeutic modalities, as some issues are better treated with more behavioural methods and some with more cognitive methods. Onc of the major strengths of CBT is that it not only helps the people to overcome the symptoms that they are presently experiencing, but also to teach the new coping skills and strategies to solve future problems. It emphasizes on the 'here and now' whilst developing a better understanding of past styles of thinking and behaviour that have developed over time.

CBT says that it is not the event which causes our emotions, but how we interpret that event—what we think or what meaning do we give to that event or situation (Figure 10.1).

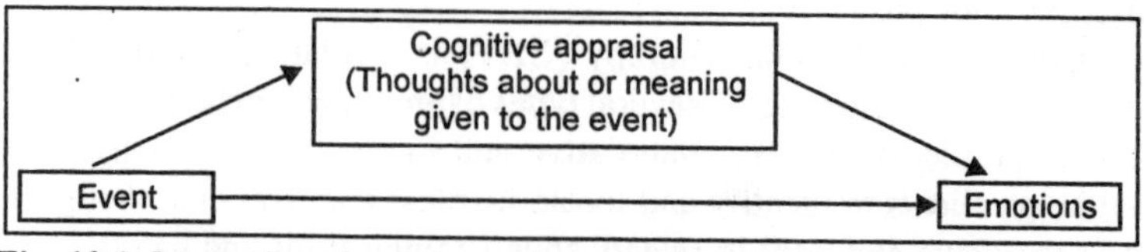

Fig. 10.1: Interaction of event, cognitive appraisal and emotion.

A person who is depressed may have the belief, "I am worthless and have no merit", and a person with panic disorder may have the belief, "I am in danger and may die." While the person in distress is likely to believe these to be the ultimate truths, with a therapist's help, the client is motivated and encouraged to monitor these irrational beliefs by improving self-control and by developing appropriate cognitive and behavioural skills. CBT is geared towards unfolding and modifying the faulty beliefs and unrealistic assumptions that can pervert our perceptions of ourselves and events that lead to depression and other disorders. It looks at the way in which our thoughts, emotions, behaviours and physical states all interact to cause and maintain difficulties. Since, we know that all of these factors interact, it follows that altering anyone of them will have an effect on the others. CBT focuses on the way we can change patterns of thinking and behaviour in order to feel better.

The theoretical origins of cognitive behaviour therapy can be traced back to the Greek Philosopher Epictetus, who in the first century AD observed that men are disturbed not by things, but by the views which take of them...when, therefore, we are hindered, or disturbed, or grieved, let us never blame anyone, but ourselves: that is our own judgements. The implication of this observation is that situations like objects in the visual world are better viewed from some angles than from others and that, at least in principle; people choose their orientations which get influenced by people's beliefs about themselves in relation to the world. Thus, if I believe myself to be a cricket umpire I will watch the cricket match from a different angle than if I believe myself to be a football spectator. The task of CBT is to relieve emotional disturbance by helping people change their maladaptive beliefs and behaviours.

From a cognitive-behavioural perspective, human experience is viewed as a product of four interacting elements—physiology, cognition, behaviour and emotion (Figure 10.2). For example, if I am tense (physiology) when I have to write an important project, this may lead me to think "I am not going to write a good project" (cognition), which in turn might lead me to feel anxious (emotion) and that might lead me to put my pen down and go for a walk (behaviour). The effect of going for a walk reduces the tension (physiology) and leads to more inclination towards reality thinking that I actually do quite well on writing good projects (cognition) and this in turn leads to relaxation of mind (emotion).

In this example, a behaviour (going for a walk) has broken down the negative chain reaction which is the prime motive of CBT. Persons (1989) has identified two levels of conceptualizing client's difficulties in distinguishing between thoughts and beliefs. The first level is one of overt difficulties, with cognitions, emotions and behaviour reciprocally interacting and second level is of covert difficulties, and it is at this level that core beliefs operate, for example, 'I am idiot'. There are reciprocal interactions between these two levels. My belief that 'I am idiot' may make it more likely that I will automatically think 'I am going to make a mess of something' when confronted with a task. But, if I can mould such automatic thoughts across a range of similar situations then core beliefs will eventually get changed (Figure 10.3).

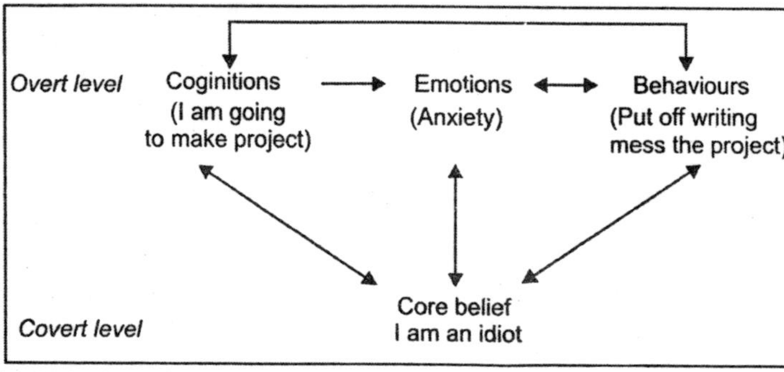

Fig. 10.2: Cognitive Behavioural Model

The **ABC Model** (Figure 9.4) is used within CBT to describe how external factors lead to subconscious thought, which has conscious effect.

- ***A:*** ***An Activating, the antecedent, trigger event or occurrence*** is the combination of a situation or moment that incites a response, either conscious or subconscious, and our perception of that situation or moment that lead to an emotional reaction. It refers to the actual event and the client's immediate interpretations of the event.
- ***B:*** ***Beliefs or thoughts*** are evaluations of reality which filter

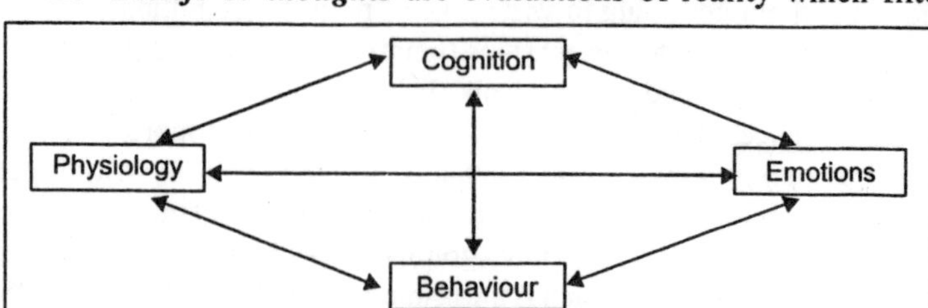

Fig. 10.3: Persons' Model of Client Difficulties

Activating Events through one's thoughts, attitudes, judgements, value, self-talk, interpretations or evaluation of that event and its possible causes and meaning." Beliefs can be rational or irrational, having a powerful impact on our perception of events, and on our reaction to them.

C: ***Consequences*** are the emotional, physiological or behavioural reactions that develop out of the evaluations of one's Activating Events. Consequences can be experienced in terms of positive or negative outcomes. Consequences often function as reinforcements for future Activating Events and Beliefs; in other words, Consequences can trigger a new Activating Event.

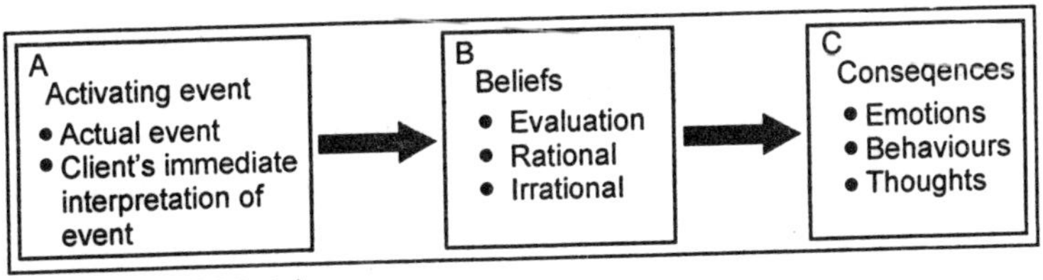

Fig. 10.4: ABC Model

The above model can be explained with the following example:

For example, you are upset because you fetched low marks in a Science test. The Activating event, A, is that you have failed in the test. The Belief, B, is that you must have good grades or you are worthless. The Consequence, C, is that you feel depressed. During CBT, the therapist identifies and challenges the client's negative thought patterns by helping the client understand the impact of those thoughts on his behaviour and feelings and the therapist and the client come up with alternative rational thoughts leading to more positive feelings and behaviours.

Characteristics of CBT: The chief characteristics of CBT are as follows:

- ***Empirical:*** CBT is highly empirical in nature as it is based on empirically testable models which provide rationale for the intervention, i.e. behaviour is the outcome of cognitive appraisal.
- ***Educational*:** The approach of CBT is educational. The therapist uses structured learning experiences that teach patients to monitor and write down their negative thoughts and mental images. The goal is to recognize how those ideas affect their mood, behaviour, and physical condition. Therapists also teach

important coping skills, such as problem solving and scheduling pleasurable experiences.

- ***Collaborative***: The client's active participation and collaboration are emphasized. The client and therapist work together to set goals and develop the treatment plan, and some clients and even create their own homework assignments. Cognitive-behavioural therapists seek to learn what their clients want out of life (their goals) and then help their clients achieve those goals. The therapist's role is to listen, teach, and encourage, while the client's role is to express concerns, learn, and implement that learning.
- ***Strong alliance***: For CBT to be effective, the therapist and the client must establish a strong therapeutic alliance. The therapist needs to be both supportive and empathetic with the client, and establishing rapport from the beginning is very important.
- ***Problem-focused***: CBT focuses on specific problems. In individual or group sessions, problem behaviours and problem thinking are identified, prioritized, and specifically addressed.
- ***Present-focused***: Since CBT is present-focused, current problems are discussed. CBT focuses on the immediate present: what and how a person thinks more than why a person thinks that way. While there may be some mention of past behaviours or thoughts, therapy takes places with a focus on here and now.
- ***Time bound***: CBT is time limited. Typically, treatment with CBT lasts for 14 to 16 weeks.
- ***Skilled based approach***: CBT builds a set of skills that enables an individual to be aware of thoughts and emotions; identify how situations, thoughts, and behaviours influence emotions; and improve feelings by changing dysfunctional thoughts and behaviours. The process of CBT skill acquisition is collaborative. Skill acquisition and homework assignments are what make CBT distinct from "talk therapies". Teaching coping skills is the core of CBT to help clients recognize the high risk situations in which they are most likely to use strategies and to develop other, more effective, means to cope.
- ***Highly structured***: Therapy sessions are highly structured. The structure of sessions will remain relatively fixed for the duration of treatment. The therapist and client will set an agenda and address all items on the list each week.
- ***Goal oriented***: CBT is goal oriented. Patients working with their

therapists are asked to define goals for each session as well as longer-term goals. Longer-term goals may take several weeks or months to achieve. Some goals may even be targeted for completion after the sessions come to an end.

- ***Cognitive Model of Emotional Response*:** Cognitive-behavioural therapy is based on the idea that our thoughts cause our feelings and behaviours, not external things, like people, situations, and events. The benefit of this fact is that we can change the way we think to feel/act better even if the situation does not change.
- ***Practice and Homework*:** Homework assignments develop new skills by teaching different ways to understand situations and their responses. The counsellor acts as a teacher and coach. Home work (including reading assignments) encourages the client to practice the techniques acquired.
- ***Cognitive restructuring and behavioural activation*:** CBT is based on two specific tasks: cognitive restructuring, in which the therapist and patient work together to change thinking patterns, and behavioural activation in which patients learn to overcome obstacles to participating in enjoyable activities.

Components of CBT: Two main components of CBT are core beliefs and automatic thoughts.

1. ***Core beliefs*** are the most central and tacit beliefs that people have about themselves, others and the world around them. A client will begin to develop these ideas in childhood as he interacts with others in his world. Some cognitive therapists also use the word **schemas** to describe core beliefs. Core beliefs can be positive or negative. **Positive core beliefs** would include thoughts like 'I am smart' or 'I am lovable and competent' and these clients are not usually seen in treatment. **Negative core beliefs** tend to fall into two categories—helplessness and unlovability. Examples of helpless core beliefs include 'I am helpless', 'I am weak', or 'I am a failure'. Examples of core beliefs that fall in the unlovable category are 'I am bad', 'I am unlovable', or 'I am unworthy'.
2. ***Automatic thoughts*** are series of spontaneous thoughts that people routinely have during the day as they make sense of their experiences and are a part of stream of cognitive processing

that is just below the surface of the fully conscious mind. These are typically secret, private, unspoken and usually occur in a rapid fire manner while evaluating the significance of events in our lives. In therapy clients can be helped to identify their automatic thoughts by asking questions such as:

- What was going in your mind then?
- What significance does it hold for you?
- What is the reaction of other people about this?

Some automatic thoughts are more important than others to understand what is going on in the client's mind. The therapist can ask clients to record their thoughts to have a better understanding of when these automatic thoughts occur.

Specific Applications of CBT

CBT has been shown to help with many different types of problems. These include: anxiety, depression, panic, phobias (including agoraphobia and social phobia), stress, bulimia, obsessive compulsive disorder, post-traumatic stress disorder, bipolar disorder and psychosis. CBT may also help if one has difficulties with anger, a low opinion of oneself or physical health problems, like pain or fatigue. CBT is one of the most established and researched psychological therapies for emotional, psychological and mental dysfunction. For some problems, such as anxiety and depression, CBT is as effective as medication and can also enhance the effects of medication. The results of CBT are long-term, and one can keep using what one has learned in therapy to approach other problems in one's life. In particular, CBT has demonstrated effectiveness with individuals experiencing the following problems:

CBT for Addiction

Dutra *et al.* (2008) in their study noted a strong evidence regarding the efficacy of CBT for cannabis dependence, with evidence for higher efficacy of multi-session CBT to that of single session or any other briefer interventions, and a lower drop-out rate compared to control conditions. Furthermore, Oakley-Browne *et al.* (2000) reported superior performance of behavioural approaches in the treatment of problematic gambling as compared to control treatments in their study.

CBT for Psychotic Disorders

Treating schizophrenia with CBT is quite challenging. It usually requires medication first. But research has shown that CBT, as an adjunct to medication, can help a patient cope with schizophrenia (Rathod *et al.*, 2008). CBT helps patients learn more adaptive and realistic interpretations of events. Patients are also taught various coping techniques for dealing with hallucinations. They learn how to identify what triggers episodes of the illness, which can prevent or put a check on relapse. CBT for schizophrenia also focuses on skill-oriented therapies, so, that clients learn skills to cope with life's challenges. The therapist teaches social, daily functioning, and problem-solving skills. This can help patients with schizophrenia minimize the types of stress that can lead to outbursts and hospitalizations. Gould *et al.* (2001) have reported the significant beneficial effect of CBT on positive symptoms of schizophrenia, viz. delusions and hallucinations. Zimmerman and associates (2005) also reported CBT to be a promising supplement to pharmacotherapy for schizophrenia patients who suffer from an acute episode of psychosis rather than a more chronic condition.

CBT for Depression

Many studies have shown that CBT is a particularly effective treatment for depression, especially minor or moderate depression. Some people with depression may be successfully treated with CBT only. Others may need both CBT and medication. CBT helps people with depression restructure negative thought patterns. CBT for depression has been proven to be more effective than control conditions (Beltman *et al.*, 2010). Whereas, some researchers reported mixed results that compared CBT to other active treatments, such as psychodynamic treatment, problem-solving therapy, and interpersonal psychotherapy (Pfeiffer *et al.*, 2011). Other studies, however, found favourable results for CBT (Jorm *et al.*, 2008; Tolin, 2010).

CBT for Bipolar Disorder

People with bipolar disorder usually need medication, such as mood stabilizers, but, CBT is often used as a supplement treatment. The medication can help stabilize a person's mood so that he or she is receptive to psychotherapy and can get the most out of it. CBT can help a person cope with bipolar symptoms and learn to recognize when a mood shift is about to occur. CBT also helps a person with bipolar disorder stick with a treatment plan to reduce the chances of relapse (Hausmann *et al.*, 2007). Beynon *et al.* (2008) also examined the efficacy of CBT for preventing relapse and found it to be somewhat effective when comparing CBT *vs.* normal treatment. Overall, Beynon *et al.* (2008) reported CBT as most effective method of preventing or delaying relapses for bipolar disorder.

CBT for Anxiety Disorders

CBT for anxiety disorders aims to help a person develop a more adaptive response to a fear. A CBT therapist may use "exposure" therapy to treat certain anxiety disorders, such as a specific phobia, post-traumatic stress disorder, or obsessive compulsive disorder. Exposure therapy has been found to be effective in treating anxiety-related disorders (Hofmann and Smits, 2008). CBT for social anxiety disorder evidenced a medium to large effect size at immediate post-treatment as compared to control or waitlist treatments, with significant maintenance and even improvement of gains at follow-up (Gil *et al.*, 2001).

CBT for Phobic Disorders

Various CBT techniques for specific phobia (systematic desensitization, exposure, cognitive therapy) were as effective as applied relaxation and applied tension, producing effect sizes in the large range, with long-term maintenance of gains (Ruhmland and Margraf, 2001).

CBT for PTSD

CBT for post-traumatic stress disorder (PTSD) has been reported to be quite effective to that of control or any other usual treatment (Bisson *et al.*, 2007; Bisson and Andrew, 2008). Clinical trials also revealed a large effect size for CBT and/or exposure response prevention for obsessive compulsive disorders (Ruhmland and Margraf, 2001).

CBT for Somatoform Disorders

Within the Somatoform Disorders category of DSM-IV, meta-analyses primarily examined the efficacy of psychological interventions for hypochondriasis and body dysmorphic disorder. Taylor *et al.* (2005) in their meta-analysis found a large mean effect size for CBT, which outperformed other psychological treatments, viz. psycho-education, explanatory therapy, cognitive therapy, exposure and response prevention, and behavioural stress management. Ipser *et al.* (2009) in their meta-analyses compared the efficacy of CBT to control treatments and found that CBT was superior in significantly reducing body dysmorphic disorder symptoms. Williams *et al.* (2006) also compared the relative efficacy of CBT *versus* pharmacotherapy on body dysmorphic disorder severity measures and found effect sizes were large for CBT, and ranged from medium to large for pharmacotherapy.

CBT for Eating Disorders

Eating disorders are highly difficult to treat. However, few studies have revealed that CBT can help reduce the risk of relapse in adults with anorexia who have restored their weight (Pike *et al.*, 2003). CBT may also reduce some symptoms of bulimia, and it may also help some people reduce binge-eating behaviour (Chen *et al.*, 2003). For bulimia nervosa, Thompson-Brenner (2002) in meta-analyses compared the efficacy of CBT to control treatments and found effect sizes in the medium range. Another meta-analysis comparing CBT with control treatments found remission response rates to be higher for CBT, with a medium relative risk ratio (Hay *et al.*, 2009). For binge-eating disorder, a recent meta-analysis found that psychotherapy and structured self-help yielded large effect sizes, when compared to pharmacotherapy, which yielded medium effect sizes (Vocks *et al.*, 2010).

CBT for Sleeping Disorders

CBT for insomnia has been proven to be more efficacious than control treatments. Okajima *et al.* (2011) in their recent meta-analysis which examined its efficacy on both subjective and objective sleep parameters in comparison to a control group for individuals with primary insomnia. Effect sizes for the efficacy of CBT *versus* control ranged from minimal (total sleep time) to large (early morning awakening at the end of treatment on subjective sleep measures). These findings were consistent with results from another meta-analysis, which examined the relative efficacy of behavioural interventions for insomnia including CBT, relaxation, and only behavioural techniques (Irwin *et al.*, 2006). This study reported effect sizes ranging from –.75 to 1.47 for CBT, –.60 to .53 for relaxation techniques, and –.82 to .91 for only behavioural techniques on subjective sleep outcomes.

CBT for Personality Disorders

Meta-analysis by Leichsenring and Leibing (2003) examined the relative efficacy of CBT *versus* psychodynamic therapy for the treatment of personality disorders and reported larger overall effect size for psychodynamic therapy compared to CBT. This was consistent with observer-rated measures, which showed a similar pattern of effect sizes: stronger for psychodynamic therapy than for CBT (although this effect size was also large). Self-report measures, however, indicated larger effect sizes for CBT than for psychodynamic therapy.

Another meta-analysis compared the efficacy of eleven different psychological therapies, including CBT, for anti-social personality disorder (Gibbon *et al.*, 2010). Results suggested that compared to control treatment, CBT plus standard maintenance was more efficacious in terms of leaving the study early and cocaine use for outpatients with anti-social personality disorder and co-morbid cocaine dependence.

CBT for Anger and Aggression

Beck and Fernandez (1998) reviewed 50 outcome studies on anger in 1640 subjects, many of whom were in programmes for violent offenders. They found a mean weighted effect size of 0.70 for cognitive behavioural therapy *versus* untreated controls. The average cognitive-behavioural therapy patients did better than 76 per cent of untreated subjects on reduction of anger. Del Vecchio & O'Leary (2004) and Saini (2009) in their meta-analytic reviews on anger control problems and aggression suggested that CBT is moderately effective at reducing anger problems. Findings from these reviews also suggested that CBT may be most effective for patients with issues regarding anger expression. CBT produced medium effect sizes as compared to other psychosocial treatments and control conditions across the two reviews that conducted quantitative analyses.

CBT for Criminal Behaviours

Considerable researches have reported the efficacy of CBT for criminal offenders (Illescas *et al.*, 2001; Wilson *et al.*, 2005). Of the various psychological interventions for sexual offenders, however, classical behavioural and CBT approaches indicated the strongest efficacy, with medium to large size effects as compared to insight-oriented and therapeutic community interventions (Lösel and Schmucker, 2005).

CBT for General Stress

For general stress, CBT interventions were more effective in comparison to other intervention types such as organization focused therapies, especially when CBT focused on psycho-social outcomes in employees (Kim, 2007). With regard to stress in parents having children with developmental disabilities, CBT yielded positive results, but the effect size was relatively small (Richardson and Rothstein, 2008).

CBT for Distress Due to General Medical Conditions

Kangas and associates (2008) in their study on the effects of CBT on cancer patients reported it to be equally effective as exercise interventions in treating cancer-related fatigue. Small to medium effect sizes were also observed in treatment of secondary symptoms (anxiety and stress) experienced by individuals who were HIV positive, with particular efficacy (particularly for stress management) in reducing anger symptoms as compared to supportive therapy (Crepaz *et al.*, 2008).

CBT was also found to be superior in the treatment of secondary symptoms of spinal cord injury as compared to controls in assertiveness skills, coping, depression and quality of life (Dorstyn *et al.*, 2011), better than placebo or diet/exercise alone (Shaw *et al.*, 2005), but equal to yoga/education in depressive symptoms (Martinez-Devesa *et al.*, 2010).

CBT Techniques

Cognitive-behavioural therapy does not exist as a distinct therapeutic technique. The term "cognitive-behavioural therapy (CBT)" is a very general term for a classification of therapies with similarities. There are several approaches to cognitive-behavioural therapy, including Rational Emotive Behaviour Therapy, Stress Inoculation Therapy and Cognitive Therapy.

1. *Rational-Emotive Behaviour Therapy:* One of the earliest developed of the behaviourally oriented cognitive therapies is the rational-emotive behaviour therapy (REBT) of Albert Ellis

in 1955. REBT is based on the belief that a person's past experiences shape their belief system and thinking patterns. People form illogical, irrational thinking patterns that become the root cause of both their negative emotions and of further irrational ideas. REBT focuses on helping patients discover their irrational beliefs that guide their behaviour and replace them with rational beliefs and thoughts in order to relieve their emotional distress.

2. *Stress-Inoculation Therapy*: A second cognitive behavioural approach to treatment is stress-inoculation therapy (SIT)—a type of self-instructional training focused on altering self-statements an individual routinely makes in stress-producing situations. Here the approach is to restructure these statements so as to improve functioning under stressful conditions (Meichenbaum, 1993). Like other cognitive-behavioural therapies, stress-inoculation therapy assumes that a person's problems result from maladaptive beliefs that are leading to negative emotional states and maladaptive behaviour. This therapy usually involves three stages. The first phase is cognitive preparation in which the client and the therapist together explore the client's beliefs and attitudes about problem situations and the self-statements to which they are leading. The focus is on how the person's self-talk can influence later performance and behaviour. In the second phase of skill acquisition and rehearsal, more adaptive self-statements are learned and practiced. The third phase is of application and practice of new coping strategies in actual situations.

3. *Cognitive therapy*: Third cognitive behavioural approach to treatment is cognitive therapy of Beck, 1960. The aim of cognitive therapy is to change the way the person thinks about the issue that is of main concern. Negative thoughts cause self-destructive feelings and behaviours. For example, someone who thinks he/she is unworthy of love or respect may feel withdrawn in social situations and behaves shyly. Cognitive therapy challenges those thoughts. Cognitive therapy seeks to help the patient overcome difficulties by identifying and changing dysfunctional thinking, behaviour, and emotional responses. This involves helping patients develop skills for modifying beliefs, identifying distorted thinking, relating to others in different ways, and changing behaviours. Cognitive therapy is a psychotherapy that is quite distinct from other mainstream forms such as

psychoanalytic or behavioural psychotherapy: rather than focusing on motivations or instincts, it is based on an information-processing model of human behaviour and psychopathology.

Strengths of CBT

- CBT is as effective as medication that can treat some psychological disorders and is also helpful in cases where medication alone cannot work.
- CBT takes a relatively short period of time for completion as compared to other related therapies.
- The highly structured nature of CBT enables it to be used in different formats, in groups, self-help books and computer programmes.
- Skills one learns in CBT are useful, practical and helpful strategies that can be used in everyday life to help one cope better with future stresses and difficulties even after the treatment is over.
- CBT has been extensively experimented in rigorous clinical trials and it supports empirical investigation.
- CBT is structured, goal oriented, and focuses on immediate difficulties as well as long-term strategies and requires by the client's active involvement.
- CBT is flexible, individualized, and can be conducted on a wide range of individuals and in different settings.

Limitations of CBT

- It requires strong commitment from the clients. To benefit from CBT, one needs to commit him/herself to the process. A therapist can only help and advice an individual, but cannot make lessen his/her problems without his/her co-operation.
- It is time consuming as attending regular CBT sessions and carrying out any other work between sessions consumes a lot of time.
- As CBT is structured, it becomes unsuitable for people with more complex mental health needs or learning difficulties.
- As CBT involves confronting one's emotions and anxieties, one may initially experience anxiety or emotional discomfort.

- According to some critics CBT only addresses current problems and focuses on specific issues, it does not address the possible underlying causes of mental health conditions, such as an unhappy childhood.
- CBT focuses on the individual's capacity to change him/herself (his/her thoughts, feelings and behaviours), but does not address wider problems in systems or families that often have a significant impact on an individual's health and well-being.

Conclusion

Cognitive-behavioural therapy integrates the cognitive restructuring approach of cognitive therapy with the behavioural modification techniques of behavioural therapy. The therapist works with the patient to identify both the thoughts and the behaviours that are causing distress, and to change those thoughts in order to readjust the behaviour. CBT is different from many other therapeutic approaches because it focuses on helping one learn to identify the relationship between one's thoughts, feelings and behaviours. While each of these are interdependent (they all serve to influence each other), CBT gives special attention to the role of cognition (automatic thoughts, rules and assumptions and core beliefs) in creating and maintaining emotional difficulties such as depression and anxiety. CBT aims to help one identify, evaluate and change one's habitual thinking patterns at each of these levels of cognition. CBT has been reported to be one of the latest effective techniques in the treatment of psychological disorders and when it is coupled with other therapies it yields wonderful results. Thus, CBT focuses on trying not to act merely in the moment but pulling back from the situation by taking a wider view and composing oneself.

References

Beck, A.T. (1970). Cognitive therapy: Nature and relation to behaviour therapy. *Behaviour Therapy,* 1, 184-200.

Beck, R., and Fernandez, E. (1998). Cognitive-behavioural therapy in the treatment of anger: A meta-analysis. *Cognitive Therapy and Research,* 22, 63-74.

Beltman, M.W., Oude Voshaar, R.C., and Speckens, A.E. (2010). Cognitive-behavioural therapy for depression in people with a somatic disease: meta-analysis of randomized controlled trials. *British Journal of Psychiatry*, 197, 11-19.

Beynon, K., Woolacott, N., Duffy, S. and Geddes, J.R. (2008). Psychosocial interventions for the prevention of relapse in bipolar disorder: systematic review of controlled trials. *The British Journal of Psychiatry*, 192, 5-11.

Bisson, J. and Andrew, M. (2008). Psychological treatment of post-traumatic stress disorder (PTSD). *Cochrane Database of Systematic Reviews*, 3.

Bisson, J.I., Ehlers, A., Matthews, R., Pilling, S., Richards, D., and Turner, S. (2007). Psychological treatments for chronic post-traumatic stress disorder. Systematic review and meta-analysis. *British Journal of Psychiatry*, 190, 97-104.

Butler, A.C., Chapman, J.E., Forman, E.M., and Beck, A.T. (2006). The empirical status of cognitive-behavioural therapy: A review of meta-analyses. *Clinical Psychology Review*, 26, 17-31.

Chen, E., Touyz, S.W., Beumont, P.J. *et al.* (2003). Comparison of group and individual cognitive behavioural therapy for patients with bulimia nervosa. *International Journal of Eating Disorders*, 33(3), 241-254.

Crepaz, N., Passin, W.F., Herbst, J.H., Rama, S.M., Malow, R.M., Purcell, D.W. and Wolitski, R.J. (2008). HIV/AIDS Prevention Research Synthesis (PRS) Team. Meta-analysis of cognitive-behavioural interventions on HIV-positive persons' mental health and immune functioning. *Health Psychology*, 27, 4-14.

Del, V.T., and O'Leary, K.D. (2004). Effectiveness of anger treatments for specific anger problems: A meta-analytic review. *Clinical Psychology Review*, 24, 15-34.

Dorstyn, D., Mathias, J., and Denson, L. (2011). Efficacy of cognitive behaviour therapy for the management of psychological outcomes following spinal cord injury: A meta-analysis. *Journal of Health Psychology*, 16, 374-391.

Dutra, L., Stathopoulou, G., Basden, S.L., Leyro, T.M., Powers, M.B., and Otto, M.W. (2008). A meta-analytic review of psychosocial interventions for substance use disorders. *The American Journal of Psychiatry*, 165, 179-187.

Ellis, A. (1962). *Reason and Emotion in Psychotherapy*. New York: Lyle Stuart.

Gibbon, S., Duggan, C., Stoffers, J., Huband, N., Vollm, B.A., Ferriter, M., and Lieb, K. (2010). Psychological interventions for antisocial personality disorder (Review). *Cochrane Database Systematic Reviews*, 6.

Gil, P.J.M., Carrillo, F.X.M., and Meca, J.S. (2001). Effectiveness of cognitive-behavioural treatment in social phobia: A meta-analytic review. *Psychology in Spain*, 5, 17-25.

Gould, R.A., Mueser, K.T., Bolton, E., Mays, V., and Goff, D. (2001). Cognitive therapy for psychosis in schizophrenia: An effect size analysis. *Schizophrenia Research*, 48, 335-342.

Hausmann, A., Hortnagl, C., Muller, M., Waack, J., Walpath, M., and Conca, A. (2007). Psychotherapeutic interventions in bipolar disorder: a review. *Neuropsychiatry*, 21(2), 102-109.

Hay, P.P., Bacaltchuk, J., Stefano, S., and Kashyap, P. (2009). Psychological treatments for bulimia nervosa and binging. *Cochrane Database of Systematic Reviews*, 4.

Hofmann, S.G., and Smits, J.A.J. (2008). Cognitive-behavioural therapy for adult anxiety disorders: a meta-analysis of randomized placebo-controlled trials. *The Journal of Clinical Psychiatry*, 69, 621-632.

Hofmann, S.G. (2011). *An Introduction to Modern CBT: Psychological Solutions to Mental Health Problems*. Oxford, UK: Wiley-Blackwell.

Illescas, S.R., Sánchez-Meca, J., and Genovés, V.G. (2001). Treatment of offenders and recidivism: Assessment of the effectiveness of programmes applied in Europe. *Psychology in Spain*, 5, 47-62.

Ipser, J., Sander, C., and Stein, D. (2009). Pharmacotherapy and psychotherapy for body dysmorphic disorder. *Cochrane Database of Systematic Reviews*, 1.

Jorm, A.F., Morgan, A.J., and Hetrick, S.E. (2008). Relaxation for depression. *Cochrane Database of Systematic Reviews*, 4.

Kangas, M., Bovbjerg, D.H., and Montgomery, G.H. (2008). Cancer-related fatigue: a systematic and meta-analytic review of non-pharmacological therapies for cancer patients. *Psychological Bulletin*, 134, 700-741.

Kim, J.H. (2007). A meta-analysis of effects of job stress management interventions (SMIs) *TaehanKanhoHakhoe Chi*, 37, 529-539.

Leichsenring, F. and Leibing, E. (2003). The effectiveness of psychodynamic therapy and cognitive behaviour therapy in the treatment of personality disorders: a meta-analysis. *The American Journal of Psychiatry*, 160, 1223-1232.

Losel, F. and Schmucker, M. (2005). The effectiveness of treatment for sexual offenders: A comprehensive meta-analysis. *Journal of Experimental Criminology*, 1, 117-146.

Martinez-Devesa, P., Perera, R., Theodoulou, M., and Waddell, A. (2010). Cognitive behavioural therapy for tinnitus. *Cochrane Database of Systematic Reviews*, 9.

Meichenbaum, D. (1993). *Stress Inoculation Training*. New York: Pergamon Press.

Oakley-Browne, M., Adams, P., and Mobberley, P. (2000). Interventions for pathological gambling. *Cochrane Database of Systematic Reviews*, 2.

Okajima, I., Komada, Y., and Inoue, Y. (2011). A meta-analysis on the treatment effectiveness of cognitive behavioural therapy for primary insomnia. *Sleep and Biological Rhythms*, 9, 24-34.

Ost, L.G. (2008). Cognitive behaviour therapy for anxiety disorders: 40 years of progress. *Nordic Journal of Psychiatry*, 62, 5-10.

Persons, J.B. (1989). *Cognitive Therapy in Practice: A Case Formulation Approach*. New York: Norton.

Pike, K.M., Walsh, B.T., Vitousek, K. *et al.* (2003). Cognitive behavioural therapy in the post-hospitalization treatment of anorexia nervosa. *American Journal of Psychiatry*, 160(11), 2046-2049.

Rathod, S., Kingdon, D., Weiden P., and Turkington, D. (2008). Cognitive-behavioural therapy for medication-resistant schizophrenia: a review. *Journal of Psychiatric Practice*, 14(1), 22-33.

Richardson, K.M. and Rothstein, H.R. (2008). Effects of occupational stress management intervention programmes: a meta-analysis. *Journal of Occupational Health Psychology*, 3, 69-93.

Ruhmland, M. and Margraf, J. (2001). EffektivitätpsychologischerTherapien von spezifischerPhobie und Zwangsstörung: Meta-Analysen auf Störungsebene/Efficacy of psychological treatments for specific phobia and obsessive compulsive disorder. *Verhaltenstherapie*, 11, 14-26.

Saini, M. (2009). A meta-analysis of the psychological treatment of anger: developing guidelines for evidence-based practice. *The Journal of the American Academy of Psychiatry and the Law*, 37, 473-488.

Shaw, K., O'Rourke, P., Del, M.C., and Kenardy, J. (2005). Psychological interventions for overweight or obesity. *Cochrane Database of Systematic Reviews*, 2.

Taylor, S., Asmundson, G.J.G., and Coons, M.J. (2005). Current directions in the treatment of hypochondriasis. *Journal of Cognitive Psychotherapy*, 19, 285-304.

Thompson-Brenner, H.J. (2002). *Implications for the Treatment of Bulimia Nervosa: A Meta-Analysis of Efficacy Trials and a Naturalistic Study of Treatment in the Community*. Michigan: University of Michigan.

Tolin, D.F. (2010). Is cognitive-behavioural therapy more effective than other therapies? A meta-analytic review. *Clinical Psychology Review*, 30, 710-720.

Vocks, S., Tuschen-Caffier, B., Pietrowsky, R., Rustenbach, S.J., Kersting, A., Herpertz, S. (2010). Meta-analysis of the effectiveness of psychological and pharmacological treatments for binge eating disorder. *The International Journal of Eating Disorders*, 43, 205-217.

Williams, J., Hadjistavropoulos, T., and Sharpe, D. (2006). A meta-analysis of psychological and pharmacological treatments for body dysmorphic disorder. *Behaviour Research and Therapy*, 44, 99-111.

Wilson, D.B., Bouffard, L.A., and Mackenzie, D.L. (2005). A quantitative review of structured, group-oriented, cognitive-behavioural programmes for offenders. *Criminal Justice and Behaviour*, 32, 172-204.

Zimmermann, T., and Heinrichs, N. (2006). PsychosozialeInterventionenfür Frauen mitKrebserkrankungen der Genitalorgane/Psychosocial interventions for women with genital cancers. *Verhaltenstherapie and Verhaltensmedizin*, 27, 14, 125.

11

Cognitive Rehabilitation of Patients with Acquired Brain Injury

Bhawna and *Tushar Singh*

Introduction

The Brain is a very crucial organ in almost every living being. It controls almost all the organs in the human body and their functioning. Brain exerts a centralized control on all kinds of behaviour involving muscular activities like walking, talking, eating, sleeping and behaviours that require use of cognitive abilities such as perception, emotions, thinking, planning, decision making, perception of time and formation of memories etc. Different areas in brain monitor our different body functions; each part of our Brain has specific functions. Apart from these activities brain controls the secretion of all the life-sustaining chemicals called hormones. It has an important role in adaptation to the ever changing environment. Thus, it would be right to call the brain a central part of human body. Any mild to severe damage to it may lead to functional, behavioural and emotional disability.

Acquired Brain Injury

Acquired Brain Injury (ABI) is a type of acquired impairment caused by damage to the brain by events that have occurred after birth. Brain damage in ABI can result due to a physical injury to head, death of the brain tissues due to lack of oxygen supply and infections. ABI does not include genetic, congenital and neurodegenerative disorders like Down syndrome, fetal alcohol syndrome, phenylketonuria, Huntington's disease, multiple sclerosis, Alzheimer's and Parkinson's.

Damage to brain in ABI could be irreversible in the absence of appropriate treatment. It could lead to various types of physical, functional and behavioural disabilities and in some cases death (Collins and Dean, 2002; Stokes, 2008). Many researches that have been done on the survivors of ABI revealed that this type of brain damage is a complex phenomenon having varied effects on different individuals depending upon the nature and severity of the injury. Various case studies have revealed that individuals with brain injury may recover physically and wounds would heal with time and medicine, but the resulting difficulties like aphasia (expressive language), indecisiveness or mental confusion, planning and organizing events and time, memory and concentration problems, depression, anxiety and other problems take time and sometimes may become permanent (Cattelani, Zattin, Zoccolotti, 2010). ABI is a life altering event and it changes individual's thinking and behaviour so radically that person becomes psychologically and behaviourally a different individual (Passer and Smith, 2013: 96). It affects almost every area of individual's life including his/her personal, professional and social life. After injury in most of the cases, the person with ABI find it difficult to go back to their normal life because in addition to physical loss, it also causes disabilities in the area of language and cognition which interfere with adaptation and adjustment to the environment. It is very difficult to predict the outcome and consequences of ABI as every case is unique depending upon the nature and severity of the damage.

The term Acquired Brain Injury (ABI) was first used and given by the Commission on Accreditation on Rehabilitation Facilities (CARF) in 1996. CARF defined ABI as "an insult to the brain that affects its structure or function, resulting in impairments of cognition, communication, physical function, or psychosocial behaviour. ABI includes both traumatic and non-traumatic brain injury" (CARF, 1996).

Non-Traumatic Injury

Non-traumatic injuries include brain damage due to stroke, brain tumors, alcohol or drug abuse, hypoxia and infections like encephalitis and meningitis. Non-traumatic brain injuries are caused by death of brain tissues due to lack of oxygen supply, disruption of blood flow to the brain, chemical poisoning and infections (Collins and Dean, 2002). Following are the causes that contribute to non-traumatic brain injury:

I. ***Stroke***: It occurs due to lack of blood supply to brain due the burst or blockage of the artery that supply blood to brain

(National Stroke Association, 2014). Lack of blood supply deprives the brain cells of blood oxygen and glucose necessary for functioning. As a result the cells may die and sometimes cause irreversible damage to the brain. A Stroke can be classified into two types: Ischemic Stroke (occurs due to blockage in artery carrying blood to brain) and Hemorrhagic Stroke (occurs when the blood vessels or artery get ruptured). Factors that contribute to the susceptibility of stroke include high blood pressure, smoking, obesity, diabetes, drug and alcohol abuse (Giustini, Pistarini and Pisoni, 2013).

II. ***Brain tumor*:** Brain tumor is a kind of new cell growth called neoplasm. It involves mass cell growth on new tissues. A Brain tumor can occur in any part of the body. It usually destroys the tissues and even affects the functioning of areas located near the origin of the tumor. Individual with a brain tumor can face symptoms like epileptic discharge, seizures, loss of sensory abilities like vision, cognitive and behavioural disabilities (Longo Dan L., 2012). This can be of two types. First type is benign tumor/treatable tumor that can be surgically removed and does not grow again. The second type is malignant tumor or non-treatable tumor which cannot be surgically removed and causes cancer. Apart from these two types there are encapsulated tumors (treatable) and infiltrating tumor (highly malignant). The most common tumors that occur in adults are meningioma, an encapsulated benign tumor that grows in meninges, and glioblastomas, a malignant and occurs on glial cells (WHO, 2014).

III. ***Viral infections*:** Some viruses like rabies and those from mosquito bite may sometimes causes brain damage and provides the basis for the development of encephalitis and meningitis that lead to functional disability and death in some cases. These viral infections produce non-specific lesion affecting widespread regions of the brain and causes disability in physical, behavioural and cognitive abilities (Big, Reineck and Aronaff, 2009). The two types of viral infections include neurotropic virus infections (includes rabies and poliomyelitis) and pantropicvirus infections (includes herpes and mums and does not have a special affinity for brain cells).

IV. ***Hypoxia and Anoxia*:** Hypoxia refers to the lack of oxygen supply to the brain due to respiratory problems, an inability of the heart to pump blood, and inability of blood to load and carry oxygen to the brain. It is a failure of oxygenation at the tissue level (Samuel and Cary, 2008). Anoxia refers to extreme loss of oxygen to brain due to suffocation, drowning, heart attack and lung problem. Lack of oxygen supply to the brain could cause the death of brain tissues in 3 to 4 minutes and produces irreversible loss of bodily functions.

V. ***Traumatic Brain Injury***: Traumatic brain injury (TBI) is caused by external factors like a blow to the head or a penetrating head injury that may require immediate hospitalization and may lead to interruption in daily life functioning of an individual (Giustini, Pistarini and Pisonic, 2013). Traumatic brain injury (TBI) is sometimes also known as head injury or cerebral injury (McCaffery, 1997). Although, head and brain injury often occur together, an individual can sustain an injury to head without the brain being injured and a brain injury can take place without injury to the head (Parikh, Koch, & Narayan, 2007). As the name suggests, traumatic brain injury is an injury to brain resulting from an external object causing temporary or permanent neurological dysfunction (Cernich, Kurtz, Mordecai, Ryan, 2010). TBI can lead to wide variety of symptoms and can cause impairment in different facets of life. TBI is one of the major causes contributing to death, impairment and disability. TBI is caused by external injury (e.g. a blow to the head or a penetrating head injury) resulting in impairments that are not only physical, but also psychosocial and cognitive in nature (Ownswoth, Tamara, McFarland and Young, 2000). Physical dysfunctions and impairments are visible and easily identifiable, but it is difficult to measure the severity of cognitive and psychosocial impairments resulting out of TBI. There are different types of treatments available that can help in the quick recovery of physical dysfunctions, but cognitive and psychosocial impairments take relatively longer time and their remediation is possible only through retraining.

It can be of two types—open and closed head injury and open head injury. Open head injury is a penetrating cerebral injury resulting from an object wounding the brain, in this case the skull and the protective lining of brain is damaged and the brain is exposed. Closed head injury results from a blow to the head without bleeding, but leading to a brain displacement is there. It can result in coup counter—coup, contusion and concussion (Sohlberg, and Catherine, 2001; Maas, Stocchetti, Bullock, 2008).

TBI can result in two type of brain damage, namely primary and secondary. Primary damage includes immediate effects like cerebral vascular damage and bleeding in the subdural area. Secondary damage is the consequences that occur as a result of the initial injury. Main causes of TBI are road accidents, fall, gun shots, sports injuries, explosive blasts and violence. These factors result in edema (intracranial pressure), ischemia (disrupted blood flow), swelling, fractures which leads to scarring of brain tissues, and skull getting partly or completely penetrated (Tyerman and King, 2008). A person with TBI have many associated problems along with these primary problems.

Effects of Acquired Brain Injury

Acquired brain injuries cause similar damage to the brain and its tissues as caused by neurological conditions. It affects cognitive, behavioural and social functioning of the individual. Both non-traumatic brain injuries and traumatic brain injuries produce somewhat similar cognitive and behavioural dysfunction, but physical impairments are different. Following are the effects that occur after traumatic and non-traumatic injury:

Physical Impairments

Physical damage due to ABI includes the death of brain cells which may cause loss of motor, sensory and behavioural functions. Common physical impairment in ABI includes problems in coordination, balance, walking, speech, taste, touch, smell, hearing, vision, and hand functions (Sohlberg, and Catherine, 2001; Dalton *et al.*, 2012). Impairment of body functions depend on the area of injury to brain. For example damage to thalamus may result in failure to process incoming sensory information. Cerebellum is considered as the motor coordinating centre of the brain, so any damage to it impairs involuntary actions, fine and motor movement, and body's balance. Similarly, damage to frontal lobe also impairs body movements as it controls all executive functions and their commands (Passer and Smith 2011). Along with these, a complete paralysis may occur in some cases leaving an individual in disabled condition. In addition to the impairments that occur in both traumatic and non-traumatic brain injury, there are some physical injuries that occur only in traumatic brain injuries like penetrating head injuries that damage skull and a large area of the brain.

TBI involves more physical damage to brain than non-traumatic brain injuries. Physical damage in TBI includes, contusion (internal bleeding but without any breakage or fracture leads to damage of cerebral circulatory system that leads to hemorrhage causing hematoma), diffused axonal injury (widespread damage to axons occur after acceleration/deceleration injuries such as road traffic accidents), hemorrhage (when the blood vessels supplying oxygen are ruptured), hematoma (localize collection of the clotted blood vessels in the subdural space) and cerebral edema (brain swelling), infections due to open injuries and wounds. All the above-mentioned injuries are accompanied by severe pain (Arciniegas and Silver, 2001; Parikh, Koch and Narayan, 2007; Crowe, 2008).

Cognitive Impairment

Cognitive impairments that occur due to ABI include ability of a person to concentrate, formulate ideas, problem solving, reasoning, remembering, emotions regulation and expression (Anderson and Bergedalen, 2002; Comper, Bisschop, Carnide *et al.*, 2005). Memory impairments include difficulty in forming new memories, retrograde amnesia (failure of memory for events that happened before the trauma that produced memory loss), post-traumatic amnesia, difficulty with acquiring new learning etc. Problems in attention and concentration are most common and found in almost every case of TBI along with impairment in information processing like reduced speed and difficulty in thought processing. Impairment of executive functioning like difficulty in planning, decision-making, self-awareness, reasoning, self-monitoring, impaired judgements, impaired ability to decide good or bad, and safety awareness are also common. Language related problem include aphasia (impairment of expression or comprehension of language caused by injury in the language centre of the brain), difficulty in naming objects, impaired comprehension, receptive or expressive dysphasia, acquired dyslexia (Cicerone, 1997; Emase, 2001; Busch, McBridge, Curtiss, Vandeploeg, 2005; Crowe, 2008; Ponsford, Draper, Schonberger; 2008; William, Wood, 2010).

Psychological, Social and Behavioural Impairments

Psychosocial impairment in ABI results from the disability faced by an individual in personal, occupational and social life. ABI leaves an individual in a dysfunctional state to interact with outside world and pursue his/her job. Thus, the person feel isolated from the rest of the world and suffer from anxiety, agitation, and depression. Damage to some areas of brain may lead to the development of delusions and mood swings as well. Behavioural changes include poor self-esteem, increased irritability, poor control on emotions, and high aggression level. Sexual problems also arise due to ABI as there might be people who may experience hyper-sexuality or hypo-sexuality. Psychological problem that are common in acquired brain injury include loss of initiative, apathy, disinhibition, insensitivity to the need of others, childishness, reduced insight, impulsivity, depression, post-traumatic stress disorder, psychosis, anxiety. Social problem that accompany ABI are lack of mobility due to physical injuries, decreased interaction with others, decreased interest in sociability, unemployment, financial hardship, difficulty in routine activity, increased dependence on other, spouse or family members, and in short, loss of pre-injury roles (Ownsworth, McFarland, Young, 2000; Eames, 2001; Kim, 2002; Tyerman and King, 2008).

Treatment of Patients with Traumatic Brain Injury

According to World Health Organization (1986) treatment implies the restoration of the patients to the highest level of physical, psychological and social adaptation attainable. It includes measures aiming at reducing the impact of disabling and handicap conditions and at enabling disabled people to achieve optimum social integration. Gopinath and Rao (1992) argued that any model of psychosocial treatment, in order to be effective, needs to focus not only on the impairment of acute stage, but also on remedying disability and compensating for handicap (Gopinath and Rao, 1992). Since terms like disability, handicap and impairment are frequently used in treatment literature; they also mentioned WHO's distinction between the three. Impairment can be physical, any loss or abnormality of psychosocial, physiological or anatomical structure or function (resulting from underlying pathology), e.g. anterograde amnesia. Disability problems arise out of impairment, any restriction or lack of ability to perform an activity, e.g. unable to recall conservations and names (Bittner and Crowe, 2006). Handicap is the problem attributing to society resulting from an impairment or disability and is a disadvantage for individual that limits or prevents the fulfilment of his/her roles (depending upon his age, sex, social and cultural factors) such as poor educational and vocational support (Gopinath and Rao, 1992).

To improve impairments due to ABI one cannot solely rely on a treatment programme that aims to improve physical injuries and damage only. A complete treatment is necessary which should focus on better recovery from cognitive, neurological, behavioural and physical impairments of patients. Before planning treatment programme, individual needs must be evaluated as every case varies in the nature and severity of the injury. Many studies have focused on holistic treatment training programme for patients with acquired brain injury. Many evidenced based reviews supported holistic treatment programmes conducted by transdisciplinary teams. It was found that holistic treatment programmes helped individual with ABI in community reintegration, awareness of deficits, regulation of behaviour and improved communication, physical and social function (Malec and Basford, 1996; Stokes, 2008). The emphasis of treatment is to help the individual to regain functional independence and return them to their community and home life. Treatment interventions can be delivered only to improve cognitive deficits earlier. But now they are offered in holistic treatment programmes that focus on cognitive, neurobehavioural and physical needs of the patients with ABI (Cappa, Benke, Clarket *et al.*, 2005, Cicerone, Dahlberg and Malec *et al.*, 2005). Thus, cognitive treatment is delivered in conjunction with other ongoing treatments.

Medicinal Approach

Lifestyle plays important role in ABI as non-traumatic injuries might be caused by drug abuse, smoking and exposure to pollutants. It is, therefore, recommended to follow a healthy lifestyle that might enhance the effectiveness of treatment programme. Dietary restrictions mainly include the use of alcohol or illicit substances because they may sometimes worsen the course of illness (Cernich, Kurtz, Mordecai, and Ryan, 2010). Some researchers have stated that some nutrients help in the improvement of neuromalfunction, synaptic plasticity, learning and memory (Vayman and Gomez-Pinilla, 2006; Gomez-Pinilla, 2008). Some alterations in one's lifestyle such as nutrient content help to improve both body and brain health (Molteni, Barnard, Ying, Roberts, and Gomez-Pinilla, 2002). Pharmacological treatments to improve cognitive impairment generally include the use of medicines like psycho-stimulant to improve attention and memory (Write and Schillerstron, 2009; Wilmott and Ponsford, 2009; Cerinch, Kurtz, Mordecai and Ryan, 2010) and dopaminergic agents to improve executive functioning (Cerinch, Kurtz, Mordecai and Ryan,

2010). Surgical interventions are also helpful to reduce the severity of intracranial pressure, treat bleeding, decreasing the likelihood of secondary injury and promoting stability of the central nervous system. However, no special surgical technique can be recommended under any treatment programme (Cerinch, Kurtz, Mordecai and Ryan, 2010).

Psychological and Cognitive Approach

ABI result in various impairments and disabilities in every area of functionality of the individual. Damage to the brain impairs many bodily as well as brain functions which bound individual to perform daily routines and their ability to think, plan and organize. Cognitive retraining programme following ABI tends to improve brain plasticity where functional areas of brain acquire the functions of the damaged area. Treatment of cognitive functions plays an important role. Thus, a good treatment programme for ABI patients should include a combination of both medicinal as well as cognitive treatment programme. Medicinal or pharmacological treatments can heal the visible physical wounds, but only cognitive treatment helps an individual to become functionally independent.

Cognitive Approaches to Treatment (Cognitive Rehabilitation)

Cognitive treatment approaches or cognitive rehabilitation focuses on intervention in the area, like memory deficits, difficulty in attention and concentration, problem in formulating ideas, solving problem and reasoning. After ABI individual becomes dependent on their caregivers as they face problem like they might not be able to recall and remember name and address or might not remember to eat. They need constant supervision or need someone to accompany them whenever they go out. Before planning cognitive treatment, an extensive neuropsychological assessment is required to define individual need as each case is different from other, having different needs depending upon the type of impairments, personality, and family support. Cognitive deficits lead to impairment in social and occupational area of one's life. Thus, by improving one's cognitive ability we can help them to go back to their normal life and help them regain those activities that have been lost (Gupta and Taly, 2012). Cognitive rehabilitation is defined as systematic and functional orientation of services for therapeutic cognitive activities based on an assessment and understanding of the person's brain behaviour deficits (Cernich, Kurtz, Mordecai, Ryan, 2010; Cicerone *et al.,* 2011). Services are directed to achieve functional changes by (1) reinforcing, strengthening/re-establishing the previously learned pattern of behaviour. (2) Establishing a new pattern of cognitive activity or compensatory mechanisms for impaired neurological systems (Alladi, Meena and Kaul, 2002; Samuel, 2008). Various tests and tools are used to enhance cognitive abilities. All of them are based one simple principle, that constant practice of one ability lead to improvement in its performance (Rees, Marshall, Hartridge, and Weiser, 2007; Cernich, Kurtz, Mordecai, and Ryan, 2010; Cicerone *et al.*, 2009). Some techniques which are used in cognitive treatment are given below:

I. *Stimulation therapy*: This therapy is based on the assumption that cognitive functions will improve through stimulation of the cognitive system. This means that constant practice or use of cognitive abilities will ultimately improve them. It includes various mental exercises using video games, computer based training programmes, paper-pencil tests and naming exercises that stimulates mental skills. It is assumed that with the help of these exercises the cognitive capacity will improve and the improvement will be transferred to the real life situations (Craine and Gudeman, 1981; Harrell *et al.,* 1992).

II. *Memory training*: Similar to stimulation therapy, but focused on specific areas of memory, these methods are designed to improve naming of objects, learning, identification and remembering objects, people, and places. Some examples may be the techniques to improve iconic memory, poor visual scanning, and visual neglect (Bracy, 1986; Raskin, Sohlberg, 2009; Rohling *et al.,* 2009).

III. *Attention training*: This training is meant to improve a person's ability to focus attention, maintain vigilance, resist distraction, and perform mental manipulations quickly and efficiently. Attention training is a very important area because attention and concentration is the base of all cognitive abilities like memory and learning, and are required to perform almost all the physical as well as higher cognitive ability tasks (Rohling *et al.* 2009; Galbaitis *et al.,* 2009; Vallat-Azouvi, Pradat-Diehl, and Azouvi, 2009).

IV. *Problem solving training*: It involves teaching an individual with brain impairment the basic problem solving skills, strategies for carrying out small daily routine activities, social skills and goal setting. Under this training therapist may use simple problems and set small goals in a controlled setting. Once the individual has learned these skills, they try to transfer them to real life (Stokes, 2008: Dalton, Farrell, Desouza, Wujanto, McKenna-Slade, Thompson, Liu, and Greenwood, 2012).

V. *External devices*: External devices are aids used to compensate the lost abilities rather than to retrain a defective process. For example—training an individual with memory loss to maintain a diary, to save reminders in phone for events or activities to be performed. External device does not cure the underlying physiological causes but helps person to improve his functional independence (Busch, McBridge, Curtiss, and Vandeplog, 2005; Stokes, 2008).

Evaluation of Cognitive Treatment Training for Patients with ABI

Cognitive treatment is not a new area. It has gradually developed and its beginning can be traced to First World War when Kurt established the first brain injury treatment programme for brain injured soldiers in Germany. Goldstein has developed facilities for psychological assessment and workshop for vocational retraining, using compensatory methods and emphasizing the importance of observing functional performance. Goldstein (1993) was also the first to describe impairment of "abstract attitude" as a basis for inappropriate social behaviour (Beers, Goldstein and Katz, 1993, Ponsford, 2004). During Second World War, Alexander R. Luria (1966) developed an approach to study the higher cerebral functions, their recovery and treatment based on his work with victims of missile wounds. This approach formed the foundation on which much of the modern neuropsychology and neuropsychological treatment is based. Luria (1966) identified the presence of functional systems mediating neurological cognitive functions, component of which might be located in different brain regions. He also emphasized the importance of detailed neuropsychological examination of the brain injured person as a means of establishing the precise nature of the cognitive impairment. This then formed the basis of an individualized treatment programme. He advocated that the uses of extensive practices are must for the retraining of impaired functions to rebuild new habits (Ponsford, 2004). In past years cognitive treatment/rehabilitation has gained much attention and many studies have been done around the globe. Cognitive treatment reduces memory failures and anxiety and improves an individual's self-concept, social interactions and personal relationships (Crowe, 2008; Ponsford, Draper, and

Schonberger, 2008). It helps in the improvement of functional outcomes in TBI and NTBI patients (Sohlber, and Catherine, 2001). Many scientific evidence based studies supported cognitive treatment in case of brain injury (Rohling, Faust; Beverly, Brenda, Demakis and George, 2009). Many studies have been done to evaluate the effectiveness of cognitive treatment in the specific area like attention, memory and executive function, and there are strong evidences that specific skill training improves cognitive functions. This type of domain-focused treatment involves training on tasks targeting selective, sustained, and divided attention and has found to be effective in ABI. Rohling, Martin, Faust and Mark (2009) in meta-analytic study originally reviewed. Cicerone *et al.* (2011) revealed sufficient evidences for effectiveness of attention training for ABI. Galbaitis *et al.* (2009) stated that less support has been found for restorative approaches to remediate memory dysfunction after TBI, although more refined researches are going on. Individuals with severe brain injuries showed less improvement than individuals with mild or moderate injuries. A meta-analytic study by Rohling, Martin, Faust and Mark (2009) found weak support for specific effects of memory training, but it could increase the use of compensatory strategies that may support improvement in day-to-day functioning.

Conclusion

To conclude, we may state that cognitive treatment is a specialized treatment programme to help individuals with acquired brain injury, to re-establish normal functioning or to reimburse lost cognitive functions. Acquired brain injury creates a lifelong burden for the individual and their families. Cognitive treatment training reduces cognitive dysfunction or assists individuals in compensating for its impact on daily living (Ponsford, Draper, and Schonberger, 2008; Gupta and Taly, 2012). Benefits of cognitive treatment are discussed in many published research studies and this technique is widely adopted by psychiatrist, neuropsychologists and neurologists to help patients with acquired brain injury and other disorders that cause cognitive and psychological impairment. However, in India patients with ABI are completely dependent on pharmacological treatment for recovery. Although in past few years, the number of published researches on cognitive treatment with acquired brain injury has increased, yet they were not able to address many important issues. Most of the studies that are done in India have focused solely on improving cognitive functions in controlled settings, but very few have focused on how well the individual is able to perform his/her daily routine functions again after receiving the treatment. Thus, the need is to conduct more studies aiming to improve performance outside hospitals, clinics and laboratories settings. More studies should focus on applying the principles of cognitive treatment to real life situations (Gupta and Taly, 2012). The use of cognitive treatment is effective only if the patient is able to transfer the learned tasks into practical life and be able to adapt to his environment once again. Thus, the techniques of cognitive treatment should be incorporated and coordinated with vocational services and special education to increase the functional independence of those with cognitive deficits.

References

Alladi, S., Meena, A.K., and Kaul, S. (2002). Cognitive rehabilitation in stroke: Therapy and technique. *Neurology India*, 50(1), S102-S108.

Anderson, S., and Bergedalin, A.M. (2002). Cognitive Correlates of Apathy in Traumatic Brain Injury. *Neuropsychiatry, Neuropsychology and Behavioural Neurology*, 15(3), 184-191.

Arciniegas, D.B., and Silver, J.M. (2001). Regarding the Search for a Unified Definition of Mild Traumatic Brain Injury. *Brain Injury*, 15(7), 649-52.

Big, C., Reinek, L.A., and Aronoff, D.M. (2009). Viral infection of CNS: A case-based review. *Clinical Medicine Research,* 7(4), 142-146.

Bittner, R.M., and Crowe, F. (2006). The Relationship between Naming Difficulty and FAS Performance Following Traumatic Brain Injury. *Brain Injury*, 20(9), 971-980.

Beers, R., Goldstein, G., and Katz, L. (1994) Neuropsychological Differences between College Students with Learning Disabilities and Those with Mild Head Injury. *Journal of Learning Disabilities,* 27(5), 315-324.

Bracy, O.L. (1986). Cognitive rehabilitation: A process approach. *Cognitive Rehabilitation*, 4(2), 10-17.

Busch, R.M., McBridge, A., Curtiss, G., and Vandeploeg, R.D. (2005). The Components of Executive Functioning in Traumatic Brain Injury. *Journal of Clinical Experimental Neuropsychology*, 27(8), 1022-1032.

Cappa, S.F., Benke, T., Clarke, S., Rossi, B., Stemmer, B., and Van Heugten, C.M. (2005). EFNS guidelines on cognitive rehabilitation: report of an EFNS task force. *European Journal of Neurology,* 12(9), 665-680.

Dalton, C., Farrell, R., De Souza, A., Wujanto, E., McKenna-Slade, A., Thompson, S., Liu, C., and Greenwood. (2012). Patient inclusion in goal setting during early inpatient rehabilitation after acquired brain injury. *Clinical Rehabilitation*, 26(2), 165-173.

Cernich, A.N., Kurtz, S.M., Modecai, K.L., and Ryan, P.B. (2010). Cognitive

Rehabilitation in Traumatic Brain Injury. *Current Treatment Options in Neurology*, 12, 412-423.

Cicerone, K.D. (1997). Attention deficits and dual task demands after mild traumatic brain injury. *Brain Injury*, 10, 79-89.

Cicerone, K.D., Dahberg, C., Malec, F.J., Langenbahn, D.M., Felicetti, M.D., Kneipp, S. (2005). Evidence based Cognitive Rehabilitation: updated review of the literature from 1998 through 2002. *Archives Physical Medical Rehabilitation*, 86, 1681-1692.

Cicerone, K.D., Azulay, J., Trott, C. (2009). Methodological quality of research on cognitive rehabilitation after traumatic brain injury. *Archives Physical Medical Rehabilitation*, 90(11), 52-59.

Cicerone, K.D., Dahlberg, C., Kalman, K., Langenbahn, D.M., Malec, J.F., and Brequist, T.F. (2011). Evidence-Based Cognitive Rehabilitation: Updated Review of the Literature from 2003 through 2008. *Archives of Physical Medical Rehabilitation*, 92, 519-530.

Collins, C., and Dean, J. (2002). Acquired Brain Injury in Turne, A., Foster M., Johnson, S.E. *Occupational Therapy and Physical Dysfunctional: Principles, Skills and Practice*, Edinburgh: Churchill Livingstone, 395-96.

Commission on Accreditation of Rehabilitation Facilities. (2012). *CARF, Medical Rehabilitation Standard Manual*, p. 317.

Cranie, J.F., and Gudeman, H.E. (1981). *The Rehabilitation of Brain Functions and Techniques of Neurotraining.* Springfield, IL: Thomas.

Crowe, S.F. (2008). The *Behavioural and Emotional Complications of Traumatic Brain Injury*, Psychology Press, Taylor & Francis: New York and London, 2.

Comper, P., Bisschop, S.M., Carnide *et al.* (2005). A Systematic Review of Treatments for Mild Traumatic Brain Injury. *Brain Injury*, 19(11), 863-880.

Eames, P.G. (2001). Distinguishing the neuropsychiatric, psychiatric and psychological consequences of acquired brain injury. In Wood, R.L., and McMillan, T. Eds. *Neuropsychological disability and social handicap following traumatic brain injury.* Psychology Press, UK.

Galbaiti, R.M., Pastore, V., Liscio, M., Bardani, A., Castelli, E. (2009). Attention remediation following traumatic brain injury in childhood and adolescence. *Neuropsychology*, 23, 40-49.

Giustini, A., Pistarini, C., and Pisonic, C. (2013). Traumatic and Non-Traumatic Brain Injury. *Handbook of Clinical Neurology*, 110(40), 1-9.

Gopinath, P.S. and Rao, K. (1994). Rehabilitation in psychiatry: An overview. *Indian Journal of Psychiatry*, 36(2), 49-60.

Goldstein, L.H., Bernard, S., Fenwick, P.B., Burgess, P.W., and McNeil, J. (1993). Unilateral frontal lobectomy can produce strategy application disorder. *Journal of Neurology, Neurosurgery and Psychiatry*, 56(3), 274-276.

Gupta, A., and Taly, A.B. (2012). Functional outcome following rehabilitation in chronic severe traumatic brain injury patients: A prospective study. *Annals of Indian Academy of Neurology*, 15(2), 120-124.

Harrell, M., Parente, R., Bellingarth, E.G., Lisica, K.A. (1992). *Cognitive Rehabilitation of Memory: A Practical Guide.* Rockville, MD: Aspen.

Kim, E. (2002). Agitation, Aggression and Disinhibition Syndrome after Traumatic Brain Injury. *Neurological Rehabilitation*, 17(4), 297-310.

Longo Dan, L. (2012). *Seizures and Epilepsy. Harrison's Principles of Internal Medicine.* (18th ed). McGraw Hill.

Luria, A.R. (1966). *Higher Cortical Functions in Man.* New York: Basic Books.

Maas, A., Stocchetti, N., and Bullock, R. (2008). Moderate and Severe Traumatic Brain Injury in Adults. *Lancit Neurology*, 7(8), 728-741.

McCaffery, R.J. (1997). Special Issues in the Evaluation of Mild Traumatic Brain Injury. *The Practice of Forensic Neuropsychology: Meeting Challenges in the Courtroom*, New York: Plenum Press, 71-75.

Malec, J.F. and Basford, J.S. (1996). Post acute Brain Injury Rehabilitation. *Archives of Physical Medical Rehabilitation,* 77, 198-207.

Molteni, Barnard, R.J., Ying, Z., Roberts, C.K., and Pinilla, G.F. (2002). A high fat, refined sugar diet reduces hippocampal brain-derived neurotropic factor, neuronal plasticity and learning. *Neuroscience*, 112, 803-814.

National Stroke Association. (2015). *Understanding stroke.* Retrieved from www.stroke.org. 4 May, 2015.

Ownsworth, T., Mcfarland, K., and Young, R. (2000). Self Awareness and Psychosocial Functioning Following Acquired Brain Injury: An Evaluation of a Group Support Programme. *Neuropsychological Rehabilitation*, 10(5), 465-484.

Parikh, S., Koch, M., and Narayan, R.K. (2007). Traumatic Brain Injury. *National Anaesthesiology Clinics*, 45(3), 119-135.

Passer, W.M., and Smith, R.E. (2011). *Psychology: the science of mind.* 5th Edition. McGraw Hill Education (India) Private Limited.

Pinilla, F.G. (2008). Brain foods: The effect of nutrient on brain function. *Nature Reviews Neuroscience,* 9, 568-578.

Pinilla, F.G., and Vayaman, S. (2006). Revenge of the sit: How lifestyle impacts neuronal and cognitive health through molecular systems the interface energy metabolism with neuronal plasticity. *Journal of Neuroscience*, 84(4), 699-715.

Ponsford, J. (2004). *Cognitive and Behavioural Rehabilitation: From Neurobiology to Clinical Practice.* The Guildford Press.

Ponsford, J., Draper, K. and Schonberger, M. (2008). Functional Outcome 10 Years after Traumatic Brain Injury: Its Relationship with Demographic, Injury Severity and Cognitive and Emotional Status. *Journal of International Neuropsychological Society*, 14(2), 233-242.

Raskin, S.A. and Sohlberg, M.M. (2009). Prospective memory intervention: A review evaluation of a piolet retrorative intervention. *Brain Impairment,* 10, 76-86.

Rohling, M.L., Faust, M.E., Beverly, B. and Demakis, G. (2009). Effectiveness of cognitive rehabilitation following acquired brain injury: A meta-analytic re-examination of Cicerone *et al.*'s (2000, 2005) systematic reviews. *Neuropsychology,* 23(1), 20-39.

Rees, L., Marshall, S., Hartridge, C., Weiser, M. (2007). Cognitive intervention post acquired brain injury. *Brain Injury*, 21, 161-200.

Samuel, J. and Cary, F. (2008). Hypoxemia and hypoxia. In Millikan, Keith, Saclarids, Theodore. (Eds). *Common Surgical Disease*. Springer, New York.

Samuel, R. (2008). Cognitive rehabilitation for reversible and progressive brain injury. *Indian Journal of Psychiatry*, 50(4), 282-284.

Sohlberg, M.M. and Catherine, A.M. (2001). *Cognitive Rehabilitation: An integrative neuropsychology approach.* The Guildford Press.

Tuner-Srokes, L. (2008). Evidence for the effectiveness of multidisciplinary rehabilitation following acquired brain injury: A synthesis of two systematic approaches. *Journal of Rehabilitation Medicine,* 40(11), 691-701.

Tyerman, A. and King, N.S. (2008). *Psychological Approach to Rehabilitation after Traumatic Brain Injury*. Blackwell Publishing Ltd.

Vallat-Azouvi, C., Pradat-Diehl, P. and Azouvi, P. (2009). Rehabilitation of central executive of working memory after severe traumatic brain injury: Two single case studies. *Brain Injury,* 23, 585-594.

William, C. and Wood, R.L. (2010), Alexithymia and Emotional Empathy Following Traumatic Brain Injury. *Journal of Clinical Experimental Neuropsychology*, 32(3), 259-267.

Wilmott, C. and Ponsford, J. (2009). Efficiency of methylphenidate in the rehabilitation of attention following traumatic brain injury: A randomized crossover, double blind, placebo controlled in-patient trial. *Journal of Neurology, Neurosurgery and Psychiatry*, 80, 552-557.

World Health Organization (2014). *World Cancer Report*. Chapter 5, p. 16.

Write, B.W. and Schillerstrom, J.E. (2009). Psychopharmacological treatment for cognitive impairment in survivors of TBI: A critical review. *Journal of Neuropsychiatry Clinical Neuroscience,* 21, 362-370.

12

Online Therapy

Current Status and Future Prospects

Smriti Sawhney Joshi

Introduction

This chapter is aimed at highlighting the current status of online psychotherapy as a treatment option and its future prospects. It will also enlist various modalities of online therapy and discuss clinical and ethical issues related to online therapy. The chapter may not give a comprehensive review of literature, but aims to raise awareness as well as ideas and issues associated with this rapidly growing field. With the internet being available at the click of a button on mobile phones and tablets, tele mental health may soon bridge the existing gap between the existing number of mental health professionals and mental health service users across the country.

Tele-psychology or delivering online psychotherapy and/or other mental health services using the World Wide Web is becoming an increasingly preferred component of mental health service delivery throughout the world. Tele-mental health can be provided *via* a range of technologies including telephone, internet and e-mail, virtual reality simulators, and video-conferencing.

Tele-psychology refers to providing psychotherapy and or other psychological services using technology media that can bridge geographical distance between healthcare providers and patients, such as telephone, e-mail, internet-based communications, and video-conferencing. It offers an innovative way to avert some of the obstacles people face in accessing and adhering to needed care. The President of the American Counselling Association, in 1998 (Lee, 1998), noted that "to think that clients in the new century would not expect to access Internet counselling services is probably foolish and short-sighted on our part". Research literature since 2003, has demonstrated that tele-mental health services are satisfactory to patients, improve outcomes, and are probably cost-effective. Tele-mental health presents an efficient treatment modality for a spectrum of mental health services so it becomes imperative to understand how this modality influences key elements of the treatment experience. It is being considered as a "bridge" between the ever increasing number of clients *vis-à-vis* the limited number of mental health professionals. In the very small number of studies that have been conducted to date, tele-mental health has demonstrated equivalent efficacy compared to face-to-face care in a variety of clinical settings and with specific patient populations. In one of the studies on jail inmates where there was limited staff catering to the mental health needs, the authors compared the subjects' perceptions of the working alliance, post-session mood, and satisfaction with psychiatric and psychological mental health services delivered through 2 different modalities: tele-mental health and face-to-face. Participants consisted of 186 inmates who received mental health services (36 *via* tele psychology, 50 *via* face-to-face psychology, 50 *via* tele psychiatry, and 50 *via* face-to-face psychiatry). Results indicate no significant differences in inmates' perceptions of the work alliance with the mental health professional, post-session mood, or overall satisfaction with services when tele-mental health and face-to-face modalities were compared within each type of mental health service (Morgan, Patrick, and Magaletta, 2008). This does give hope that geographical locations that have a lower number of professionals providing face-to-face psychotherapy, tele-video-conferencing as a mode of providing psychotherapy can be a viable option.

Various Modalities for Conducting Online Therapy

Long distance management of problems and maintaining contact with clients or therapists due to change in either party's geographical location has been in practice ever since writing letters to stay in touch has been in practice. Freud utilized letters as a means to communicate and stay in touch with his clients. Necessity is the mother of all invention and one can imagine the rising need for online therapy due to demands for more time and cost-effective, convenient methods for receiving and providing therapy. It is considered as a platform where the user could maintain anonymity and yet receive the help he/she needed. Self-help web sites, e-mail and text based therapies were the first to surface as service modalities in the field of tele-psychology.

People have been writing e-mails and participate in social forums online to vent out and share emotionally disturbing experiences as a way to seek emotional support from professionals or people with similar people. Mental health professionals had probably started using telecommunication like e-mails for follow-ups fairly early (1990s) in their practice. Clients who had formally terminated therapy or shifted base kept in touch through e-mails with updates about their progress or wrote for advice in times of crisis. Later, e-mails and chats became a formal mode of therapy with their own code of conduct. Frequency of sessions through e-mails would be charted out and a predefined fee would be charged.

But now, with the advent of video-conferencing options like skype or google hangout, it is being considered a more efficient modality for online therapy as compared to e-mails or chats. This may be due to the multi-sensory output and real-time quality of video-conferencing as compared with other tele-mental health modalities, which access a narrower range of sensory modalities when assessing or intervening in mental health setting like texting or just e-mailing. Thus, two main kinds of service delivery modalities have been recognized based on time and format of delivery of service—asynchronous and synchronous. Synchronous (chat and video-conferencing) and more popularly asynchronous (e-mail) communication have been used by client(s). Asynchronous communication refers to communication that is stored and forwarded at a later time, like an e-mail. This is often used when the provider does not need to interact face-to-face with the patient. Some web-based self-administered treatments for a variety of disorders have included online counselling support, usually in the form of asynchronous post-sessions feedback, which appears to increase adherence and yield enhanced outcomes (Newman, Szkodny, Llera, and Przeworski, 2011).

Synchronous communication encompasses live, real-time interactive two-way communication like texting, voice or video-conferencing. VTC, as in other forms of live two-way interactions allows live interaction to happen in real time between multiple parties. Most providers use video-conferencing along with other formats like e-mails and chats for communication.

These online therapy programmes delivered *via* the internet have adapted evidence-based psychological interventions (e.g. cognitive behavioural therapy) delivered using e-mail; chats or video-conferencing or self-help applications depending on the degrees of therapist contact required. For example, some are pure self-help programmes while the others are predominantly self-help with therapist involvement restricted to diagnostic assessments and instruction in the use of the programme. There are therapeutic programmes involving minimal contact with communication done using e-mail, while there may be some programmes based predominantly on therapist administered interventions requiring regular video-conferencing along with some e-mail 'sessions' plus self-help tools.

Online Therapy: Current Status and Issues

The field of online counselling emanated only recently, supported by rapid technological developments. Online psychotherapy is a term that has been coined to describe the process of interacting with a therapist online in ongoing conversations over time when the client and counsellor are in separate or remote locations and utilize electronic means to communicate with each other. Online psychotherapy can come in many formats like *via* e-mail, video-conferencing, virtual reality technology, chat technology, or any combination of these (Manhal-Baugus, 2001).

There are several factors which differentiate among the different therapeutic methods delivered online. One of these has to do with the kind and purpose of the therapeutic intervention selected for service delivery—whether it includes human communication (termed here e-therapy) or is a self-help, website-based therapy (termed here web-based therapy). Another major factor has to do with the time of service delivery—whether an intervention is delivered in "real-time" (synchronously) or is delayed (asynchronously). Online therapy services could be delivered to and received by individuals or a group mode and this also is a major differentiating factor amongst therapeutic methods delivered online. Another differentiating factor has to do with the mode of communication used to deliver the online therapy—text, by audio only, or by video (webcam).

Recent researches in this field consider aspects of delivering therapeutic interventions online. These include, but are not limited to, the potential effectiveness of online counselling, establishing a therapeutic alliance, potential benefits and challenges of using the technology, client suitability for online counselling, therapists' and clients' attitudes and experiences of online counselling, professional training for working online with clients, and its very nature and definition as a therapeutic intervention

(Richards and Viganò, 2012). Researchers have also been exploring the psychology of online behaviour, including the effects of perceived anonymity, inhibition, writing and emotional expression and ethical behaviour in the virtual world, to name a few, as it applies to online counselling.

A qualified online psychologist or psychotherapist is often the primary person providing direct care to individuals using the various online or internet based modalities to access mental health services. The role of an online psychotherapy provider includes, but is not limited to:

- Providing counselling and treatment services using distance technologies, including telephone, internet chat, e-mail, and web/ video-conferencing.
- Maintaining a secure distance delivery system that ensures client informed consent, confidentiality, and safety.
- Conducting client screening and assessment and developing and implementing treatment plans based on the client's individual strengths, needs, abilitics, and preferences.
- Following all laws, statutes, regulations and standards applicable to comparable on-site services when delivering distance-based services.

The focus of e-therapy will differ for each client. The kind of issues that clients may bring in for an online therapy session will range from interpersonal relationships, or learn new ways of dealing with stress to e-therapy as an adjunct to other types of real-world services, or to get help with serious psychological or emotional disturbances they are currently experiencing. Some others may make use of online therapy for a more objective third-party professional opinion about various issues in their lives and work on more philosophical life issues.

There are several technical and ethical difficulties one may encounter in our efforts to transform the traditional face-to-face therapeutic relationships into online formats across Internet-facilitated boundaries and modalities. Given below is a discussion of some of these issues associated with providing and receiving online therapy that have been experienced both providers and receivers and also researched. This is not an exhaustive list of the practice issues associated with online therapy but would surely give the reader an idea about the key points to keep in mind while planning to be a provider for online therapy:

Therapeutic Alliance

Therapeutic alliance is the key to having a positive outcome for the client receiving therapy services. One of the main issues in the counselling or psychotherapy practice, especially online therapy is whether a working therapeutic alliance can develop when the provider and the client are geographically separated. There are some obvious concerns related to therapeutic alliance in online therapy.

Even though the client and therapist seem to look at each other's faces on a computer screen, it cannot be termed as an eye-to-eye contact, which can lead to missing out important cues in the non-verbal feedback. While using voice call or e-mails or chats there may be a complete lack of non-verbal cues which may lead to poor therapeutic relationship. Technical issues may arise like the screen going blank during the therapy process, or problems with voice and visual clarity or background noise. Thus, even though some degree of emotion can be easily communicated in online transactions be it in writing or face-to-face when using video-conferencing, can a deep, non-judgemental sustained sharing of emotion considered necessary for many forms of psychotherapy be effectively maintained in an online environment?

There are many factors which may influence therapeutic alliance in online psychotherapy and most important of them is the modality used for service delivery. It may take longer for therapeutic alliance to develop while using e-mail as a therapy providing mode, due to the obvious lack of physical contact, unless the therapist is already known to the client. But e-mail as an adjunct to face-to-face therapy or if used along with therapy sessions using video-conferencing, say for providing and monitoring homework given during therapy, enhances the therapeutic alliance. A review done recently indicates that a positive therapeutic alliance can be established regardless of the medium of communication. The therapeutic alliance was rated equally satisfying as in conventional face-to-face therapy (Klasen, Knaevelsrud and Böttche, 2013).

Therapeutic alliance needs to be studied from both the client and the provider's perspective while using internet as a means to provide therapy to avoid any gaps and enhance the outcomes. Even though tele-psychology has been seen as a mode that can reduce barriers to psychotherapy not many psychologists offer or provide it as an option. It is possible the traditional understanding of the therapeutic alliance, and the environment in which it is created (face-to-face), prompts caution in psychologists regarding the use of e-mails or video-conferencing as a means to provide psychotherapy.

To evaluate this Rees and Stone (2005) hypothesized that psychologists would rate therapeutic alliance as being higher when psychotherapy is provided face-to-face *versus* via video-conferencing. Thirty clinical psychologists were randomly assigned to watch a twenty minute excerpt from a therapy session conducted in one of two formats: face-to-face or video-conferencing. The psychologists viewing the video-conferencing session rated the bond from the client's point of view as significantly lower than those who viewed the face-to-face session. However, there was not a significant difference between the session formats on the psychologists' ratings of how well the therapist and patient worked together. This study was conducted in 2005 and today when many mental health professionals are resorting to using technology to aid the therapeutic process and even to use it as a main medium to provide therapy, it would be interesting to re-examine the psychologists perceptions of therapeutic alliance and whether or not these results have changed with the rapid growth in technology use since 2005. Therapists should also have an openness and belief in the therapeutic benefits of online counselling (Fenichel *et al.*, 2002).

Yet, given the importance attributed to therapeutic alliance as a predictor of treatment response and compliance, psychologists using video-conferencing for psychotherapy may want to use some form of client assessment or rating of the therapeutic alliance. Therapists should also focus in particular to the client's opinion and impression of the therapist to assess the therapeutic alliance so as to maximize treatment response. Thus, it is also of extreme importance to know if the client felt at ease, felt heard and a rapport could be established between the client and therapist, satisfactorily when receiving online therapy. In an early study (Hufford, Glueckauf, and Webb, 1999) that compared the alliance in video-conferencing and face-to-face counselling for teenagers, clients reported significantly higher levels of alliance in face-to-face. Yet, despite the lack of social signalling, another early study (Cohen and Kerr, 1998) reported similar ratings between online therapy services and face-to-face counselling regarding clients' perceptions of therapists' expertness, attractiveness, and trustworthiness. In a study done in 2002, working alliance scores were compared between a small, primarily, female sample of online therapy consumers and a representative sample of traditional face-to-face therapy clients. The results revealed significantly higher means on the goal subscale and composite score of the Working Alliance

Inventory in the online sample. This suggested that a working alliance can be adequately established in therapy delivered online. Also, no significant differences in the level of working alliance were found within the online therapy sample with respect to modality of communication, client presenting problem, or therapist (Cook, and Carol Doyle, 2002).

Client Suitability

The debate continues regarding the suitability of individuals and the types of presenting issues that are appropriate for online therapy. It has been observed that the use of anyone particular modality say e-mail or video-conferencing may not suit everybody and that individual factors may be important in determining the success of online counselling (Fenichel *et al.*, 2002). "Suitability refers to a variety of factors, including the person's preferences regarding online therapy, how suggestible the person is within a particular communication modality, his or her skills in communicating within that modality, and the potentially therapeutic aspects of that modality for the person" (Suler, 2001).

Ability for written expression and reading, as well computer-literacy are examples of factors that constitute suitability for online counselling, for clients especially if the therapist will be working with the client using e-mail or chat based therapy. A person's reading and writing skills, both, are necessary for text-based therapy (Suler, 2001; Fenichel *et al.*, 2002; Rochlen, Zack *et al.*, 2004). In his article on client suitability John Suler mentions the following points to be kept in mind while assessing client suitability for online therapy (Suler, 2001):

- Does the person demonstrate adequate knowledge of his or her computer system and internet technology?
- Is the person motivated and capable to experiment with new communication environments and techniques?
- Is the person's computer system compatible with that of the clinician?
- What kind of internet access does the person have?
- Where is the client accessing the internet (home, work), and does this present any problems regarding privacy or any technological difficulties (e.g. firewalls that limit internet activities)?
- If the client's internet access is problematic, are there viable alternatives (e.g. a web-based e-mail account)?
- What kinds of experiences has the person had with reading and writing?

- What do reading and writing mean to the person?
- Are there any known physical or cognitive problems that will limit the ability to read and write?
- How well can the person type?
- Does the person enjoy in-person and phone conversations. Why?
- How does the person feel about instant, at the moment, spontaneous communication of chat as opposed to compose or edit an e-mail?

The presenting complaints or the issues that the clients bring in for online therapy is another factor to keep in mind while assessing client's suitability for online therapy or counselling. Apparently there exists no difference between the presenting issues in online counselling as compared to face-to-face counselling (Leibert *et al.*, 2006; Richards, 2009). The Department of Defence (DoD) Task Force on Mental Health reports in its tele-mental health guidebook that there are no absolute contra indications to patients being assessed using tele-mental health. Very limited empirical research exists about the issues presented by online clients. As a rule of thumb, serious psychological disorders with complex psychopathology and clients with risky behaviours such as suicidal ideations or intentions to harm others may be considered inappropriate for online work. In a study of 55 e-therapy Websites (Recupero and Rainey, 2006) it was found that some sites specified criteria that would render prospective clients ineligible to receive services (e.g. suicidal tendency).

Some online therapy providers advocate online medium thus to be restricted to less serious issues (Haberstroh *et al.*, 2008) whereas there are others who note specific advantages for specific populations and presentations (Simpson *et al.*, 2005), while others advocate that the online medium is adequate to address most issues at any level of severity (Fenichel *et al.*, 2002). Going by one's clinical judgement clients who seem to require any form of hospitalization, say an active substance abuser, or those requiring observation and supervision may not be suitable for online therapy. The online therapist may need to assess the client's history of level of functioning, and then periodically reassess the client during the therapy as the level of functioning may change over time. Age of the client would also be of some importance when discussing client suitability factors. Many therapists prefer their clients to be at least 18 or stepping into their youth to be able to make the best use of online psychological services. Barack *et al.* (2008) reported that while all age-groups showed benefits in online interventions individuals in the 19-39 age range appeared to benefit the most.

Outcome

There is a large assortment of internet interventions that has been developed and tested for common mental disorders, and the evidence from client ratings and researches show that these treatments often have similar outcomes as in face-to-face psychotherapy. Clinical researchers have studied whether online psychotherapy and conventional face-to-face therapy are equally effective in experiments. Based on earlier studies, researchers at University of Zurich assumed that the two forms of therapy were on a par. Their theory was confirmed and the results for online therapy even exceeded their expectations (Birgit, Horn, and Andreas, 2013; *Science Daily*). Most studies support and reflect the attractiveness of the online mode of service deliver as it can be adapted for many uses including administrative and managerial tasks, patient intervention and psychotherapy, assessment and evaluation, psycho-education and counselling and professional supervision and training (Glueckauf and Ketterson, 2004; Godleski, Nieves, Darkins, and Lehmann, 2008). A research at University of Zurich on two groups of patients with depression, of which one group was given face-to-face treatment and the other was given online therapy, revealed that online medium of providing therapy was more effective than the face-to-face therapy as patients showed more motivation in doing online assignments as they could monitor their own progress personally (Birgit, Horn, and Andreas, 2013). The most commonly and consistently reported outcomes for online mental health services research are satisfaction and acceptance, which are virtually always high (Browne, Reilly and Bradley, 2006). There was evidence of success with tele-mental health in the areas of child psychiatry, depression, dementia, schizophrenia, suicide prevention, post-traumatic stress, panic disorders, substance abuse, eating disorders, and smoking prevention. Some of the clinical disorders that have been treated *via* online therapy include panic disorder (e.g. Richards, Klein, and Austin in press), phobias (Kenwright, Liness, and Marks, 2001), obsessive-compulsive disorder (Clark, Kirkby, Daniels, and Marks, 1998), post-traumatic stress symptoms (Lange, van de Ven and Shrieken, 2003) and depression (*e.g.*, Christensen, Griffiths and Jorm, 2004). In another research on online therapy, the clients presented a variety of issues, including weight issues and personality disorders. The most common complaints, the clients reported were body image or weight, family relationships, other relationships, and work or school. The clients were provided online counselling services using three modes of services deliver—Video-conferencing, face-to-face and audio conference. The authors reported that "the similarities among the three treatment groups—face-to-face, video-teleconference, and audio conference—came through more strongly than any differences" (Day and Schneider, 2002).

An investigation of reliability of distance neuropsychological evaluation of patients, using the online medium, with alcohol abuse suggested comparable outcomes to face-to-face consultation with patient satisfaction listed as "good" (Kirkwood, Peck and Bennie, 2000). There is also some evidence pointing to possible cost saving of this format (Kennedy and Yellowlees, 2003). The patient may be able to save both money and time, particularly if the patient has to travel. This would also mean less drop-out rates from therapy. Hailey, Roine and Ohinmaa (2008) reviewed the evidence of benefit from use of tele-mental health in studies that reported clinical or administrative outcome and noted that those treated with distance methods had a higher attendance rate and that follow-up visits were shorter than in face-to-face encounters discarding fears that online modalities leads to drop-outs. Overall, the results for online psychotherapy appear to be promising.

Ethical Issues While Providing Online Therapy

It is obvious there is a need for thoughtful consideration about professional, ethical practice, with particular concern about risk management for particular types of client situations which one may not have encountered in the traditional face-to-face therapy situation. The online medium brings to the psychotherapists and counsellors an innovative modality through which they can provide psychological interventions which can be delivered appropriately through this medium. But like with any new invention that brings in loads of benefits to its users along with challenges in its use, online therapy also offers new ethical challenges for therapists and counsellors interested in providing online services.

The lack of non-verbal cues in interactive text-based communication and in-person verbal communication or the increased risk of misinterpretations while using web telephony or video-conferencing may create new ethical challenges not previously encountered in face-to-face therapy. Ethical issues such as confidentiality, lack of awareness of location of the client, inadequacy of counsellor interventions, misuse of computer applications, privacy concerns, credentialing, and relationship development issues were identified early in the literature (Sampson, Kolodinsky and Greeno, 1997) and are still being debated upon.

American Psychology Association Ethics Board in 1995 made one of the first attempts to address the ethical concerns by issuing a general statement that described the ethics code applicable to psychologists and therapists using telephone and internet services (Shapiro and Schulman, 1996). This was followed by development of standards for online practice by the National Board for Certified Counsellors (NBCC) (Bloom, 1998). International Society for Mental Health Online (ISMHO) was formed in 1997 with a clear objective to promote the understanding, research and development of online communication in mental health. As a result of continuous research ISMHO produced guiding principles for the ethical practice of online counselling (ISMHO, 2000) and is now widely followed by the providers. Many more psychology and counselling associations across the globe, especially in the US, UK and Australia, came up with their own practice guidelines to ensure that ethical concerns were addressed while providing online mental health services. In India we still lack research as well a body to govern the provision of online therapeutic services even though one can see a rapid rise in Indian websites providing mental health services.

Informed Consent, Confidentiality and Security, competency in using the technology that psychotherapists are using and a clear communication about the process and fees involved are some of the ethical issues that arise in an online therapy practice. For a competent practitioner who is providing mental health services online adhering to the following minimum standards and practices will make sure that they are working in an ethical manner (reproduced under the creative commons licence from, Dee Anna Merz Nagel and Kate Anthony (2009) on Online Therapy article abstract.docx).

Practitioners have a Sufficient Understanding of Technology

Technology basics are required for practitioners who choose to deliver therapeutic services *via* technology. Practitioners will possess a basic understanding of technology as the technology relates to delivery of services:

- ***Encryption***: Practitioners understand how to access encrypted services to store records and deliver communication. Records storage can be hosted on a secure server with a third-party, stored on the practitioner's hard drive utilizing encrypted folders or stored on an external drive that is safely stored.

- ***Backup Systems***: Records and data that are stored on the practitioner's hard drive are backed up either to an external drive or remotely *via* the Internet.
- ***Password Protection***: Practitioners take further steps to ensure confidentiality of therapeutic communication and other materials by password protecting the computer, drives and stored files or communication websites.
- ***Firewalls***: Practitioners utilize firewall protection externally or through web-based programmes.
- ***Virus Protection***: Practitioners protect work computers from viruses that can be received from or transmitted to others, including clients.
- ***Hardware***: Practitioners understand the basic running platform of the work computer and know whether or not a client's hardware/platform is compatible with any communication programmes the practitioner uses.
- ***Software***: Practitioners know how to download and operate software and assist clients with the same when necessary to the delivery of services.
- ***Third-party services***: Practitioners utilize third-party services that offer an address and phone number so that contact is possible *via* means other than e-mail. This offers a modicum of trust in the third-party utilized for such services as back-up, storage, virus protection and communication.

Practitioners Work within their Scope of Practice

Scope of Practice indicates the specific area to which a practitioner may practice. Scope of practice in many geographic areas also defines where a practitioner may practice; whether the practitioner may practice across various geographical boundaries and within what parameters a practitioner may practice. Practitioners also follow local and regional laws and codes of ethics as applicable.

- ***Understanding of boundaries and limitations of one's specific discipline:*** Practitioners understand which assessments and interventions are allowed within their specific discipline. For instance, career counsellors who have no training in mental health issues generally do not provide psychotherapy services.

- ***Understanding of specific laws or ethics within one's own discipline or geographic location:*** Practitioners understand the limits set forth by laws or ethics within the applicable geographic location. For instance, in the United States, Licensed Professional Counsellors cannot call themselves Psychologists, and in the UK the term 'Chartered Psychologist' is reserved by law for use only by those with proper recognition from the appropriate authorities.
- ***Respect for the specific laws of a potential client's geographic location:*** Practitioners understand that different geographic regions may offer additional limits to practice, particularly with regard to jurisdiction. For instance, a counsellor in the UK should be cognizant of the laws of a client who resides in a U.S. state such as California in which the law prohibits consumers residing in California from engaging in counselling from a practitioner who is not licensed in California.

Practitioners Seek Out Training, Knowledge and Supervision

Training, knowledge and supervision regarding mental health and technology is paramount to delivering a standard of care that is considered "best practice" within one's geographic region and within a global context. Practitioners are encouraged to demonstrate proficiency and competency through formal specialist training for online work, books, peer-reviewed literature and popular media. Clinical and/or peer supervision and support are mandated for practitioners who cannot practice independently within a geographic region and is highly recommended for all practitioners:

- ***Formal Training*:** Practitioners seek out sufficient formal training whenever possible through college, university or private settings. Formal training is displayed on the practitioner's website.
- ***Informal Training*:** Practitioners seek out continuing education and professional development and conferences, conventions and workshops.
- ***Books*:** Practitioners read books written by the general public and professionals.
- ***Peer-reviewed Literature*:** Practitioners read peer-reviewed

literature that includes the latest theories and research.

- ***Popular Media***: Practitioners are informed through popular media such as magazines, newspapers, social networking sites, websites, television and movies and understand the impact of mental health and technology on the popular culture.
- ***Clinical/Peer Supervision***: Practitioners seek clinical supervision whenever the practitioner cannot practice independently within his or her geographic location. Clinical and/or peer supervision is sought by all practitioners who deliver services *via* technology. Clinical and peer supervision is delivered either face-to-face or *via* encrypted methods.

Example Topics of study related to Training, Knowledge and Supervision (not an exhaustive list): Online Therapy; Online Clinical Supervision; Online Peer Supervision; Cyberpsychology; Text-based Therapy; Tele-health; Behavioural Tele-health; Tele-psychiatry; Internet Addictions; Social Media; Online Relationships; Online Peer Support; SMS Text Messaging; Mental Health and Technology.

Practitioners Display Pertinent and Necessary Information on Websites

Websites provide access to information for the general public, potential clients, clients and other professionals.

- ***Crisis Intervention Information***: People may surf the internet seeking immediate help. Practitioners display crisis intervention information on the home page. Practitioners understand that people in crisis may visit the website from anywhere in the world. Offering global resources such as Befriender's International or The Samaritans is the best course of action.
- ***Practitioner Contact Information***: Practitioners offer contact information that includes e-mail, post address and a telephone or VOIP number. While it is not recommended that post addresses reflect the practitioner's home location, clients should have a post address for formal correspondence related to redress, subpoenas or other mailings requiring a signature of receipt. Practitioners state the amount of time an individual may wait for a reply to e-mail or voice mail. Best practice indicates a maximum of two business days for therapeutic inquiries.

- ***Practitioner Education, Licence and/or Certification Information***: Practitioners list degrees, licences and/or certifications as well as corresponding numbers. If the licence, certification board, or professional body offers a website that allows the general public to verify information on a particular practitioner, the licence and certification listings should link directly to those verifying body websites. Practitioners consider listing other formal education such as college or university courses, online continuing education and professional development courses, and conference/convention attendance directly related to mental health and technology.
- ***Terms of Use and Privacy Policy***: Terms of Use, often all or in part, synonymous with a practitioner's informed consent, is available on the website either as a page on the website or a downloadable document. The practitioner's privacy policy is also available in the same way and offers information about if or how e-mail addresses, credit card information and client records are used, shared or stored. Practitioners must ensure that they comply with the requirements of the Data Protection Act and other aspects of applicable law, and in the United States, practitioners display the Notice of Privacy Practices to indicate compliance with HIPAA. Applicable information regarding privacy and confidentiality that are required for patient consent in the geographic location of the practitioner should be posted on the website as well.
- ***Encrypted Transmission of Therapeutic and Payment Information***: Practitioners offer secure and encrypted means of therapeutic communication and payment transactions. Payment methods are explained as well through merchant information or information provided by the practitioner.

Practitioners Conduct an Initial Intake and Screening Process

The initial screening and intake process begins with the potential client's first contact. The practitioner implements formal and informal measures for screening a client's suitability for delivery of mental health services *via* technology.

- ***Client's Technology Skills***: Practitioners screen potential client's use of technology through questions at the outset. Questions include but are not limited to an inquiry about the client's experience with online culture, e.g. e-mail, chat rooms, forums, social networks, instant messaging and online purchasing, mobile texting, VOIP or telephones.

- ***Client's Language Skills***: Practitioners screen for language skills from the initial contact through the first few exchanges. Assessing for language barriers, reading and comprehension skills as well as cultural differences is part of the screening process.
- ***Presenting Issue, Client Identity and Clinical Concerns***: Practitioners screen to ensure the presenting issue is within the scope of practice and knowledge base of the practitioner. Screening around issues of suicidal and homicidal tendency and immediate crisis are formally addressed through an intake questionnaire or first exchange.
- ***Practitioners incorporate***: A mechanism for verifying identity of clients by asking for a formal identification number such as Driver's Licence or other satisfactory method. The client must not be anonymous, offering at a minimum: first and last name, home address, and phone number for emergency contact. Minors must be identified through parental consent. If client identity is not required, such as is the case with crisis hotlines and triage settings, limitations of the service are stated clearly. Other concerns regarding mental stability are addressed—e.g. client currently hallucinating or delusional; actively using drugs and alcohol so, that insight-oriented interventions would not be suitable; and any other medical or physical issues that might impede the intervention or require a different method of delivery, e.g. disability that impairs typing, rendering a chat exchange cost-prohibitive. Any assessment instruments that are utilized should be approved for online or computer-assisted use according to the test author/publisher.

Practitioners Offer an Informed Consent Process

The informed consent process begins when the client contemplates accessing services. It includes a formal acknowledgement from the client to the practitioner and is received *via* encrypted channels. The following topics are addressed within Informed Consent:

- ***Possible Advantages and Disadvantages of Online Therapy***:

Information is disseminated about the pros and cons of online therapy including such disadvantages as lack of visual and auditory cues and the limitations of confidentiality *via* technology, and advantages that include easy scheduling, time management and a no need to incur transportation costs.

Confidentiality and Technology

- ***Encryption***: An explanation about the use of encryption for therapeutic exchanges and lack of encryption if/when unencrypted methods (standard e-mail, forum posts, mobile telephone, SMS texting, social networking) are used for issues such as appointment changes and cancellations.
- ***Therapist as Owner of the Record***: Unless otherwise specified through law in the practitioner's geographic location, the therapist remains the owner of the therapeutic record including all transcripts, notes and e-mails. The client is informed that posting direct information about the therapist or verbatim information from sessions is prohibited.
- ***File Storage Procedures***: The client is informed about how records are stored (web-based, third party or hard-drive/external drive) and for how long the records are maintained. All procedures conform to the standards laid down in applicable law and as required by any relevant authority (such as professional body) and, at least, include encryption and password protection and a commitment to destroy all records after a given period as required by law/regulation/best practice.
- ***Privacy Policy***: The practitioner's privacy policy is also included in the Informed Consent process including information about how e-mail addresses, credit card information and client records are used, shared or stored.

Other Informed Consent Issues

- ***Practitioner's Geographical Jurisdiction***: The physical location of the practitioner is offered in the Informed Consent and if the practitioner is licensed within a specific jurisdiction, the Informed Consent states client understands services are rendered under the laws or jurisdiction of the relevant country, state or region.

- ***How to Proceed during a Technology Breakdown***: The client is informed about how to proceed if a technology breakdown occurs during a session, e.g. "If we disconnect, try to reconnect within 10 minutes. If reconnection is not possible, e-mail or call to reschedule an appointment."
- ***Emergency Contact***: Practitioners offer specific information about who to contact in case of an emergency and set specific rules about emergency e-mails that the practitioner may not be privy to e.g. (suicidal e-mails in the middle of the night, threatening posts on a support forum). Practitioners research local resources within the client's geographic area as emergency backup resources.
- ***Cultural Specifics that May Impact Treatment***: Practitioners discuss varying time zones, cultural differences and language barriers that may impact the delivery of services. Practitioners should also ensure at or prior to the start of therapy, that the client's expectations of the service being offered (such as the meaning of the term 'counselling' etc.) is sufficiently close to their own understanding and should take into account that different cultures around the world can have very different understandings of these matters.
- ***Dual Relationships***: Practitioners discuss with clients the expected boundaries and expectations about forming relationships online. Practitioners inform clients that any requests for "friendship", business contacts, direct or replies, blog responses or requests for a blog response within social media sites will be ignored to preserve the integrity of the therapeutic relationship and protect confidentiality.
- ***Insurance, Subsidy or Reimbursement Information***: If the client resides in a geographic area that generally accepts insurance or other forms of reimbursement for therapy services, the practitioner informs the client of this information. Conversely, services delivered *via* technologies that are not covered at all or at the same rate, the practitioner informs the client of this information also.

Advantages of Online Psychotherapy

Technology has made our lives easier and it definitely is one of the reasons for online therapy to become so popular. There are obvious advantages like saving on time and travel, fee and office rent as have been experienced by both service providers and end users. Yuen and colleagues summarize some of the latest professional literature and highlight challenges and opportunities for psychologists in the realm of telepsychology (Yuen, Goetter, Herbert and Forman, 2012).

It is often the real advantages as perceived by clients who make therapist venture into using the online mode of service delivery as there are fewer sessions cancelled due to physical ailments, work pressures or child care. People who have been in long-term therapy with one particular therapist need not worry if the therapist changes location as therapy and contact can still be maintained using the online modalities.

Mental health professionals realize that it is essential to reach out to people such locations that are suffering from lack of service avenues due to either their geographical location or lack of trained professionals. Web based services have the potential to increase accessibility of mental health services for people by overcoming hurdles posed by transportation, physical disabilities or life threatening illnesses, location and lack of services and stigma. Online therapy and counselling is beneficial to individuals residing in place where face-to-face service providers are not available and with individuals who are unable to leave home due to ill-health or familial responsibilities. Online counselling has the potential for 24 hour service provision and makes it easy for those with a hectic work schedule to seek help. Due to use of various modalities, even if the therapist is not accessible on phone or face-to-face, therapy or ability to be contacted using the e-mail is an option available for end users thus making it easier for a client to communicate without having to wait, as they may have to in a face-to-face setting.

Stigma associated with psychiatric illness and emotional disturbances is a major reason due to which clients and families of those suffering with emotional or psychological disturbances do not seek in their own community. Therapy offered online offers a more "stigma free" way to seek help for mental health issues. It provides a platform to seek help without having to meet venture out of their house or any other comfort zones and also reduces the chances of the client meeting neighbours or relatives or acquaintances at a clinic or a hospital. Also, in cases of severe psychiatric disturbances or a crisis where a person may be hesitating or not finding enough motivation to go to a hospital or a clinic, online therapy offers a good option to at least make a contact with mental health professional and get psycho-educated as well as appropriate guidance about managing their condition. This would be effective in eliminating the social stigma of receiving therapy especially in the rural areas. If online therapy services are provided at primary healthcare centres in rural areas, help-seeking for mental health services may improve as people there may perceive primary healthcare centres less stigmatizing as compared to visiting a mental care set-up. Again, this would only help reducing the mental barrier to help-seeking and indirectly enhance seeking help at mental care set-ups. In the West, the long distance healthcare model has been in use for some time for delivering online consulting to remote healthcare centres and helping disseminate skills to primary healthcare providers in handling of even difficult cases. This model has been tried and tested in hospital and prisons where healthcare workers conducted counselling with inmates under close supervision of specialists in distant locations (Morgan, Patrick, Magaletta, 2008).

Only those services are demanded for that turn out to be cost-effective with regard to time and energy and money spent by both the service providers and of course, more so for the end service users. Online therapy and counselling may appear more economical for those who offer their services using a clinical set-up due to an absence of overhead costs like rent for renting a commercial space or having a in-house team and bearing their expenses. It also eliminates travelling expenses for the client and therapist. A lot of time and energy is also saved when using online therapy service as it saves on the travel as well as waiting time which a client would have to when using a face-to-face service. A lot of time is also saved as communication is more goal directed when using various e-therapy modalities. Research done reveals that when communicating using the voice or video modality "small talk" is almost absent since both side involved address relevant issues faster. Another example of how online therapy is cost-effective is that follow-up and monitoring of chronically ill or those with physical disabilities can be done using video or voice modality. Compliance to therapy may be enhanced as clients can track their own progress on a regular basis using self-help tools and homework that can be accessed online. This again saves time and energy spent in visiting clinics or therapist offices. Even supervision and training of mental healthcare workers can be done online assuring sustained support to workers or clinicians in remote areas. Continuing medical education on mental health issues can be provided to primary health workers present in rural areas reducing costs involved in onsite training as well as increasing the number of trained mental healthcare workers. Health workers in far off geographical locations/areas can be provided with video-conferencing for case consultations on routine and urgent mental health cases (Roine, Ohinmaa, Hailey, 2001). This has enhanced service delivery speed and efficiency of service provided at the same reducing client's travel costs.

Even though ethical and legal codes require client identification as necessary, the element of being able to maintain anonymity especially while using e-mail or chat based therapy is a factor that attracts users to try it. To cite an example, even though the end user of a mental health service providing portal may be required to provide their name or location or both, the World Wide Web is a platform where the perceived sense of psychological safety helps them transcend all barriers of location, caste, disabilities or religion. Features of apparent anonymity and geographical distance in online interactions have been theorized to facilitate psychological safety, disinhibition and increased self-disclosure (Suler, 2000, 2004). This is one of the main reasons for increasing demand on online mental health services. In 1986, Cornell University started one of the first online counselling services called "Dear Uncle Ezra". It allowed queries from anonymous students the counsellor would respond using a public internet post. This programme was successful, due to its anonymous format as reported by students who used it and, is still active now. In a qualitative study, analysis of clients' experiences of online counselling found that clients typically reported experiencing disinhibition, which helped them express themselves more openly and honestly (Cook and Doyle, 2002).

Another advantage of availability of online mental health services is that it offers the clients a greater selection of therapists or counsellors to choose from. It also offers them accessibility to specialized services like a client may not find an eating disorder therapist near his or her residence but may find one easily on the internet. Thus, online mental health services may be especially beneficial for people looking for a therapist with experience in a specific area or with a specific disorder, or belonging to a specific community or culture or religion. There are also online support groups and forums dedicated to a variety of emotional problems which offer a lot of emotional support and alternate ways of coping with a particular issue to people and help them connect with others dealing similar issues from across the world.

Disadvantages of Online Therapy

Every coin has two sides. Things or practices considered beneficial by some may be considered unhelpful or even harmful by the others. Not only opponents, but practitioners of online therapy realize the presence of following hurdles or loopholes while offering mental health services over the internet. These hurdles are mainly to do with ethical and legal issues around online clinical practice, its clinically efficacy and if it is financially viable to the end users and the providers.

Ethical and legal guidelines are a must in all kinds of services catering to any living being. Be it a face-to-face setting or an online portal offering therapy there are numerous and almost similar ethical and legal issues. We have discussed most of them above. Areas of particular concern which may be ethical front on the online medium include confidentiality, dealing with clients in a crisis situation or those who are suicidal or dangerous client and taking side the realm of one's clinical practice, geographically. There were serious concerns regarding issues of informed consent, duty of care, confidentiality of records and privacy due to apprehensions raised regarding anonymity, distance, and the lack of cues in online therapy (Bloom, 1998; Childress, 1998; Shapiro and Schulman, 1996). There is also a risk of clients accessing people who pose as therapists or counsellors but are unlicensed or unregulated and who may not have the training or education that is essential to ethical practice.

Lack of visual and verbal cues as well as time delay in sending responses from the client or therapist are some of the criticisms and perceived limitations of mental health services that are offered online. Also these are mainly perceived with the usage of asynchronous modalities like chat or e-mails for offering therapy or support. Both the client and therapist often do not know much about each other and the visual and verbal cues that convey subtle yet pertinent information about the client and their current affect in face-to-face interactions are missing (Suler, 2000). This may delay the process of rapport formation or lead to an early drop-out. Also, while using e-mails or forums or chat for receiving or providing support the time delay in receiving a response from either side may lead to misinterpreting the unexplained delays. Suler (2004) calls this the "black hole phenomenon", i.e. the ambiguity in the no-reply can become a blank screen where easily we can project our own expectations, emotions, and anxieties (Suler, 2004). This can easily arouse anxieties in an already anxious patient or can feel a patient with depressive symptoms to feel rejected again hampering rapport formation or even exacerbating the presenting complaints.

Clinical efficacy of online therapy is a much debated area and there still seems to be more research needed to comment on this one conclusively. While many studies reveal efficacy to be inferior to in-person sessions, others have found client improvement with various online and telephone modalities to be equal, and in some cases greater, than in-person services (read the section on outcome of online therapy above for studies). Also, unlike traditional psychotherapy, online counselling cannot provide formal diagnosis and treatment which means a referral to a face-to-face set may have to be made ultimately.

Financial issues surrounding provision of online mental health services include the cost of beginning and maintaining an online practice, advertising and marketing, receiving training to be equipped to provide therapy using online modalities and receiving payment. There is a lack of literature on if maintaining a online practice is financially viable or not for a psychotherapist or a counsellor.

Conclusion: Prospects for India

As discussed above under various sections, technology's rapid growth brings with it the opportunity to bridge the various gaps between mental health professionals and those in need of mental health services. One can now reach people at residing in the remotest areas of the world and administer consultations, treatments, assessments, and even supervision and training for mental health professionals *via* video-conferencing, websites, and mobile devices. People are willing to experiment with new ways of managing their health, especially those that can fit in their busy schedules or help them access expert help not easily accessible to them due to various reasons.

With the growth in the online mental health sector, effective, affordable, computerized mental health interventions can be delivered to the end users at reduced costs and shorter waiting lists along with an increase in mental health literacy. As the burden of lifestyle related chronic diseases increase, such services are being perceived as the need of the hour globally and in India. In a recent pilot study done in India with the objective of exploring people's perceptions about using online lifestyle counselling services among individuals living in rural settings in India, nearly 47 per cent of the individuals were interested in obtaining online lifestyle counselling (Laxmi, Sharma, Singh, Amadi, Mohan, and Joshi, 2014). A lot of web portals and websites offering mental health services have mushroomed up recently in India. Psychologists, therapists, counsellors and life coaches are now making their presence felt online for the urban population, but with the major objective of increasing their face-to-face clientele. There is an urgent need for evaluating the role of an online therapy and counselling intervention and other mental health services among individuals living in urban as well as rural settings.

These interventions could become an important part of primary healthcare services in both urban and especially rural settings, providing a useful first step toward psychological care for some patients and a full treatment programme for others. Since a large number of people with mental illnesses approach their general physician in urban settings or their primary healthcare centres in a rural setting, computerized mental health interventions in these settings could provide a large proportion of the population with access to psychological treatments. This would be very beneficial for a large number of people in both urban and rural settings who are currently unable to attain the psychological care they need. A study done by Grubaugh, Cain, Elhai, Patrick and Frueh (2008) demonstrated that both rural and urban primary care patients were generally receptive to using medical and tele-mental health interventions *via* video-conferencing if offered; and they did not believe that video-conferencing technology would be overly sophisticated or complicated. The results also revealed that rural patients expressed a willingness to use tele-psychiatry if it improved their access to services they would not otherwise receive. The Institute of Medical Quality healthcare in America reports that rural based E-Systems are on the rise and are being integrated effectively into healthcare programmes and behavioural medicine provided through long distance mediums has already proved to be effective. Such studies are the need of the hour in India, where there is an extreme imbalance in the number and geographical distribution of trained professionals between urban and rural areas. Video-conferencing as a modality to deliver mental health services can be used to deliver specialized services to rural and remote areas as it can surpass educational and technical literacy hurdles assumed to be present in the rural population.

Online resources can also be used for training healthcare workers in the remote areas for aiding an early diagnosis leading to early intervention as well as creating awareness about the importance of mental health and disorders. This can bring staff with various medical expertises together as well as reduce the time, cost, and effort associated with travelling from one place to another for training or consultation. With video-conferencing, long-term and continued support can be provided to health workers and it gets easier for them to access continuing educational training through mentoring and supervision from the best experts in mental health from their own location. Clients can also be provided psycho-education and teaching patients about medications and assessing compliance with individual treatment plans.

Researches need to be encouraged in this field to be able to establish a working model of provision on mental health services and for imparting training on mental health issues for rural areas as well as those areas deprived of adequate number of mental health professionals. The Telemedicine Society of India along with the various psychologist and counsellor associations have this immensely important task of setting clearer legal and ethical guidelines to be used by those setting up online practices as well as to keep a check on any kind of malpractice.

References

Barak, A., Hen, L., Boniel-Nissim, M., and Shapira, N. (2008). A comprehensive review and a meta-analysis of the effectiveness of internet-based psychotherapeutic interventions. *Journal of Technology in Human Services,* 26(2), 109-160.

Bloom, J.W. (1998). The ethical practice of WebCounselling. *British Journal of Guidance and Counselling,* 26(1), 53-59.

Browne, D., Reilly, M., Bradley, O. (2006). Telepsychiatry in a child and adolescent psychiatric service. *Irish Journal of Psychological Medicine.* 23, 21-23.

Childress C.A. (2000). Ethical issues in providing online psychotherapeutic interventions, *J Med Internet Res 2000,* 2(1). Retrieved from http://www.jmir.org/2000/1/e5.

Christensen, H., Griffiths, K.M., and Jorm, A.F. (2004). Delivering interventions for depression by using the internet: randomised controlled trial. *British Medical Journal,* 328, 265-275.

Clark, A., Kirkby, K.C., Daniels, B.A., Marks, I.M. (1998). A pilot study of computer-aided vicarious exposure for obsessive-compulsive disorder. *Australian and New Zealand Journal of Psychiatry,* 32, 268-275.

Cohen, G. and Kerr, B. (1998). Computer-mediated Counselling: An empirical study of a new mental health treatment. *Computers in Human Services,* 15, 13-26.

Cook, J.E. and Doyle, C. (2002). Working alliance in online therapy as compared to face-to-face therapy: Preliminary results. *Cyber Psychology and Behaviour,* 5(2), 95-105.

DeeAnna, M.N. and Kate, A. (2009). Ethical framework for use of technology in mental health. Retrieved from http://onlinetherapyinstitute.com/ethical-training/doi: 10.1207/s15327019eb0602_3.

Fenichel, M., Suler, J., Barak, A., Zelvin, E., Jones, G., Munro, K., and Walker-

Schmucker, W. (2002). Myths and realities of online clinical work. *Cyber Psychology and Behaviour,* 5(5), 481-497.

Glueckauf, R.L. and Ketterson, T.U. (2004). Telehealth interventions for individuals with chronic illness: Research review and implications for practice. *Professional Psychology: Research and Practice.* 35, 15-627.

Godleski, L., Nieves, J.E., Darkins, A., and Lehmann, L. (2008). VA Telemental health: Suicide assessment. *Behavioural Sciences and the Law.* 26, 271-286.

Grubaugh, A., Cain, G.D., Elhai, J.D., Patrick, S.L., and Frueh, B.C. (2008). Attitudes toward medical and mental healthcare delivered *via* telehealth applications among rural and urban primary care patients. *Journal of Nervous and Mental Disease,* 196, 166-170.

Haberstroh, S., Parr, G., Bradley, L., Morgan-Fleming, B., and Gee, R. (2008). Facilitating online counselling: Perspectives from counsellors in training. *Journal of Counselling and Development,* 86(4), 460-470.

Hailey, D., Roine, R., and Ohinmaa, A. (2008). The effectiveness of telemental health applications: a review. *Canadian Journal of Psychiatry.* 53(11), 769-78.

Hufford, B.J., Glueckauf, R.L., and Webb, P.M. (1999). Home-based, interactive video-conferencing for adolescents with epilepsy and their families. *Rehabilitation Psychology,* 44(2), 176-193.

Kennedy, C., and Yellowlees, P. (2000). A community-based approach to evaluation of health outcomes and costs for telepsychiatry in a rural population: preliminary results. *Journal of Telemedicine and Telecare,* 6(1), 155-157.

Kenwright, M., Liness, S., and Marks, I. (2001). Reducing demands on clinicians by offering computer-aided self-help for phobia panic: a feasibility study. *British Journal of Psychiatry,* 179, 456-459.

Kirkwood, K.T., Peck, D.F., and Bennie, L. (2000). The consistency of neuropsychological assessments performed *via* telecommunication and face-to-face. *Journal of Telemedicine and Telecare,* 6, 147-151.

Klasen, M., Knaevelsrud, C., and Bottche, M. (2013). The therapeutic alliance in internet-based therapy procedures: an overview. *Nervenarzt,* 84(7), 823-31.

Klein, B., Richards, J.C., and Austin, D.A. (in press). Efficacy of internet therapy for panic disorder. *Journal of Behaviour Therapy and Experimental Psychiatry.* Retreived from http://www.epsychologist.org/

Lange, A., Van de Ven, J.P., and Shrieken, B. (2003). Interapy treatment of post-traumatic stress *via* the Internet. *Cognitive Behaviour Therapy,* 32, 110-124.

Laxmi, V., Sharma, S., Singh, A.K., Amadi, C., Mohan, K., and Joshi, A. (2014). Perceptions of online lifestyle counselling among individuals living in rural India. *Journal of Technology Healthcare,* 22(4), 597-606.

Lee, C. (1998). Counselling and the challenge of cyberspace. Retrieved from http://www.counselling.org/ctonline/sr598/lee498.html.

Leibert, T., Archer, J., Munson, J., and York, G. (2006). An exploratory study of client perceptions of internet counselling and the therapeutic alliance. *Journal of Mental Health Counselling,* 28(1), 69-83.

Lisa, K., Richardson, M., Christopher, F., Anouk, L., Leonard, E., and Jon, D.E. (2009). Current Directions in Video-conferencing Tele-Mental Health Research. *Clinical Psychology* (New York). Sep. 1, 2009; 16(3), 323-338.

Manhal-Baugus, M. (2001). E-therapy: practical, ethical, and legal issues. *Cyber Psychology and Behaviour,* 4 (5), 551-63.

Morgan, R.D., Patrick, A.R., and Magaletta, P.R. (2008). Does the use of tele-mental health alter the treatment experience? Inmates' perceptions of tele-mental health *versus* face-to-face treatment modalities. *Journal of Consulting Clinical Psychology,* 2008 Feb., 76(1), 158-62.

Newman, M.G., Szkodny, L.E., Llera, S.J., and Przeworski, A. (2011). A review of technology-assisted self-help and minimal contact therapies for anxiety and depression: Is human contact necessary for therapeutic efficacy? *Clinical Psychology Review,* 31(1), 89-103.

Recupero, P.R., and Rainey, S.E. (2006). Characteristics of e-therapy web sites. *Journal of Clinical Psychiatry,* 67(9), 1435-1440.

Rees, C.S., and Stone, S. (2005). Therapeutic alliance in face-to-face *versus* video-conference psychotherapy. *Professional Psychology: Research and Practice,* 36(6), 649-653.

Richards, D. (2009). Features and benefits of online counselling: Trinity College online mental health community. *British Journal of Guidance and Counselling,* 37(3), 231-242.

Richards, D. and Viganò, Online Counselling, chapter-59 in Zheng Yan (2012). *Encyclopedia of Cyber Behaviour*. Retrieved from http://books.google.co.in/books?id=gLqYYFoVoR8C publisher Information Science Reference.

Rochlen, A.B., Beretvas, S.N., and Zack, J.S. (2004). The online and face-to-face Counselling Attitudes Scales: A validation study. *Measurement and Evaluation in Counselling and Development,* 37(2), 95-111.

Sampson, J.P., Kolodinsky, R.W., and Greeno, B.P. (1997). Counselling and the information highway: Future possibilities and potential problems. *Journal of Counselling and Development,* 75(3), 203-212.

Shapiro, D.E., and Schulman, C.E. (1996). Ethic and legal issues in e-mail therapy. *Ethics and Behaviour,* 6(2), 107-124.

Simpson, S., Bell, L., Knox, J., and Mitchell, D. (2005). Therapy *via* video-conferencing: A route to client empowerment? *Clinical Psychology and Psychotherapy,* 12(2), 156-165.

Sinha, M. (2012). Telemental Health: The Growth of Video-conferencing. *Bihar Psychological Association ISPS,* 5(1), 3-11.

Suler, J. (2000). Psychotherapy in cyberspace: A 5-dimensional model of online and computer-mediated psychotherapy. *Cyber Psychology and Behaviour,* 3(2), 151-159.

Suler, J. (2001). Assessing a persons suitability for online therapy: The ismho clinical study group. *Cyberpsychology and Behaviour,* Volume 4(6). Retreived from http://construct.haifa.ac.il/~azy/AssessingSuitability.pdf

Suler, J. (2004). The online disinhibition effect. *Cyber Psychology and Behaviour,* 7(3), 321-326.

University of Zurich. (2013, July 30). Psychotherapy *via* internet as good as if not better than face-to-face consultations. *Science Daily*. Retrieved November 22, 2014 from *w.ww.sciencedaily.com/releases/2013/07/130730091255.htm*

Yuen, E.K., Goetter, E.M., Herbert, J.D., and Forman, E.M. (2012). Challenges and opportunities in internet-mediated telemental health. *Professional Psychology: Research and Practice,* 43(1), 1-8.

13

Play Therapy with Children

Theory, Research and Practice

Neelam Verma

Importance of psychological Interventions is well recognized for dealing with psychological, emotional and developmental problems of children. There is now plenty of work available describing impact of such treatments and helping children suffering from various mental health issues. Play Therapy is one such treatment that has gained attention of researchers and mental health practitioners/professionals in some past years and has been found to be one of the major interventions to deal with mental health issues of children. Play Therapy is an effective treatment modality for children that offer psychological help using "play". It is a way of helping troubled children to come out of the difficult situations. In Play Therapy, child uses objects or toys symbolically for people who are absent in that situation and child's interaction with objects is observed by the therapist. It is said that children do not have adequate vocabulary to express feelings. Play works as a mode of communication by which a therapist can listen to child's sensitive words that are unsaid. Plethora of researches conducted in this field reveal significance of this treatment modality and its utility. Current chapter focuses upon Play Therapy from the very beginning, i.e. history and emergence of this valuable technique. This chapter discusses theoretical models and approaches of this technique and their utility in clinical practice. Discussion will lead describing various practical aspects of Play Therapy such as importance of play in therapeutic settings, what set-up is required for Play Therapy, what all one needs to observe while seeing a child playing for therapeutic purposes and how play can be approached more creatively in clinical set-ups. The chapter would cover a wide range of researches and evidence based practical approach to throw light on its utility and developments. In a nutshell, the chapter would cover this treatment ranging from its emergence and history, its development, theoretical approaches, major methods of play or practice guidelines, focus of researches and practical approach to treatment using Play Therapy with children.

Introduction

Play has been identified and explained as a mean of social interaction for children. It is said and well recognized that children lack the capacity to communicate their thoughts and feelings through verbal means. Play activities have been an interest area of researchers since long and its relation to child development is very evident. One major theory of child development given by Piaget represents play as a part of child's intellectual development and relates play to the processes of assimilation (when child relates to the new elements of environment as a result of experiences encountered in past) and accommodation (when child is changed by the current/present environmental circumstances). Play is well recognized as a universal language for communication and it provides a context for social relationships and spontaneous learning. Researchers have described that through play activities children learn to gain control and mastery of their world, they develop more accurate ways of problem solving and releasing tension (Broding, 2005; Landreth, 2002; Schaefer, 1993).

Importance of play and its relation to child development lead to the researchers discovering its importance in deeper ways when play emerged as an immense intervention tool for children suffering from various psychological issues. *Association of Play Therapy* (2008) described play therapy as "the systematic use of a theoretical model to establish an interpersonal process wherein trained therapist uses the therapeutic powers of play to help clients prevent to resolve psycho-social difficulties and achieve optimal growth and development."

Emergence of Play as a Therapeutic Modality

Play as a full blown therapeutic technique has recently gained attention of researchers, however, its use and importance can be seen way back in the work of *Sigmund Freud* in the year 1909. This year turned out to be a major milestone in the history of Play therapy when Freud was treating a five years old boy *"Little Hans"* displaying symptoms of Phobia. This case was the first documented case where play was used as a mean of therapy. Following is the brief summary of how Play developed and achieved further milestones in the field of psychotherapy with children:

- ***1932***: *Klein* (Freud's student) used play for free association in therapy sessions.
- ***1933***: *Taft* created relationship play therapy where past events were de-emphasized and present relationships were focused to bring about healing.
- ***1938***: *Levy* created Release Therapy; a structured approach that aimed at releasing emotions of children experienced in a troubling situation.
- ***1942***: *Allen* expanded *Taft's* work done in 1933.
- ***1946***: *Anna Freud* used play therapy for rapport formation with children.
- ***1947***: *Axline;* Roger's student applied Rogerian constructs and pioneered Non-Directive or Child Centred Play Therapy.
- ***1955***: *Hambridge* expanded *Lavy's* work by developing Structured Play Therapy: A Directive Approach.
- ***1964***: *Guerneys* developed Filial Therapy; a time limited form of therapy focused on teaching parents effective ways of working and playing with their children.
- ***1983***: *Schaefer* pointed out variations and creative applications of Play Therapy. Later in the same year *O'Connor* increased awareness about systemic issues.
- ***2001***: *Kottman* advanced Play Therapy beyond initial child centred perspectives.
- ***2002***: *Landreth* expanded upon *Axline's* work and advocated that Play Therapy should involve a kind of interaction between child and therapist that the child has never experienced before.
- ***2005***: *Gil* and *drewes* expanded Play Therapy based upon multicultural and diversity domain and made it used worldwide in the field.

How Play Works as an Intervention Tool

In play therapy children interact with some external objects that are offered by the therapist. These external objects may involve variety of toys, blocks, pattern matching games, clay, craft material, colours, drawing materials etc. While playing children formulate their own world which is different from the real one and most importantly they hold control on. Activities done by the child during play are imaginary and their interaction with play material is symbolic in nature. Play help troubled children express and obtain relief from their conflicts symbolically and it also facilitates children's growth. If minutely observed, play serves following functions when used as therapy:

- ***Emotional function***: It allows cathartic release of tension and anxiety.
- ***Cognitive function:*** It allows child to symbolically review play activities such as what happened in play, what has to be planned further, how to solve hazards of play; thereby consideration of different outcomes at the end.
- ***Behavioural function:*** Play permits role rehearsal that allows enlarging child's perspective beyond the current situation.

Play has numerous benefits. It gives pleasure and enjoyable time; it helps in building rapport and forming social relationships, releasing stress and anxiety; offers restorative functions when dealing with grief; helps in adapting and identifying with new roles, leadership, cooperation skills and releasing conflicts through catharsis (Hart, 2010).

Approaches to Play Therapy

1. ***Psychoanalytic Play Therapy***: This is the oldest approach to play therapy and as discussed earlier Sigmund Freud was the first one to use play as therapy with his client Little Hans. Freud's daughter Anna Freud took this to another level and became the forerunner of psychoanalytic play therapy. In psychoanalytic perspective play facilitates communication and therapeutic relationship. It helps the therapist gathering information and understanding of child's conflicts. According to Lee (2009), play is seen as a way of free association for children where they can verbalize their thoughts as much as they can in quantity and quality. During play activity therapist participates in play in direct or indirect manner and observes the child. The therapist avails guidance while playing if required and interpret the play behaviour for therapeutic purposes. Insight is the key to play therapy and a major premise behind play therapy of psychoanalytic nature (O'Connor and Braverman, 2009; Schaefer and O'Connor, 1983).

2. ***Adlerian Play Therapy***: The key feature of Adlerian Theory describes people's primary "*need to belong*" as they are social beings. This approach sees clients/child as unique and creative that holds the ability to make decisions about their growth and goals. Adlerian play therapy describes "discouragement" as unhealthy and maladjustment and it occurs when people lack belongingness. Adlerian play therapy sees the child as "Discouraged" when a child lacks belongingness and significance in the world or relationships, when s/he faces inability to cope with feelings of inferiority (Kottman, 2009). This approach works on building that belongingness and decreasing discouragement by increasing insight and awareness. This approach emphasizes on developing four C's: Courage, Connect, Capable and Count. Kottman advocated that a child is able to increase his/her courage, connect with others, feel s/he is capable and s/he counts to others, self and life. Overall it is all about feeling encouraged and enhancing social interests that leads to increased state of mental health. In Adlerian Play Therapy, the therapist-child relationship fosters positivity in child to develop healthy relations outside the therapy, i.e. real life settings. It is assumed that whatever child learns during the therapy would apply in the actual world. Psycho-education of parents in this condition gives best results when child gets consistent encouragement from their side to develop relationships in more healthy ways.
3. ***Jungian Play Therapy***: Jungian Play Therapy was also developed on formative theory of Freud's Psychoanalysis, however, the role of therapist in Jungian Play therapy differs from the Psychoanalysis. The therapist does not lead the sessions in this type of play therapy; rather s/he facilitates the therapy process (Green, 2009). The child himself/herself leads the therapeutic process and achieves growth in the therapy by connecting to others. Oden and Johnson (2010) suggested that the goal of Jungian play therapy is to strive for greater self-realization. In Jungian view *Self* has been described as the central organizing principle of the "collective unconsciousness" and self-leads to the emergence of "Ego" to form "I" which is described as the centre of consciousness. The whole process of formation of "I" emerged from "Ego" helps the child to deal effectively with real world. At this stage of therapy child understands what

directions are available and therapist helps the child to follow them. As the child achieves increased self-awareness through play, the self-achieves growth and ego reaches maturity (O'Connor and Braverman, 2009). Jungian play therapy includes reflections, questions and interpretations during play to enhance self-awareness and follow leads of the child towards healing and health.

4. ***Gestalt Play Therapy***: Gestalt Play Therapy is widely attributed to the author of "*Windows to Our Children and Hidden Treasure*" Violet Oaklander. In her book Oaklander explains her goal to help the child to become aware of her existence in the world. Carroll (2009) describes Gestalt Play Therapy as an experiential therapy which is process oriented and majorly concerned with the integrating functioning of one's senses, body, emotions and intellect. Basically this type of play therapy is all about helping the child to get engaged in his/her own world and feel their "existence". During the therapy process, a fully engaged, genuine and congruent relationship is formatted between the therapist and the child and a collaborative alliance is formed as goals of therapy are designed with the child and his/her family. Carroll (2009) further elaborates that in Gestalt Play Therapy, the therapist uses games, drawing, colouring, storytelling, symbolic and imaginative play and use of sandtray to facilitate the child creating meaningful life narrative that helps in enhancing integration, building support and restoring functions of self-regulation.

5. ***Child-Centred Play Therapy***: Child Centred Play Therapy is a non-directive therapy which is most widely associated with the book titled as "*Play Therapy and Dibbs in Search of Self*" by Virginia Axline. This type of play therapy allows the child to strive for more mature behaviour and health believing that the child possesses the ability to solve them at his/her own. McCalla (1994: 5) explains Axline's perspective of "drive for self-actualization". According to Axline, every child has an instinct and capacity to achieve growth by exploring his/her self and a child centred therapist helps the child in exploring and achieving his/her actual self. McCalla (1994) denotes that a child needs acceptance from himself and from others to walk on the path of self-actualization. Play is a process of healing itself (Axline; 1969; McCalla, 1994; Carroll, 2009). McCalla (1994) explains

that Self-awareness need not to be interpreted to the child. The therapist only observes the play behaviour and non-judgementally reflects back to the child. This reflection itself becomes a path of self-awareness for the child and s/he gradually reaches a place of healing from self-directed play. During self-directed play child experiences different emotions such as love, anger, joy, fear, sadness etc. It is known that emotions are abstract in nature and for a young child it is difficult to express them the way they are. Play works as a concrete medium to experience and express abstract things in more meaningful ways and helps in self-exploration, self-direction and self-growth. The child strives to remove hurdles obstructing the process of self-actualization and gradually learns to face the emotions, control them and abandon them.

6. ***Cognitive Behaviour Play Therapy***: Unlike Child Centred Play Therapy, Cognitive Behaviour Play Therapy is a directive, structured and focused therapy. This type of play therapy is highly precised and problem oriented that avoids a long process. This therapy works on traditional principals of cognitive behaviour therapy following the idea that beliefs shape the perception. Classically, as we study that an event leads to the thoughts, thoughts influence the feelings and feelings lead to particular behaviour. According to this theory faulty thinking and cognitive distortions lead to problematic behaviours. Play works as a medium of communication between child and therapist and they both establish the goals of therapy together; whether it is about choosing the play activity or the play material (McCalla, 1994). During therapy the therapist models the ways to remove cognitive distortions such as making positive statements through puppet play, building self-esteem and encouragement etc. Gradually, the child learns how to control emotions and how to interpret events. One task of the therapist also includes educating child's parents about such positive statements and encouraging the child so that nothing contradictory happens at home or communication between child and parents. Similar messages from parents lead to faster learning and better outcomes in therapy.
7. ***Theraplay***: It is based on attachment theory (Bundy-Myrow and Booth, 2009). It is different from most of the other approaches of play therapy and focuses on healthy communication and interaction between child and his caregivers/parents. Theraplay

is more relationship focused, more playful and more engaging type of play therapy. The goal of theraplay is to build more healthy relationship between child and parents and other significant people of child's life by fostering attachment and connection between them. The process also aims at enhancing child's self-esteem with more involvement of parents in the sessions. Bundy-Myrow and Booth (2009) further explain that unlike other approaches of play therapy, theraplay has no toys in the therapy room accept some props like lotion for handprints, blanket for the child to swing in, bubbles, clay, drawing material and dress-up items. Adult is the primary object for play in theraplay and it teaches the child that the adult present in the room would ensure safety, focus and regulation. Major motive behind primary object being adult in theraplay is to develop a secure attachment pattern between child and parent and helping the child meet previously unmet needs. The process helps at attaining positive self and replacing negative feelings with positive ones.

8. ***Ecosystemic Play Therapy***: Ecosystemic play therapy is a hybrid model that combines biological science and many models of developmental theory and child therapy (O'Connor, 2009). This therapy focuses on the individual and the series of nested systems s/he is a part of, not only on one system as it believes to value and preserve diversity in every possible way. The goal of this approach is to maximize child's ability to get his/her needs met without interrupting other's ability to get their needs met. Secondary goal of this play therapy is to facilitate the assumption of optimal growth and attaining better developmental functioning.

In ecosystemic play therapy child as a basic unit works in three critical domains, i.e. (a) as physical body, (b) as child engaging in his/her interpersonal relationships, and (c) representational through child's own internal working models of the world. Largely the model starts with child's individual functioning, and then it goes on another level such as child's primary and significant relations like family, peers etc. and other systems of child's surroundings in which s/he may be directly involved such as school, medical system, mental health system, legal and religious system etc. Here, it is important to learn that all these mentioned systems influence the child in two ways: (a) directly, through child's interactional experiences with these systems and (b) indirectly, through the interpretation drawn by the child about these systems. During the therapy process therapist creates a context where curative element of the pathology could take place. Task of the therapist is to help the child learn about alternative views about their life situations. This is done by the therapist during play by sharing alternative cognitive and verbal experiences with the child. The child himself takes active participation in this task and experiences perceiving his or her own life experiences in different ways. Regular practice of this task helps the child being reflective and also helps him/her in discovering more effective and appropriate ways of problem solving and getting their needs met.

In a nutshell, Ecosystemic play therapy is an integrative theory that incorporates individual and family (Developmental), dyadic, familial, social and other systems (Systemic), socio-cultural metasystems (Contextual) and intrapsychic (Representational) variables from the perspective of child's functioning in his/her ecosystemic world.

Above mentioned are the most widely studied and well established models of play therapy. Many times the therapist learns about the client during assessment phase and then chooses anyone type of therapy which is best suited for that particular child is also considered to be a form of play therapy. This type of play therapy is known as "*Prescriptive Play Therapy*". This type of therapy does not combine various approaches of play; it rather works on a single model and shifts to another if the previous one does not work. According to Jensen-Hart (2010) choosing a particular model of play majorly depends on emotional needs of the child and being creative and flexible, the therapist chooses one model to use in the therapy. According to Gill and Shaw (2009) this is a child-led, therapist informed way of choosing and implementing a play therapy approach. It is evidence based treatment that aims at reducing symptoms and provides relief to the child. This type of play therapy allows the therapist to use change the play approach as per child's need in the current condition; therefore, the technique is said to be flexible and client oriented.

Process of Therapy: Initiating, Forwarding and Ending Therapeutic Play

1. ***The Beginning of Session and Playing***: First session aims at making contact with the child. Therapist helps the child to explore possibilities of play in the given situation with the available play material. Beginning of the play is always an

awkward situation for both child and therapist and it might take some time to move on. It is difficult to get the task started with very young children and they might require a lead from therapist such as saying that this is a place where children come to play, you could also play whatever and however you want. This gives a lead to the child to explore the possibilities of play. On the other hand, with a little older children task may be initiated in more direct ways. Therapist might start it by saying that people around you are worried about your worries and difficulties in life and many times children like to play and draw about those difficult situations. Many times children start playing spontaneously and therapist ensures them that they will be there just to share what they are doing and make sure that they don't do anything which is harmful. The child may stop playing suddenly and here the therapist has to judge that why playing has been stopped. If it seems that child's problems are hindering his/her playing behaviour, it is necessary for the therapist to probe/facilitate and help the child to start playing again. It is very important to keep in mind that no direct prompting is required. Therapist has to reflect only through his body language and resist asking questions at this stage. If child welcomes the therapist in play it is a good sign and therapist must take part in that; however, there should be no direct leading. Therapist is supposed to concentrate only on eliciting and facilitating play rather than directing and prompting the play. Observation of the play behaviour gives great leads to the therapist to understand child's problem behaviours, his/her anxieties, conflicts and insecurities. It is also important to make notes of all important observations and making a summary after the session is over so that it can help you preparing for the next session. In view of the next session, it is important to prepare the child also and give him/her an idea about the activities of next session.

2. ***Control and Limits***: Some children might be messy and destructive while playing. Therapeutically, it gives a direction to the therapist to interpret child's internal world; however, it is always better to explain to the child at the beginning of the session that therapist will be there every time to look after the child and see that nothing dangerous happens to him/her, to the therapist or to the material being used for play. Many like the idea of setting limits as the play progresses. Limits are also supposed to

be settled about the time of sessions. Sometimes, a child may start playing late and it can lead to a late ending of the session. It depends on the situation how much extra time can be allowed to the child and how many times. There are times in therapy when something very important is about to come. In such conditions, it is necessary to tolerate some amount of mess and allow extra time to the child to allow ventilation of feelings. On the contrary, it is not appreciable if it happens because child likes to spend more time with therapist or she/he does not want to leave the play room at all. Sometimes, children might get stubborn about staying at the play room and not leaving the play material or carrying it with them to their place. In such conditions, it is important for the therapist to be firm and focused about explaining to the child that play material is used only for an amount of time and returning it safely after allowed amount of time would be appreciated. The child need to be alarmed before ending of the session so, that game achieves its end and also they get some time to clear up the room. This preparation also helps the child to adjust back in the original world and cope with the feelings aroused during the play.

3. ***Recording and Observation***: It is always helpful to note down each observation immediately the session is over. Observation is an important part of recording as you record what you observe. According to Oaklander (1978) following are the major things that need to be observed and recorded during play session:
    - Approach to the play material; spontaneous or delayed?
    - What is being chosen?
    - What is being avoided?
    - What is the general style of playing; destructive, messy, peaceful, soothing?
    - Is there any difficulty in shifting from one material to the other?
    - Play is organized or disorganized?
    - Content and theme of play such as loneliness, aggression, nurturance etc.
    - Contact with play objects.
    - Use of social skills.
4. ***Preparation and Planning for Coming Sessions***: Planning of further sessions is based on the information and time available for therapy. Also, it depends on the type of play therapy chosen

for the child. In some cases therapist might choose to work with a single approach where in other cases therapist may require shifting the approach time to time as per the child's need. In cases where therapists are ready with a well planned structured programme, it takes less time to accomplish the task. On the contrary, shifting the approach consistently as per client's need takes longer time to finish the sessions. Both approaches are different from each other in terms of time, content and progress yet found to be equally effective.

5. ***Child's Emotional State at Every Step of Therapy*:** Emotional outbursts are obvious during the therapy and therapist must reflect it to the child. Reflection of feelings would make the child-therapist relationship more compact and trustworthy. There can be different phases of child's mood as the therapy progresses and it can heavily contribute to the outcome of each session and overall therapy. Moustakas (in Howorth; 1964) has described following four stages of child's mood and changes in the mood conditions:

   Stage 1: On the first stage child's mood and feelings affect almost everything in therapy as they are diffused and pervasive. They might get frightened with every object or start destroying everything. Through therapist's containment, child's feelings become more focused.

   Stage 2: At this stage feelings are more focused and specific. Anger might be more directed towards particular things and objects including the therapist and fears become fears of specific things rather than being generalized. Acceptance of these feelings in genuine way by the therapist helps the child to grow his/her self-esteem.

   Stage 3: At the third stage child may exhibit contradictory feelings on same occasion such as showing positive and negative feelings together. For example: a child may be playing with the doll and showing nurturing feelings towards it like tying her hair and at the same time child might tie hair so tightly so, that it hurts the doll. These feelings are often expressed intensely; however, they come down gradually.

   Stage 4: This is the state of therapy where child has learned to differentiate between positive and negative feelings and at the same time expressing them adequately in a particular situation.

6. ***Breaks during Therapy***: Sometimes, the child may feel insecure when the therapist is away. It can reinforce the feelings of abandonment, loss and containment. In this condition, the therapist needs to prepare the child for the break or the gap prior to the next session. Therapist might give a task to the child to complete during the break. Drawing tasks may also be given and asked to keep safely and show when the therapist is back.
7. ***Termination of Therapy***: Termination of therapy is a sensitive issue in all cases and requires more preparation if being conducted with children. During the low phases of child therapist supports him/her non-judgmentally. Most of the times children perceive their therapists as real life persons rather than perceiving them only as a therapist or as a mediator who is resolving their life issues. Most play therapists believe that therapy with children cannot be carried or ended like adults. With adults it is easier to terminate a session and conveniently conveying the fact that there would be no meetings further unless any problem persists or occurs. On the other hand, it is not so easy with children doing the same task. Children may not be accepting the fact that they are not going to meet the person anymore they have been meeting for long. It may also create bouts of anxiety and intense emotional reaction in the child. Sometimes, it becomes hard for the therapist also to control such situations. Play therapist "Jenet West" believes that the sessions can be terminated without any hard feelings and not necessarily clearing up all relationships completely. She believes that there is no harm planning occasional short meetings after therapy is over. Phone numbers can be exchanged so that child is able to contact the therapist whenever required. Occasional phone calls are of no harm especially on child's special days and festivals. For preparation of termination both child and therapist may go out of the play room and talk about it. Some children may accept it gracefully yet their emotions should be considered. They may be brought back to the play room and told that they have got their own play room which is inside them. They have got all the favourite things to eat, they have their loving family members with them and now they have a friend too with whom they shared a lot of good moments. There is no need to end up the relationship with child

absolutely and provoking feelings of separation. Most children start taking it normally after some amount of time and they remain with pleasant feelings of working and learning together with their therapist.

What is Needed for Play Therapy?

A well equipped play room is desirable, however, not essential for play therapy. The idea behind keeping toys, blocks, clay, drawing material etc. is not to engage the child in play rather help him/her to explore and experience his/her own feelings at his/her own pace. Not everything kept in the play room is required for the child. Most children need specific material for expressing their feelings. The idea is to select the material not collect the material before initiating the play therapy. Basically play therapy is all about letting the child select material as per his/her wish and task of the therapist is to arrange the room in a way so, that everything is nearby and easily approached by the child including drinking water, snacks to eat and toilet to use if required. Age and culture appropriate toys are desirable as they better elicit the play behaviour. Major chunk of material includes soft toys, cars, puppets, dolls of different types like male, female and baby dolls, clothes, wild and domestic animals made of plastic, domestic things like tea cups, cook wares, other kitchen wares, very few dress up and grooming materials like comb, ribbon, hair bands etc., cushions, blanket, small easy chair, mattress, swing etc. are also required. Walls are best if painted in different shades and knowledge enhancing drawings like stories, shapes, objects etc. and carpet on the floor is always good. Drawing sheets, colours of different types, playing dough or clay, colourful paper should also be provided. Scissor, sticking gum, water colours and any other material that requires careful handling should be provided only in the vigilance of the therapist. Block games, picture completion games, educational games, computer, puzzles can also be kept in the play room. The room should be spacious and should allow easy accessibility of things kept around.

Extending Play Therapy to Families and Other Forms of Play

Engaging child's family in the play therapy sounds interesting and have been found to be a preferred mode of intervention currently. Schaefer and Carey (1994) have extensively spoken about family play therapy explaining it as an action oriented intervention. Creatively using play by family members can give very good outcomes and results in increased attachment and bonding between child and other family members. After a long study period Guerney introduced "Filial Therapy" in 1964. Filial Therapy incorporates basic child centred play therapy skills that are taught to the parents of the child and they are trained in using and applying those skills in daily life. In the year 2006, Landreth and Bratton formally introduced a ten-session model based on Guerney's work which was known as "Child Parent Relationship Therapy (CPRT)". Using this model in therapy, a trained mental health professional trains the parents in a weekly parent child play session to strengthen parent-child ties and reduce problem behaviours of children. Parents are supervised to learn empathy and reflect to the child in more genuine ways and give them unconditional positive regards.

When this CPRT model was introduced there was already an existing model which was chiefly developed by clinical psychologist Sheila M. Eyberg, named "Parent Child Interaction Therapy (PCIT)". Brinkmeyer and Eyberg (2003) found this model very effective for disruptive behaviours in preschoolers. This therapy basically focuses on improving parent child interactions to improve the quality of their relationship. PCIT works in two phases. In phase one, the parents learn to give attention to the child's desirable behaviours while playing and in phase two they learn to praise child's desirable play behaviours and ignore small undesirable play behaviours. More recently in 2013, Aletha Solter has developed a comprehensive treatment programme called Attachment Play. This programme includes evidence based forms of play and several laughter producing activities to strengthen emotional connection of parents with their children. Parents are encouraged to use these playful activities to connect better with their children. These activities also help in resolving discipline issues at home and children experiencing trauma, hospitalization and parental separation/divorce.

Art Therapy has been a very close part of all play therapies such as using drawings, colours, clay, music, dance etc. Sandtray Therapy, a form of play using miniature figures and a tray full of sand has become an important and effective approach of this treatment. Dora Klaff advanced this technique in Switzerland in 1950s and 1960s. She gave this technique the name "Sandplay" and it became so popular worldwide. Sandtray therapy gives the children an opportunity to speak through the scenes they create or build in the sand. This process was beautifully spoken out by Lowenfield (1935), as "speaking with hands". This therapy has been found to be effective in treating behaviour problems in preadolescents and improving self-concept of adolescent girls.

Play Therapy: "Psychological First Aid"

Some very important trends characterize play therapy for children in current era and one of the most important is disaster relief. It works as a crisis intervention resulting in relief from feelings of trauma. The term "Psychological first aid" differs from traditional play therapy and was given by Jennifer N. Baggerly. Baggerly and Nadine D. Mescia (as cited in Baggerly, 2006) developed a model, named "Child C^3ARE" to train play therapists for helping children in disaster situations. Play based crisis interventions have been included in the "psychological first aid (PFA) field operation guide". Several mental health professionals used this technique in Sri Lanka to help children who suffered in Indian Ocean Tsunami in 2004.

Efficacy of Play Therapy: A Glimpse of Empirical Studies

There has been a wide range of researches proving efficacy of play therapy in various mental health conditions of children and adolescents. This section of the chapter would include empirically tested trials of this dynamic intervention.

A case study conducted by Gold Steanberg and Logan (1999) showed significant contribution in treating children with symptoms of Obsessive Compulsive Disorder (OCD). While behavioural and psycho-pharmacological treatment approaches have been found to be most promising for such conditions, psychodynamically oriented play therapy can result in better treatment adherence, lowering the feelings of shame associated with symptoms of OCD, improve self-concept and issues related to social adjustment. The study concluded that play therapy can contribute to the treatment of OCD in children in secondary ways.

Another research conducted by Kasari, Freeman and Paparella (2006) proved efficacy of this treatment on two most important developmental problems of autistic children, i.e. joint attention and symbolic play. Play therapy was applied on the experimental groups for 6 weeks daily for about thirty minutes. Pre- and post-assessment results differed significantly and both groups showed much improved behaviours than the control group. In a similar diagnostic category Josefi and Ryan (2004) conducted a case work using non-directive play therapy. This single case study included a six years old boy diagnosed with severe autistic symptoms. He was provided with 16 sessions of play therapy and all the sessions were video recorded. Video recordings of each session were analysed qualitatively and quantitatively. Later sessions in the therapy indicated improvement in child's behaviour in terms of attachment towards therapist and initiation of play. Ritualistic behaviours also showed mild improvement. The study indicated that non-directive play therapy can accelerate emotional and social development of children with autism.

It is well recognized that children suffering from psychiatric disorders need special care and immediate attention; however, children in palliative care need much more than symptoms management and pain control. Play therapy can be very effective with these children also as they reveal their hopes and fears through play. Van Breeman (2009) found this therapy effective to understand mental condition of a dying child in palliative care. It facilitates communication between parents and child and the treatment turns to be effective as it clears the parent-child connection thus promotes the healing during dying process.

Sometimes psychological well-being of children may be affected by various reasons and one may suffer through issues with self-esteem. A study conducted by Baggerly and Jennifer (2004) on 42 homeless children showed efficacy of child centred play therapy in improving self-esteem and significantly decreasing level of depression and anxiety in children. Hill (2006) found prominently positive results of play therapy with children who suffered from childhood sex abuse (CSA). This study included parents of sexually abused children in the play sessions and found to be effective in modifying psychological and physical apprehensions of children caused by the painful experience of sexual abuse in childhood. Paone, Tina, Douma and Kara (2009) conducted a case study on a seven years old boy diagnosed with intermittent explosive disorder. This child was given sixteen sessions of Child Centred Play Therapy (CCPT) and significant improvement was noted in problem behaviours as the outcome of this study. Another research was conducted by Brinkmeyer and associates (2003) on children with disruptive behaviour disorder. In this study parent-child interaction therapy was used and key element included involvement of parents and child together in the play sessions, actively coaching the parents in relationship and behaviour change skills, assessing family's progress and continuing treatment until parents mastered the skills and behaviour of their children came within the normal range. The study resulted in improved parent-child ties and decreased disruptive behaviours in the child. Ginsburg and

Kenneth (2007) showed importance of play in promoting healthy child development and improving quality of parent-child relationship. This report provides guidelines on how paediatricians can advocate for children by helping parents, family, school, and community/society. They make sure that play opportunities are protected for every child as it works as a balancing agent in optimal developmental milieu.

Filial therapy has been found to be effective for children experiencing a wide range of social, emotional and behavioural difficulties. Jones, Leslie, Tammy, Rhine, and Bratton (2002) had examined the efficacy of filial therapy on 32 high school children. Parents of these children were trained in child centred play therapy. Outcome of the study indicated significant improvement in empathic reactions. Another part of the research indicated that the children being provided only play therapy without involvement of parents showed significant reduction in problem behaviours.

Post (1999) advocated importance of child centred play therapy as a precautionary method. Students of 4th, 5th and 6th grade were taken for the study that were at risk of decreased self-esteem and locus of control and increased anxiety. Participants were divided into two groups. One group received play therapy and other group received no treatment. Above mentioned parameters in post assessment findings were found to have no effect on the group that received play therapy. On the contrary, the group that received no treatment was found to have decreased self-esteem and locus of control and high anxiety. The study concluded that play interventions can prevent children going at risk of such problems and can also improve their academic performance.

Morrison and Newcomor (1975) tested efficacy of play therapy on intellectually dull children. Eleven sessions of directive play therapy and eleven sessions of non-directive play therapy were conducted and one group was given no treatment. Compared to the non-treatment group both directive and non-directive play therapy groups showed significant improvement in fine motor skills and scored better on Denver Developmental screening test. A study conducted at AIIMS (All India Institute of Medical Sciences) by Renuka Dutta and Manzju Mehta (2006) showed efficacy of play therapy in treating children with Somatoform disorder. In this study 15 children diagnosed with Somatoform disorder were provided 25 sessions of non-directive play therapy and their parents received three sessions of reflective counselling. Pre- and post-results of the study were compared on children's global assessment scale, interview schedule for children and adolescents and child behaviour checklist. Post-assessment results showed increased scores on global functioning and social competence and decreased scores on symptom severity. Thus, the study proved efficacy of child-centred play therapy along with reflective parent counselling in treating somatoform disorder in children.

Remarkable contribution of play therapy is not limited to the above mentioned conditions. There are studies available that prove significance of play therapy in treating alcohol abuse, elimination disorders, attention deficit hyperactivity disorder, and conduct disorder and so on. Despite of a wide range of literature available advocating efficacy of play therapy; the field is in need for more recent studies with more controlled trials. There is a bunch of researches conducted in outer countries that contribute to the field a lot. More researches are required to be conducted in Indian settings to enrich the literature and also to understand closely children being treated in our own country. Well controlled randomized treatment studies and small series of single case studies can contribute a lot to the said purpose.

Conclusion

Play therapy has bright future as a well established treatment in the field of clinical psychology. Professionals who work in this field believe that play therapy allows children not only to express their unsaid thoughts and feelings, but also helps in understanding and interpreting emotions in more meaningful ways. Organizations are becoming aware of this immense treatment and focusing on training and supervision of play therapy to enhance competency in the field. Play therapy is being effectively used and tested on various populations and proven to be the most natural way of healing minds of children.

References

Aletha J. Solter (2013), *Attachment Play: How to Solve Children's Behaviour Problems with play, Laughter, and Connection*. Shining Star Press, California, U.S.A.

Allen, F. (1942). *Psychotherapy with children*. New York: Norton Association for Play Therapy. http://www.a4pt.org/ps.index.cfm

Ann Cattanach (2003). *Introduction to Play Therapy*. Brunner-Routledge, Taylor & Francis Group, Hove and New York.

Athena, A., Drewes, Sue C. Bratton, Charles E. Schaefer, (2011). *Integrative Play Therapy*. John Wiley & Sons, Inc, Hoboken, New Jersey.

Axline, V. (1947/1969) *Play Therapy*. New York: Ballantine Books.

Baggerly, J.N. and Mescia, N.D. (2005). Disaster Behavioural Health First Aid Specialist Training with Children (CFAST). Paper presented at the *19th Annual Governor's Hurricance Conference*, Tampa, FL.

Baggerly, Jennifer N. (2006). Preparing play therapists for disaster response: Principles and practices. *International Journal of Play Therapy* 15, 59-81.

Baggerly, Jennifer. N. (2004). The Effects of Child-Centred Group Play Therapy on Self-Concept, Depression, and Anxiety of Children Who Are Homeless. *International Journal of Play Therapy*, Vol. 13(2) 31-51.

Brinkmeyer, Mary Y., Eyberg, Sheila M. Kazdin, Alan E. (ed.); Weisz, John R. (Ed), (2003). *Parent-child interaction therapy for oppositional children. Evidence-based psychotherapies for children and adolescents*. New York, NY, US: Guilford Press.

Bundy-Myrow, S., and Booth, P.B. (2009). Theraplay: Supporting attachment relationships. In K.J. O'Connor, and L.D. Braverman (Eds.), *Play Therapy Theory and Practice: Comparing Theories and Techniques*, (pp. 315-366), Hoboken, NJ: John Wiley Sons.

Carey, Lois J. (1998). *Sandplay Therapy with Children and Families*. Centre for Play Therapy, University of North Texas. The world of play therapy literature. http://cpt.unt.edu/researchpublications/literature-index.

Carroll, F. (2009). Gestalt play therapy. In K. O'Connor and L. Braverman (Eds.), *Play Therapy Theory and Practice: Comparing Theories and Techniques* (2nd ed., 283-314). Hoboken, NJ: Wiley.

Dale-Elizabeth Pehrsson, and Mary E. Aguilera, (2007). Play Therapy: Overview and Implications for Counsellors. *Professional Counselling Digest, American Counselling Association.*

Dutta R., Mehta M., (2006). Child-centred play therapy in management of somatoform disorders. Brief report. *J. Indian Assoc. Child Adolesc. Ment. Health;* 2(3): 85-88.

Freud, A. (1946). *The Psychoanalytic Treatment of Children*. London: Imago.

Gil, E. and Shaw, J. (2009). Prescriptive Play Therapy. In K.J. O'Connor and L.D. Braverman (eds.) *Play Therapy Theory and Practice: Comparing Theories and Techniques* (Chapter 10). Hoboken, NJ: John Wiley & Sons, Inc.

Gill, E., and Drewes, A. (2005). *Cultural Issues in Play Therapy*. New York, NY: Guilford Press.

Ginsburg, Kenneth R. (2007). The importance of play in promoting healthy child development and maintaining strong parent-child bonds. *Paediatrics,* 119, 182-91.

Gold-Steinberg S., Logan D. (1999). Integrating play therapy in the treatment of children with obsessive-compulsive disorder. *American Journal of Orthopsychiatry*, 4, 495-503.

Green, E. (2009). Jungian analytical play therapy. In K. O'Connor and L. Braverman (eds.), *Play Therapy Theory and Practice: Comparing Theories and Techniques* (2nd ed., 83-121). Hoboken, NJ: Wiley.

Guerney, B. (1964). Filial therapy: Description and rationale. *Journal of Consulting Psychology*, 28, 304-310.

Hambridge, G. (1955). Structured Play Therapy. *American Journal of Orthopsychiatry*, 25, 304-310.

Hill, A. (2006). Play therapy with sexually abused children: Including parents in therapeutic play. *Child and Family Social Work*, 11(4), 316-324.

Jensen-Hart, S. (2010). Prescriptive play interventions: Connecting fundamentals with creativity. *Play Therapy*, 5 (4), 14-17.

Jones, Leslie, Tammy J. Rhine, and Sue C. Bratton (2002). High school students as therapeutic agents with young children experiencing school adjustment difficulties: The effectiveness of a filial therapy training model. *International Journal of Play Therapy*, 11, 43-62.

Josefi, O. and Ryan, V. (2004). Non-directive play therapy for young children with autism: a case study. *Clinical Child Psychology and Psychiatry*, 9(4), 533-551.

Kasari, C., Freeman S., and Paparella, T. (2006). Joint attention and symbolic play in young children with autism: a randomized controlled intervention study. *Journal of Child Psychology Psychiatry*, 47(6), 611-620.

Kevin, John, O'Connor and Sue, Ammen (1997). *Play Therapy: Treatmet, Planning and Interventions: The Ecosystemic Model and Workbook.* Academic Press, California, USA.

Klein, M. (1932). *The Psycho-Analysis of Children*. London: Hogarth Press.

Kottman, T. (2001). *Play therapy: Basics and Beyond*. Alexandria, VA: American Counselling Association.

Kottman, T. (2009). Adlerian Play Therapy. In K. O'Connor and L. Braverman (Eds.), *Play Therapy Theory and Practice: Comparing Theories and Techniques* (2nd ed., 237-282). Hoboken, NJ: Wiley.

Landreth, G.L., and Bratton, S.C. (2006). *Child Parent Relationship Therapy (CPRT). A 10-Session Filial Therapy Model*. New York/Abingdon (UK): Routledge.

Landreth, G.L. (2002). *Play Therapy: The Art of Relationship* (2nd ed.). New York: Taylor & Francis Books, Inc.

Lee, A.C. (2009). Psychoanalytic Play Therapy. In K.J. O'Connor and L.D. Braverman (eds.) *Play Theory and Practice* (2nd ed.), (pp. 25-81). Hoboken, N.J.: J. Wiley & Sons.

Levy, D. (1938). Release therapy for young children. *Psychiatry*, 1, 387-389.

Homeyer, L.E., and Morrison, M.O. (2008). Play therapy: practice, issues and trends. *American Journal of Play*, Volume 1, Number 2, Fall 2008, http://www.journalofplay.org/issues/1/2

Linnet McMohan, (2005). First published in 1992. *The Handbook of Play Therapy*. Taylor & Francis e-Library.

Lowenfeld, M., (1935). *Play in Childhood*. Cambridge University Press.

McCalla, C.L. (1994). A comparison of three play therapy theories: Psychoanalytical, Jungian, and Client-Centred. *International Journal of Play Therapy*, 3 (1), 1-10.

Moustakas, C. (1964). The Therapeutic Process. In M. Haworth (eds.) *Child Psychotherapy,* New York: Basic Books.

O'Connor, K.J. and Braverman, L.D. (Eds). (2009). *Play Therapy Theory and Practice* (5th ed.). Boboken, NJ: John Wiley & Sons, Inc.

Oaklander, V. (2006). *Hidden Treasure: A Map to the Child's Inner Self.* Karnac Books.

Oaklander, V. (2007). *Hidden Treasure.* London, UK: Karnac Books.

Oaklander, V. (1988). *Windows to Our Children: A Gestalt Therapy Approach to Our Children and Adolescents.* Highland, NY: The Centre for Gestalt Development.

Oden, K.A.; Johnson, Q.S. (2010). An Exercise in Values Exploration for Play Therapists, *International Journal of Play Therapy,* Vol. 19 (2), 117-128.

Paone, T. and Douma, K. (2009). Child-centred play therapy with a seven-year-old boy diagnosed with intermittent explosive disorder. *International Journal of Play Therapy,* 18(1), 31-44.

Post, P. (1999). Impact of child-centred play therapy on the self-esteem, locus of control, and anxiety of at-risk 4th, 5th, and 6th grade students. *International Journal of Play Therapy,* 8(2), 1-18.

Schaefer, C.E. and O'Connor, K.J. (eds). (1983). *Handbook of Play Therapy.* New York: John Wiley & Sons, Inc.

Schaefer, C.E., and Carey, L. (eds.). (1994). *Family Play Therapy.* Northvale, NJ: Jason Aronson.

Schaefer, C.E. (1983). Play Therapy. In C.E. Schaefer and K.J. O'Connor (eds.), *Handbook of Play Therapy.* New York: Wiley.

Schaefer, C.E. (ed.). (1993). *The Therapeutic Powers of Play.* Northvale, NJ: Jason Aronson.

Schaefer, C.E. (2001). Prescriptive play therapy. *International Journal of Play Therapy,* 10(2), 57.

Solter, A. (2013). *Attachment Play: How to Solve Children's Behaviour Problems with Play, Laughter and Connection.* Goleta, CA: Shining Star Press.

Taft, J. (1933). *The Dynamics of Therapy in a Controlled Relationship.* New York: MacMillan.

Van Breeman C. (2009). Using play therapy in paediatric palliative care: listening to the story and caring for the body. *International Journal of Palliative Nursing,* 15, 510-514.

14

Relevance of Existential Therapy in Present Scenario

Radha Maddhessia and *Anubhuti Dubey*

Introduction

This chapter reviews Existential therapy as acting on one's conviction in order to arrive at personal truth. Existentialism deals with the problems of meaning and purpose of life on earth, finding the world at hostile in nature. Perspectives of Existential Therapy as a client centred therapy in treating anxiety, feeling meaninglessness and emptiness. It emphasizes a responsibility on both the therapist and client, to understand our position in the world and to evaluate the consequences in the light of truth and reality. Prevalence of existential therapy in India and shortcomings in practicing Existentialism in India has been focused.

An Overview of Existential Therapy

Human birth is natural. At birth one is placed in a concrete and historical environment. While living in this logically ordered society one is subjected to distorted reality of himself and others (Herbert, 1975), though in reality one's presence is subjective and is beyond theorizing (Manfred, 1968; Srinivasan, 1967). Estrangement in modern man is connected with changes in society (Heinman, 1953), and his total involvement in interpersonal (social) existence to cope with his anxieties and universal fear of death (Fuller, 1969; Srinivasan, 1967). However, from social context the emphasis should not be on "what causes suffering, but on the kind of world experience by the suffering person" (Herbert, 1975). The ultimate goal is to come to grips with frustrations and become conscious and responsible of an individual's own idiosyncratic existence.

Maslow has classified Existential therapy or counselling as a humanistic theory due to its focus on helping people to achieve their full potential in life (Maddi, 1978). As it is loosely based on existential philosophy and it is not tied to any particular therapeutic technique, it has been viewed more as an attitudinal or philosophical approach to counselling rather than a theory of therapy. Existential therapy encourages clients to develop comprehension of their personal meaning of life and purpose of their existence in the universe (Frankl, 1997; Yalom, 1980).

Existential theory grew out of existential philosophical movement of the nineteenth century which reflected human existence in the universe. Existential psychotherapy was primarily developed after Second World War as a reaction against determinism of Freud's psychoanalysis and the mechanistic approach of behaviourism (Frankl, 1997; Yalom, 1980). Existential theory was developed by many theorists throughout world of whom four of the best known are James, Bugental, Viktor Frankl, Rollo May and Irving Yalom (Corey, 2009; Szasz, 2005).

Existentialism has four main themes—death, freedom, isolation, and meaninglessness. Each person must confront in his or her quest to answer the question of "What is the ultimate meaning of human existence?" (Frankl, 1997; Yalom, 1980). Existential therapists believe that failure to resolve these ultimate questions or conflicts results in the creation of an 'existential vacuum' that leads to existential anxiety which is ultimately the root of many psychological problems that people face (Frankl, 1997). Existential conflict is caused by the ultimate concern of death because people know that life is finite and there is the desire to continue to be (immortality). Death and life are interdependent, and though physical death, destroy us, the idea of death saves us (Yalom, 1980). The conflict presented in the freedom is the existential belief that, freedom means absence of external structure. That means, a human does not enter into a well structured universe that has an 'inherited design', but instead he must create (responsible for) his or her own world, life design, choices, and actions. In existential sense freedom comes with responsibility. The existential concern with isolation is not being separated from parts of oneself. In existential isolation the fact remains that doesn't matter how much interpersonal contact a person has, he or she enters and leaves this world alone. The conflict arises between the awareness of one's isolation and the wish for contact, protection and to be part of a large whole. The ultimate conflict is between a creature seeking meaning that is thrown into a meaningless universe (Yalom, 1980).

According to existentialism, a human body has no (a prior) essence, only to their existence. A general definition of existence might be that it contains those given (existential conditions) that are due to our being. Based on their freedom—it is up to an individual how he take a position in regard to self and being-in-the-world: "The person must create his own essence by throwing himself into the world, by suffering in it, by fighting in it, he defines himself gradually" (Satre, 2000).

Existential therapy is the practical application of philosophy to everyday living. It is an understanding and therefore living productively and creatively within the constraints and possibilities of life. It is a contemporary form of practical and applied philosophy that seeks to assist people in acquiring the wisdom to understand and live their lives with greater awareness and understanding. Therapy helps people in doing so through a process of judicious questioning and shifting through feelings, experiences and intuitions in order to come to clarity of reflection and insight.

Van Deurzen (2002) writes that existential counselling is not designed to "cure" people of illness in the tradition of the medical model. She does not view client as being sick but as "sick of life or clumsy at living" and unable to live a productive live. In existential therapy attention is given to clients' immediate ongoing experience with the aim of helping them develop a greater presence in their quest for meaning and purpose (Sharp and Bugental, 2001). Existential therapy grew out of an effort to help people resolve dilemmas of contemporary life such as alienation, isolation, and meaninglessness.

The existential path seeks a balance between recognizing the limits and tragic dimensions of human existence on one hand and the possibilities and opportunities of human life on the other hand. Humans are in a constant state of transition, emerging; evolving and becoming.

A general map of human existence can be drawn of the way a person is in the world at any particular time of their life (Yalom, 1980; Deurzen, 2010) which basically falls into four basic dimensions, or world of human existence. The four dimensions are—the physical dimension, the personal dimension, the social dimension and the spiritual dimension. They entangle in different ways for different people. It is useful in the client simultaneous multi-dimension of existence and the aspects of their existence clients are talking about and they are not talking about.

Yalom (1980) portrayed four thematic areas as existential givens, which form a fundament for existence: death, freedom, existential isolation and search for meaning. There are few other terms as defining features of existential psychotherapy: freedom, inter-subjectivity, temporality, becoming, existential anxiety and existential guilt, authenticity, therapeutic relationship, understanding, psychotherapeutic relationship and flexibility.

Application of Existential Counselling

Assisting clients in moving towards authenticity and learning to recognize when they are deceiving themselves is an aim of therapy (Van Deurzen, 2002). The existential orientation holds that there is no escape from freedom as we will always be held responsible. We can relinquish our freedom, which is the ultimate in-authenticity. Existential therapy aims at helping clients face anxiety and engage in action that is based on the authentic purpose of creating a worthy existence. Existentialist usually deal with people who have what could be called a restricted existence. These clients have a limited awareness of themselves, and are often vague about the nature of their problems. They may see few, if any, options for dealing with life situations, and they tend to feel trapped, helpless and stuck.

Due to the fast pace of life in this modern impersonal technological world now-a-days, Existential Therapy may be more applicable. As such more people are having feeling of meaninglessness and emptiness. These feelings of emptiness and meaninglessness constitute what Frankl terms an '*existential vacuum*' and manifests itself in boredom and apathy. Boredom expresses a loss of interest in the world and apathy portrays a lack of initiative to do something that matters to be done in the world (Frankl, 1997). Satisfaction of all persons' needs and wants are part of this technological society, but instead it creates the need to find and fulfil an authentic meaning of life. It does not give opportunity to find that authentic meaning in life (Miars, 2002; Frankl, 1997).

According to Frankl (1997), addiction, aggression, and depression are all the result of this sense of futility. Today society appears to be more existentially minded due to this feeling of being lost and the feeling that life is meaningless (Bliar, 2004; Yalom, 1980). Furthermore, existential therapy is more applicable today because more people are dealing with end of life issues faced in terminal illness (Frankl, 1997). By facing a fate a person cannot change, one can 'transcend oneself' and grow beyond his or herself by changing oneself. By involving in as existential therapy a person can turn suffering into achievement and accomplishment, deriving change from guilt, and seeing in death an incentive to take action while one is still alive (Frankl, 1997).

Existential therapy is appropriate for counsellors to use because it is a client centred therapy and suggests a collaborative counsellor-client relationship. The counsellor in this process should listen empathetically and enter the phenomenological world of the client. In entering the world of the client, the counsellor should 'be present' as the client attempts to define his or her view of the world in this interrelational worldview of therapy (Spinelli, 2002). In addition the medical model is not supported by existential theory and is more closely associated with the wellness model of counselling (Halling, McNabb and Rowe, 2006). Furthermore, the counsellor is encouraged to self-disclose himself at times when he or she has 'stared into the existential' void of pain, suffering and meaninglessness. Then the clients will feel that the counsellor knows how what he or she really feels. In other words, counsellors would be able to help their clients who are facing these same universal questions (Heilminiak, 2001).

Existential psychotherapy puts emphasis on the exploration of clients' consciousness and experience of being-in-the-world. In this way, clients' various embodied attitudes, values, beliefs, choices or assumptions regarding what it means and how it is for them to exist in and engage with themselves, others and the world in general can be explored, examined, challenged and reconsidered in relation to the problems encountered throughout their lives, and the limits imposed upon the possibilities inherent in being-in-the-world.

According to Rollo May, existential psychology strives to understand human beings in their world and the capacities they bring to therapy. Therapists mostly guide their clients to become indulge in use of their capacities and aid them to discover newer approaches for engaging life problem (May, Angel and Ellenberger, 1958).

Existential psychology is concerned with the science of being, seen as expression and influence of societal, cultural and individual reflections that capture the most personal of experiences. It is focused on understanding people, their capacities to be in the world, and the barriers that are preventing them from fully experiencing their capacities.

Bugental presupposes about self as a process that significantly influences his perspective on the central aim of existential therapy. He focused that the sense of being is recovered, when there is internal wholeness, people are freed from the bonds of 'fear, guilt, shame and conflict'. A person who does this work is able to live in their 'true nature' (Bugental, 1978).

The existential therapy emphasizes a different kind of basic conflict within an individual. It is neither a conflict with suppressed instinctual strivings nor one with internalized significant adults, but instead a conflict that flows from the individual's confrontation with the givens of existence. By givens Yalom refers to certain facts of human existence which he calls concerns: death, isolation, freedom and meaninglessness. "An individual's confrontation with these facets of life constitutes the content of the existential dynamic conflict."

Unlike other therapeutic approaches, the existential stance argues that the sources of conflict in an individual's life are not due to instinctual demands that are not being sufficiently met or that are in conflict with opposing demands, nor are they directly due to conflicts with significant others, or to misunderstood, incomplete or improper learning experiences, but rather, they lie with the ontological 'given' of human interrelational existence such as temporality, freedom, encounter and meaning/ meaninglessness and the degree to which each individual responds to these either to minimize or to deny the anxiety they provoke *via* the construction and adoption of his or her worldview. For people, who are coping with developmental crises, experiencing grief and loss, confronting death, or facing a major life decision, existential therapy is especially appropriate. Some examples of this critical turning point that mark passages from one stage of life into another are the struggle for identity in adolescence, coping with failures in marriage and work, and dealing with increased physical limitations as one ages. Uncertainty, anxiety, and struggling with decisions are all part of this process. It tends to work well with people who are at crossroads and who question the state of affairs in the world and are willing to change the *status quo*.

Anxiety is a result of trying to cope with the painful realities of suffering and death, not because of depressed desires or childhood traumas (Yalom, 1980). Yalom posits that there are essentially two modes of defending against the most basic form of anxiety—death anxiety. One way is to convince oneself of one's special and personal inviolability (Yalom, 1980). That is we might logically accept that, like everyone else, we will die at some point, but this rational understanding may be met with a powerful, opposite belief that, whereas others may be doomed to die, we are somehow different, more important, special and such will be spared this fate. In order to convince themselves of their unique status, some individuals will enact all manner of 'death-defying' symptoms.

According to the existential theory, "anxiety results from having to face choices without clear guidelines and without knowing what the outcomes will be and from being aware that we are ultimately responsible for the consequences of our actions" (Corey, 2008). Deurzen (2002) further identifies the purpose of anxiety as a marker of living with the awareness that we are fully alive, and though the feeling of anxiety may not be initially welcome by the individual, it is necessary in order to challenge ourselves to become what we are capable of becoming. In short, challenging ourselves to grow creates unavoidable anxiety. The goals then becomes identifying personal strengths that can be utilized to welcome and manage levels of anxiety that can if "unmanaged", create barriers to personal growth and experiencing life to its fullest.

Existential psychotherapists take the experience of anxiety to be a fundamental 'given' of being-in-the world. The responses that individuals raise up in order to minimize, deny or repress intolerable levels of anxiety are in themselves, central factors in subsequent experiences of sedimentation and dissociation, confusion, learned helplessness and denial of freedom. In other words, the great variety of unwanted and unpleasantly experienced "symptoms" that clients want to be cured of are themselves defense against the acceptance of the various existential anxieties of being-in-the world: nothingness, meaninglessness, isolation and so forth. As we begin to understand anxiety as an unavoidable component embedded within any life event that signifies change, we can assume that anxiety is present in all life events including, but not limited to work, school, home, interpersonal interactions, and daily living. Therefore, it can be interpreted that individuals who seek to gain better understanding of anxiety and how it interplays within their life will gain insight as how this natural force can be managed as a resource for interpersonal growth.

The workaholic, as being motivated by desires of 'getting on top of things', is convinced that no one else is capable of doing the work as successfully or knowledgeably as he or she can. If no one else can match these set standards, the workaholic individual becomes more convinced of his—her indispensability—the world could not possibly survive their death.

Like the compulsive hero and the workaholic, the narcissist, the autocratic controller, the aggressor, all place their desires and abilities to control, determine, manipulate their world at centre stage. The power they convince themselves they have acts as a means to a deeper conviction: the more 'god-like' they appear to be others and to themselves, then, like 'god', the more they can view themselves as immortal.

Self-alienation, as Bugental says, leads a person to that of a prisoner who is driven by suspicious and relentless keeper. The person is split into a tyrannical boss and an untrustworthy worker who continually strives to do more, to do it better, to prove self against an impossible standard (Bugental, 1978).

Clients in existential therapy are encouraged to take seriously their own subjective experience of their world. They are challenged to take responsibility for how they now choose to be in their world. They are expected to go out into the world and decide how they will live differently. It can be reminded that the journey towards freedom began by putting on foot in front of the other to get to office.

Existential therapy helps clients to face the fear of death and non-being or confront the problem of personal freedom, searching of courage to live and dealing with the self-alienations and estrangement from others. By making clients aware of what they are doing and to get them out of the victim role and find the motivation to live. Existential therapy will also help client to be aware that they have the power to change the situation and grow towards maturity and independence. The client will have the courage to confront the creativity, anxiety, despair, fear, dread, guilt, nothingness, meaninglessness and isolation that they are facing (Corey, 2009).

As such it is not the 'treatment' of these symptoms that is central, but rather it is the reconsideration of one's defensive, limiting beliefs that is the focus of existential psychotherapy. The existential focus does not dispute that an individual's fears, denials and anxieties are likely to be operating at different levels of awareness. Nevertheless, its primary interest lies in the exploration and clarification of current conscious experience and the perceived conflicts inferred from this experience.

Methods of Existential Therapy

Existential Therapy can be conceptualized in three general phases. During the initial phase of counselling, therapists assist clients in identifying and clarifying their assumptions about the world. Clients are supposed to define and question the ways in which they perceive and make sense of their existence. They examine their values, beliefs and assumptions to determine their validity. They may initially present their problems as resulting almost entirely from external causes. They may focus on what other people "make them feel" or on how others are largely responsible for their actions or inaction. The counsellor teaches them how to reflect on their own existence and to examine their role in creating their problems in living.

During the middle phase clients are encouraged to more fully examine the source and authority of their present value system. This process of self-exploration typically leads to new insights and some restructuring values and attitudes. Individuals get a better idea of what kind of life they consider worthy to live and develop a clearer sense of their internal valuing process.

The final phase of existential counselling focuses on helping people take what they are learning about themselves and put it into action. The therapeutic hour is a small contribution to a person's renewed engagement with life, or a rehearsal for life (Van Deurzen, 2002).

Existential Therapy helps clients elucidate their personal meaning of life. One approach to counselling from an existential phenomenological perspective has been described by Spinelli (2002). This theory requires the counsellor to:

(1) Set aside or bracket any preconceived beliefs, theories, biases or assumptions;
(2) Explore the client's immediate conscious experience of "being with another" (the counsellor); and
(3) Focus on the descriptive components of the client's life not driven interpretations of them.

The existential counsellor's function in the therapy process is to help the client clarify, evaluate and possibly change the implicit, explicit and assumptions, values, and beliefs of the client's interrelational world. Spinelli (2002) suggests that clients and the therapist interactions with can be seen through three realms based on Biswanger's 'Unwelt', 'Mitwelt' and 'Eigenwelt', with the fourth 'Uberwelt' added by Van Deurzen-Smith. The Unwelt can be described as the unique set of interpretations and meanings each us makes on unique physical world we inhabit. The Mitwelt dimension focuses on how we interact with others in our world and how societal messages on age, race, gender, culture, language, and rules influence our development of differing attitudes and values, basically our perception of our interactions with the public world. The Eigenwelt describes the intimate relationship each of us has with both ourselves and significant others in our lives. How we view ourselves in the areas of self-confidence, self-acceptance and individuality and how these views affect the relationships with significant others, families and friends in our lives. These relationships with people whom we are intimate in our lives can affect whether we feel our lives are meaningful, secure, or anxiety filled. The Uberwelt describes our absolute and abstract constructs on life and how these are incorporated into our outlook in life—the beliefs about life, death, and existence which are basis for all our subsequent beliefs and interpretations in life.

The most widely used technique in Existential Therapy is *Logo Therapy* developed by Viktor Frankl. It is based on the concept that having a reason for living or having a purpose (meaning) for life is necessary for the development of a worthwhile existence. Logotherapy is concerned with both the 'being' as well as the meaning. Logotherapy is based on three fundamental assumptions which provide the order for finding meaning in life. These three assumptions are:

(1) Freedom to will,
(2) Will to meaning, and
(3) Meaning of life.

The first tenet of 'freedom to will' is based on the concept that a human's freedom of will is based on the human capacity to choose how one responds to external circumstances. Although people cannot always influence the biological, sociological or psychological conditions they may face, people can choose how they respond to those conditions. A technique used by Frankl to get people deal with their predicaments was paradoxical intention. In this technique he would suggest to the client to do the opposite of the behaviour the client was struggling with. Humour is the upmost importance to help a person arise in his or her own predicament and be able to view himself/herself in a more detached manner. According to Frankl this ability to choose remains intact under even the most dismal choices (including death) and even where does not appear to be a freedom to choose there still a choice (Frankl, 1967). Based upon the pioneering work of Frankl (e.g. 1975), Goldstein and Chamblers (1978), along with Ascher (1989) and Heide and Borkovec (1984), had proposed that the elements of paradoxical intention employed as in the vivo component in treatment programmes for social anxiety associated with fear or recursive anxiety.

With the second assumption, 'The will to meaning' Frankl (1967 and 1997) argues that it is the most basic of human motivations. The key impetus of this concept is that it allows people to choose to search for meaning they desire. This meaning can only be realized in relation to others or through a cause greater than himself or herself. "Existence falters unless it is lived in terms of transcendence towards something beyond itself" (Frankl, 1967). The essence of meaning is that humans are responsible for fulfilment of their specific meanings of their personal lives. However, human beings are also responsible to something whether it be society, humanity, mankind, one's own conscience or a spiritual

"Higher Power". According to Frankl, with meaning comes responsibility. An existential vacuum can be exhibited by apathy and boredom.

The third and final assumption of Logo Therapy is 'The meaning of life'. Frankl postulates that life can become meaningful in threshold way. First through what we give through our creative works. Secondly, through what we take from life in terms of our values, and thirdly by our willingness to confront a fate we can no longer can change such as an incurable disease, an inoperable cancer or any life threatening condition. Life has meaning under all circumstances including intense unavoidable suffering. The challenge of life is to find that unique meaning for each of us in our lives. The most basic of human motivation is to find purpose in life, is unique in each and every human being, which enables the individual to sustain through pain and suffering with dignity. From this viewpoint, self-actualization and fulfilment of happiness are not goals of life instead are the result of finding one's purpose (Frankl, 1967 and 1997).

Another method of existential counselling described by Miars, is based on Bugental's self-in-the-world construct system (Miars, 2002). This self-in-the-world construct system is described as the conception each person has of who and what one is and how the world operates. Each person answers the existential question of "How shall I live?" by the way each person constructs life each day. In counselling, the self-in-the-world constructs system is delineated by exploring at a subjective level, the personal meaning structures (beliefs) and self-perceptions due to the fact that these form the client's fundamental way of being in the world. Even though these constructs are central to a person's functioning they can operate at an unconscious level and as a result not to be recognized by the client as the source of life's problems and resulting emotional distress. The self-in-the-world construct system allows a person to operate in world that existentially has no absolute structure and meaning which is the source of existential anxiety (which Frankl described as existential vacuum). The client must become aware of his or her self-in-the-world construct system so that the systems can be modified to enable the client to have a more satisfying and adaptable life. Authenticity which is an existential concept that refers to autonomous self-creation of whom and what individuals are to become. To become authentic individuals must transcend enculturation and re-invent themselves from within. Bugental claims that by reclaiming authentic contact with their inner experiencing selves, client can reduce existential anxiety which is causing them emotional distress (Miars, 2002). All clients, except for those experiencing extreme psychotic symptoms do have the will to power to choose how to think, feel, and act in the world (Frankl, 1997 and Miars, 2002). The pursuit of such choice and responsibility is the essence of being an authentic human being in the world (Miars, 2002).

Prevalence of Existential Therapy in India

Though existentialism is Western it has enough Eastern thoughts and therefore can easily be in Eastern perspective in general and Indian in particular as evidenced by scholarly comparison of existentialism with Hindu philosophy by Srinivasan (1967). In some researches, some patients during this form of psychotherapy expressed the view that most of the concepts were familiar to them—but they had not understood its full dimensions. Further, existentialism deals with basic questions of existence—birth, life, death and miseries, which are common to all human beings in whatever culture they are. Once the central concepts are suitable for any culture the details can be added or subtracted according to cultural beliefs and patient's acceptance and expectation. As regards the technique in existentialism, there is scope to make it directive and assertive for less intelligent and introspective and analytical for more intelligent persons.

It has been revealed that Jean Paul Sartre, considered existentialistic education essential for creating awareness about man's existence and preparing for life's struggle. It is necessary for ensuring freedom—the freedom of making a choice. We can strike a balance between spiritualism and materialism in the Indian context. Social problems such as drug addiction, gangsterism, running away from home and others can be prevented by philosophy of existentialism. Rao (1990) reported a case that was treated with existential therapy in anxiety neurosis without medication.

Existential cries is a deep questioning about life and its meaning in an individual's life that arises from angst, despair or failure or due to any event that triggers our hearts and minds, to a level where our existence become dilute, apparently. In a study, Verma and Ghosh (1975) found that the Indian psychotherapist led a relatively more active role than the Western counterpart, suggesting, sympathizing, manipulating the environment, teaching and reassuring. The Indian psychotherapists, in suggesting departures from the Western model, pleaded for greater flexibility, greater activity on the part of psychotherapist and greater use of suggestions and reassurance.

Some similarities lies between the viewpoints of Radhakrishnan and the existentialist thinkers. The philosophy of Radhakrishnan is an attempt to reinterpret and reconstruct the *Advaita Vedanta* of Sankara in the light of scientific knowledge and techniques of modern time. Existentialism is an attitude and outlook that emphasizes human existence. For Radhakrishnan, the human is essentially subject, not object. The existentialists assert that the human is not an object to be known, but a subject. Both the Radhakrishnan and the existentialists emphasize the immense potential and present day condition of humanity. Radhakrishnan acknowledges the reality of suffering and misery of worldly existence. The existentialists maintain that there are antinomies, contradictions and distress at the root of existence. Radhakrishnan is concerned with liberation as a state of freedom. Freedom is the central concept around which the existential enquiry revolves.

Existential Therapy in India—Shortcomings

Neki (1995) feels "Western psychotherapy as it is, hardly applicable to the multitudes in India—except for a handful of Westernized Indians living in large cosmopolitan cities." Surya and Jayaram (1964) comment "As compared to his Western counterpart, the Indian patient is more ready to accept dependency relationship,...less ready to seek intra-psychic explanations,...more ready to discard ego-bounds and involve the therapist in direct role relationships; and finally his ideal or idealized support is the good joint family elder... (Indian patient) more readily alludes to conceptual references like *karma*, *dharma* and traditional figures for orientation..."

In India considering the suitability of psychotherapy or at least its classical Western model, the significant differences in socio-cultural beliefs and practices; specially in terms of apparent lower sophistication of our patients; greater dependency needs of the Indian population; their inability to enter into a professional as opposed to a filial relationship, the impediment created by a greater social distance perceived between the doctor and the patient; the possible implications of the Hindu philosophical beliefs of transmigration of soul, re-birth, and fatalism, the different nature and quantum of guilt feeling in our own culture and the differences in the need for confidentiality and inactivity exercised by the therapist especially with regard to decision-making for the patient and environmental manipulation. Neki (1992) discussed confidentiality and privacy in the Indian context and opined that these terms do not even exist in Indian languages and, in the socio-cultural context; the concept of privacy could severe people from interdependent society.

Conclusion

There are strengths to counselling from an existential basis. It focuses on the choices available to the client in development 'purpose or meaning in life' (personal growth). The client defines his or her way of being in the world and subsequently the client defines his or her own meaning in life (personal autonomy) (Frankl, 1997; Heilmiak, 2001; Spinelli, 2002). There is evidence that existential counselling is effective in treating depression, addiction, developmental issues, grief and loss, changes in life, facing death, and life's existential anxieties (Coery, 2009; Blair, 2004; Helminiak, 2001; Frankl, 1997). Existential therapy can be effective in working with a multi-cultural population since it does not prescribe a particular way relating to the universe and because of its broad perspective (Corey, 2009). Existential therapy may be used more effectively when a client has access to emotional experiences or when obstacles must be overcome to facilitate a client's entry into or continuation of recovery. (e.g. to get someone insists on remaining helpless to accept responsibility for her actions.)

Existential approach help in bringing the client back into central focus. It emphasize on the central fact of human existence which is self-conscious and client's subsequent freedom. Human refer their sense of being controlled by external forces. It helps clients to reflect on life and recognize their range of alternatives and to decide among them to start on a new path that consciously shaping their own life. Therefore, it has brought the positive and healthy way for human being (Corey, 2009). One of the contributions of existential approach is its focus on the human quality of therapeutic relationship. This will decrease the chances of dehumanizing psychotherapy by making it a mechanical process. Existentialists reject the philosophy of the therapeutic objectivity and professional distance thus viewing themselves as unhelpful (Corey, 2009).

Limitations of Existential Therapy

There are some disadvantages of using existential theory in counselling. According to Cooper (2003), existential practitioners generally reject the idea that the therapeutic process can be measured and evaluated in quantitative and empirical ways. There is a distinct lack of studies that directly evaluate and examine the existential approach. Existentialism makes use of techniques from other theories and approaches, making it difficult to apply research to this approach to study its effectiveness.

According to Van Deurzen (2002), the main limitation of this approach is that of the level of the maturity, life experiences, and intensive training that is required of practitioners. Existential therapists need to be wise and capable of profound and wide ranging understanding of what it means to be human. Authenticity is a cardinal characteristic of a component existential practitioner, which is certainly more involved than mastering a body of knowledge and acquiring technical skills.

References

Akhter, R. (2014). Existentialism and its relevance to contemporary system of education in India: Existentialism and present scenario. *Hamburg, Anchor,* Academic Publishing. ISBN: 978-3-954, 5-17.

Ascher, L.M. (1989a). Paradoxical intention: Its clarification and emergence as a conventional behavioural procedure. *The Behaviour Therapist,* 12, 23-28.

Ascher, L.M., and Schotte, D.E. (1999). Paradoxical intention and recursive anxiety. *Journal of Behaviour Therapy and Experimental Psychiatry,* 39, 73.

Barry, K.L. (1999). Brief interventions and brief therapies for substance abuse. Treatment Improvement Protocol, Series 34, *DHHS* Publication No. (SMA) 99-3353, 11-12.

Blair, R. (2004). Helping older adolescents search for meaning in depression. *Journal of Mental Health Counselling,* 26(4), 333-347.

Boss, M. (1958). The role of psychotherapy in schizophrenia. *Indian Journal of Psychiatry,* 1, 4-12.

Bugental, J. (1978). *Psychotherapy and Process: The Fundamentals of an Existential-Humanistic Approach.* Boston: McGraw Hill, 8-15.

Bugental, J.F.T. (1999). *Psychotherapy isn't what you think: Bringing the psychotherapeutic engagement into the living moment. Phoenix:* Zeig, Tucker & Co., 83-92.

Bugental, J. and Yalom, I. (2009). Two masters of existential therapy cultivate presence in the therapeutic encounter. *Journal of Humanistic Psychology.* Sage Publication, Vol. XX, No. 4, 8-14.

Cooper, M. (2003). *Between freedom and despair: Existential challenges and contributions to person-centred and experiential therapy. Person-centred and experiential psychotherapies.* London: Sage, 2 (1), 43-56.

Corey, G. (2008). *Theory and practice of group counselling* (8th edition). Brooks/ Cole, Belmont, pp. 223.

Corey, G. (2009). *Theory and practice of group counselling* (9th edition). Brooks/ Cole, Belmont, pp. 132-155.

Deurzen, E. Van. (2002b). Existential therapy. In W. Druden (ed.), *Handbook of Individual Therapy* (4th ed.). London: Sage Publication, pp. 179-208.

Deurzen, E. Van. (2010). *The Framework of Existential Therapy: Skills in Existential Psychotherapy*. Sage Publication, pp. 9-19.

Flanagan, J.S. and Flanagan, R.S. (2004). *Counselling and Psychotherapies Theories in Context and Practice*. John Wiley & Sons, Inc., Hoboken, New Jersy, p. 7.

Frankl, V. (1967). *Psychotherapy and Existentialism*. New York: Simon and Schuster, 138-142.

Frankl, V. (1975). Paradoxical intention and dereflection. *Psychotherapy: Theory, Research and Practice*, 12, 226-237.

Frankl, V. (1997). *Man's Search for Ultimate Meaning*. New York: Plenum Press, 84.

Fuller, M. (1969). *A History of Philosophy* (3rd edition). New Delhi: Oxford and IOH Publishing Company, 603-612.

Glassman, W.E. and Hadad, M. (2004)). *Approaches to Psychology* (4th edition). Open University Press, Berkshire, England, 282.

Goldstein, A.J. and Chambless, D.L. (1978). A reanalysis of agoraphobia. *Behaviour Therapy*, 9, 47-59.

Halling, S., McNabb, M., and Rowe, J.O. (2006). Existential-Phenomenological Psychotherapy in the trenches: A collaborative approach to serving the underserved. *Journal of Phenomenological Society*, 37 (2), 171-196.

Heide, F.J., and Borkovec, T.D. (1984). Relaxation induced anxiety: Mechanism and Theoretical Implications. *Behaviour, Research and Therapy*, 22, 1-12.

Heinman, F.H. (1953). *Existentialism and the Modern Predicament*, New York: Harper and Brother Publishers, 1-13.

Helminiak, D. (2001). Treating spiritual issues in secular psychotherapy. *Counselling and Values*, 45 (3), 163-189.

Herbert, H. (1975). *Existential Philosophy. In comprehensive textbook of psychiatry*, (2nd edition) Freedman, A.M., Kaplan, H.J., Sadock, B.J., Vol. I, Baltimore: Williams and Wilkins, 661-668.

Maddi, S. (1978). Existential and Individual psychologies. *Journal of Individual Psychology*, 34 (2), 182-190.

Manfred, S.F. (1968). Heidegger and the Quest for truth. Chicago: *Quadrangle Books*, 13-19.

Marappan, D., Mustaffa, M.S., and Ahmad, R. (2010). Existential approach in treating self-harming behaviour. *International Journal of Fundamental Psychology and Social Sciences*. Publication 81310 UTM Skudai, Johor, Malaysia, p. 3.

Miars, R. (2002). Existential authenticity: A foundational value for counselling. *Counselling and Values*, 46 (3), 218-225.

Neki, J.S. (1992). Confidentiality, Secrecy and Privacy in Psychotherapy: Socio-Dynamic Considerations. *Indian Journal of Psychiatry*, 34(3), 171-173.

Pitchford, D.B. (2009). The Existentialism of Rollo May: An influence on trauma treatment. *Journal of Humanistic Psychology*, Vol. 49, Sage Publication, pp. 442-446.

Rao, K.N. (1990). Practical steps in existential psychotherapy and one year follow-up of a case. *Indian Journal of Psychiatry,* 32, 244-250.

Sartre, J.P. (2000). Der Existentialismus ist ein Humanismus. In JP Sartre, *Der Existentialismus ist ein Humanismus and andere Essays*. Reinbek: Rowohlt, 145-192.

Sharp, J., and Bugental, J.F.T. (2001). Existential-Humanistic psychotherapy. In R. Corsini (Ed.), *Handbook of Innovative Therapy* (2nd Edition) (pp. 206-217). New York, NY, Wiley.

Spinelli, E. (2002). The therapeutic relationship as viewed by existential psychotherapy: Re-evaluating the world. *Journal of Contemporary Psychotherapy,* 32(1), 111-118.

Spinell, E. (2006). Existential psychotherapy: An introductory overview. Vol. 24. In chapter of the interpreted world: An introduction to phenomenological psychology, 2nd edition 2005. *Analise Psicological,* 3, 312-318.

Srinivasan, G. (1967). *The Existentialist Concept and the Hindu Philosophical Systems*. Allahabad: Udayan Publishers, 1-270.

Stumm, G. (2008). The person centred approach from an existential perspective. *Ubersichtsartikel Existenzanalyse,* p. 7.

Szasz, T. (2005). What is existential therapy not? *Existential Analysis,* 16(1), 127-130.

Surya, N. and Jayaram, S. (1964). Some basic considerations in the practice of psychotherapy in Indian setting. *Indian Journal of Psychiatry,* 6, 153.

Varma, V.K. and Ghosh, A. (1976). Psychotherapy as practiced by Indian psychiatrists. *Indian Journal of Psychiatry,* 18, 177.

Varma, V.K. (1982). Present state of psychotherapy in India. *Indian Journal of Psychiatry,* 24 (3), 210-215.

Yalom, I. (1980). *Existential psychotherapy*. New York: Basic Books (1989). *Existentielle Psychotherapie*. Koln: Edition Humanistische Psychologie, 5-115.

15

Holistic Treatment Approach of Trauma

Rape

Narendra Singh Thagunna

Introduction

A trauma can be any painful experience, physical or emotional, that can pose a threat of injury or death to oneself or others. In this chapter, treatment issues in psychotherapy/counselling survivors of trauma rape are reviewed, including socio-cultural influences on a woman's response to rape, a survivor's history of victimization, the specific nature of the assault, and a survivor's experiences with victim-blame. 'Rape trauma syndrome' is the medical term for the response survivors have to rape. It is similar to traumatic stress disorder. People who are defiled and people who get sodomized also experience this syndrome. Significant psychological and physical symptoms can emerge in the aftermath of rape. Women are hesitant to seek counselling until their symptoms are chronic, and counsellors' lack formal training in assisting survivors in their recovery. The purpose of this chapter is to provide an overview of treatment considerations for survivors of rape, and to describe a multimodal treatment approach for women who are experiencing chronic symptoms of Rape trauma syndrome, post-traumatic stress disorder in the result of rape is also presented. The model incorporates four empirically supported techniques based upon expert consensus guidelines for treating survivors of trauma: psycho-education, exposure therapy, cognitive therapy, and anxiety management (Foa *et al.*, 1999).

A trauma can be any painful experience, physical or emotional, that can pose a threat of injury or death to oneself or others. Trauma can make an individual feel terrified and helpless. There can be at least two parts of trauma, one is what actually happened, the Physical effect of the trauma; the other is the experience that takes place inside an individual, the psychological experiences. *Trauma-* and *Stressor-Related Disorders* a new category for DSM-5, trauma and stress disorders emphasize the pervasive impact that life events can have on an individual's emotional and physical well-being. Diagnoses include reactive attachment disorder, disinhibited social engagement disorder, post-traumatic stress disorder, acute stress disorder, and adjustment disorders. Any powerful events such as an MVA, war, refugee/migrant may or may not turn out to be a traumatic experience for any individual. If an accident dispute the person's life and causes a significant physical and/or emotional (Psychological) reaction, then it can be called traumatic. How each individual perceives and reacts to an event determines whether an event turns out to be seen a traumatic or not.

Epidemiological Studies

Violence against women is a significant social problem, as there is a high probability that any woman will experience some type of violence in her lifetime. According to the National Violence Against Women Survey, more than half of all women report an experience of attempted or completed rape and/or physical assault (Tjaden and Thoennes, 1998).

The World Health Organization (WHO) has estimated that in the year 2000, 1.6 million worldwide died from self-inflicted, interpersonal or collective violence (Krug, Dahlberg, Mercy, Zwi, and Lozano, 2002). Women who are physically assaulted in intimate relationships (including dating relationships) are often psychologically abused and/or sexually assaulted by their partners as well (Krug *et al.*, 2002). In various countries around the world, approximately 25 per cent of adult women report sexual assault by an intimate partner and up to 33 per cent of teenaged girls report that there first sexual experience was forced (Krug *et al.*, 2002). Fifty per cent of Canadian women have experienced at least one incident of physical or sexual after age 16 (Johnson, 2005).

Childhood sexual abuse is documented in many countries and this form of childhood abuse is associated with a wide variety of long-term adverse effects. The mean lifetime prevalence of childhood sexual abuse (involving contact forms of abuse) is estimated at 20 per cent for females and 5-10 per cent for males (Krug *et al.*, 2002). While both men and women are victims of rape, women are disproportionately affected by this crime; 1 in 6 women compared with 1 in 33 men report having experienced an attempted or completed rape in their lifetimes. About half of global sexual trafficking occurs in Asia (Huda, 2006). The special rapporteur on trafficking in persons reports that approximately 30 million Asian women and children have been trafficked over the past 30 years (Huda, 2006). The best known forms of sexual violence against women include sexual assault and child sexual abuse, though other forms including violence against sex trade workers, genital mutilations, forced virginity examinations, war related rape, forced marriage (including child marriage), forced abortion, and sexual trafficking (Brack, 2006).

The Diagnostic and Statistical Manual of Mental Disorders—Text Revision (DSM-IV-TR; American Psychiatric Association, 2000) groups PTSD symptoms into three clusters: (i) Intrusion (re-experiencing of the trauma, including nightmares, flashbacks, recurrent thoughts) (ii) Avoidance (avoiding trauma-related stimuli, social withdrawal, emotional numbing), and (iii) Hyperarousal (increased emotional arousal, exaggerated startle response, irritability). While most women experience these symptoms in the immediate aftermath of rape, PTSD continues to persist in survivors at lifetime rates between 30 per cent and 50 per cent (Foa, Hearst-Ikeda, and Perry, 1995; Meadows and Foa, 1998; Resnick *et al.*, 1999). When symptoms persist for 3 months or longer and meet DSM-IV-TR diagnostic criteria for chronic PTSD, there is likelihood that survivors will also experience co-morbid disorders including anxiety, depression, and substance abuse (Foa, Davidson and Frances, 1999; Koss and Kilpatrick, 2001; Resnick, Acierno, Holmes, Dammeyer, and Kilpatrick, 2000). Further, they are likely to experience greater physical distress (e.g. chronic pain, sexual dysfunction, headaches, upset stomach, back pains, acne, indigestion) in the year following rape and utilize medical services at higher rates than do women who have not been raped (Clum, Nishith, and Resick, 2001). Women who are particularly at risk for chronic PTSD include those who were injured during the attack, were threatened by the perpetrator that they may be hurt or killed, have a history of prior assault, or have experienced negative interactions with family, peers, or law enforcement systems (Regehr, Cadell, and Jansen, 1999).

The research suggests that there is no one type of perpetrators of domestic violence, violent behaviour may be result from loss of control, dependency, fear, anxieties, frustrations, and threat to self-esteem, personality disorders (especially borderline and antisocial) are often common to batterers, and many have a history of attachment disorders that originate within their own families of origin (Kantor and Jasinski, 1998). Male who perpetrate violence against their female partners tends to hold traditional beliefs regarding gender role (Krug *et al.*, 2002). The dynamics and patterns of abuse on same-sex relationships are similar to those seems in the abusive heterosexual relationships (Harway *et al.*, 2001).

When women remain in abusive relationships, people may question why do they not leave? The reasons why women remain in abusive relationships are complex, and often involve traumatic bounding (Dutton and Painter, 1981). Traumatic bounding refers to a particularly strong attachment bond that develops between victims and perpetrators in abusive relationships. The victim often feels quite ambivalent knowing that the relationship is unhealthy but unable to break the attachment due to the traumatic bond.

Sexual violence against teenage girls may result in pregnancies, and rates vary between countries. Approximately 5 percentages of rape victims in USA become pregnant, compared to up to 18 per cent in Ethiopia and Mexico (Krug *et al.*, 2002).

Significant psychological and physical symptoms can emerge in the aftermath of rape. Women are reluctant to seek counselling until their symptoms are chronic, and counsellors lack formal training in assisting survivors in their recovery. A significant proportion of women who are sexually assaulted or raped experience symptoms of post-traumatic stress disorder (PTSD) within 2 weeks following the assault (Resnick, Acierno, Holmes, Kilpatrick, and Jager, 1999). Survivors do not typically seek formal mental health services in the year following rape (Kimerling and Calhoun, 1994). Mental health professionals can serve as a primary source of support in a survivor's recovery, yet many practitioners report a lack of training in this area during their programmes of study. Campbell and colleagues also found that when training does occur, it takes place through continuing education and does not include information regarding the significant legal and medical issues that can impact a woman's recovery (Campbell, Raja, and Grining, 1999). Mental health counsellors' lack of training may become particularly problematic if they are not adequately prepared to assist survivors of rape who are experiencing chronic PTSD symptoms and comorbid disorders.

The purpose of this chapter is to focus upon women's experiences and treatment needs following sexual assault and rape and describe a multimodal treatment approach for women who are experiencing chronic PTSD symptoms resulting from rape-related trauma. The model incorporates four empirically supported techniques based upon expert consensus guidelines for treating survivors of trauma: psych education, exposure therapy, cognitive therapy, and anxiety management (Foa *et al.*, 1999).

Rape

Several authors have observed (e.g. Bourque, 1989; Estrich, 1987; Koss, 1993) that many people still believe that rape occurs only when a stranger attacks an adult woman using overwhelming force. Using this definition, boys or men cannot be raped; girls and adolescents cannot be raped; no one can be raped by someone they know; and forced oral or anal sex does not constitute rape. Early feminist scholars (e.g. Brownmiller, 1975) argued that rape is not a crime of sex but should be conceptualized as a crime of power. Brownmiller asserted that rape is a tool of a patriarchal system that serves to perpetuate gender inequality and the devaluation of women. According to this theory, fear of rape limits women's freedom and use of power. This inescapable fear operates to maintain gender inequality, as women's "actions and movements, self-expression, self-presentation, and agency within relationships are constrained by the fear of sexual assault" (Low and Organista, 2000: 132). While feminists have examined rape through the lens of gender and power, cultural variables such as ethnicity and class also affect women's responses to and recovery from rape-related trauma (Low and Organista, 2000).

Thus, attempts to discuss the topic are often frustrating because many people define rape differently. Very often after a rape, people will say things to the survivor, such as "It's over now, you must get on with the rest of your life." Or they will not understand why, six months after the rape, the survivor is still suffering. Rape begins with the physical act, during which the victim concentrates on surviving. After the assault, the struggle to comprehend what has happened begins. Its meaning floods over the survivor, who must find a way to return to life, body and self. Rape is as much a destruction of 'self' as a physical invasion. The battle between 'mind rape' and the will to find self again is called survival.

Rape Trauma Syndrome

'Rape trauma syndrome' is the medical term for the response survivors have to rape. It is similar to traumatic stress disorder. People who are defiled and people who get sodomized also experience this syndrome.

Physical Symptoms of Rape Trauma Syndrome

- Shock, in which the survivor feels cold, faint, confused and disoriented, trembles, nauseous and sometimes vomits.

- Resulting pregnancy.
- Gynaecological problems include irregular, heavier and painful periods, vaginal discharge, bladder infections and sexually transmitted diseases.
- Bleeding and infection from tears or cuts in the vagina or rectum.
- A soreness of the body, bruising, grazes and cuts.
- Nausea and vomiting.
- Throat irritation and soreness from forced oral sex.
- Tension headaches.
- Pain in the lower back and in the stomach.
- Sleep disturbances, including difficulty in sleeping or feeling exhausted and needing more sleep than usual.
- Eating disorders, including not eating, eating less or eating more than usual.

Behavioural Symptoms of Rape Trauma Syndrome

- Crying more than usual.
- Difficulty in concentrating.
- Restless, agitated and unable to relax or feeling listless and unmotivated.
- Not wanting to socialize or see anybody or socializing more than usual, to fill-up every minute of the day.
- Not wanting to be alone.
- Stuttering and stammering more than usual.
- Avoiding anything that reminds victim of the rape.
- More easily frightened or startled than usual.
- Very alert and watchful.
- Easily upset by small things.
- Problems with family, friends, lovers and spouses from irritability, withdrawal and dependence.
- Fear of sex, loss of interest in sex or loss of sexual pleasure.
- Change in lifestyle.
- Increased substance abuse.
- Increased washing or bathing.
- Denial, behaving as if the rape did not occur, trying to live life as it was before the rape.

Psychological Symptoms of Rape Trauma Syndrome

- Increased fear and anxiety.

- Self-blame and guilt.
- Helplessness, no longer feeling in control of life.
- Humiliation and shame.
- Lowered self-esteem, feeling dirty.
- Anger.
- Feeling alone and that no one understands.
- Losing hope for the future.
- Emotional numbness.
- Confusion.
- Memory loss.
- Constantly thinking about the rape.
- Having flashbacks to the rape, feeling it is happening again.
- Nightmares.
- Depression.
- Developing suicidal ideas.

Marital Rape

Most studies of marital rape have included couples who are legally married, separated, divorced or cohabiting with the understanding that the dynamics of sexual violence in a long-term cohabiting relationship are similar to those of a married couple (Mahoney and Williams, 1998). Researchers estimate that 10 to 14 per cent of married women experience rape in marriage (Finkelhor and Yllo, 1985; Russell, 1990). Diana Russell's (1990) landmark study of sexual assault that involved interviews with 930 women in a randomly selected representative community sample in San Francisco established that marital rape is a serious problem that millions of women face each year. Rape in marriage is an extremely prevalent form of sexual violence, particularly when we consider that women who are involved in physically abusive relationships may be especially vulnerable to rape by their partners. Studies using clinical samples of battered women reveal that between one-third and one-half of battered women are raped by their partners at least once (Bergen, 1996; Browne, 1993; Campbell, 1989). When researchers have examined the prevalence of different types of rape, they have found that marital rape accounts for approximately 25 per cent of all rapes (Randall and Haskall, 1995; Resnick, Kilpatrick, Walsh, and Vernon, 1991).

It appears that marital rape is most likely to occur in relationships characterized by other forms of violence. This has led some researchers to argue that marital rape is "just one extension of domestic violence"

(Johnson and Sigler, 1997: 22). On one hand, viewing rape in marriage as a form of domestic violence is logical given that researchers have found that the majority of women who are raped by their partners are also battered. In "battering rapes", women experience both physical and sexual violence in the relationship (Finkelhor and Yllo, 1985). Women who are raped and battered by their partners experience the violence in various ways—e.g. some are battered during the sexual violence or the rape may follow a physically violent episode where the husband wants to "make up" and coerces his wife to have sex against her will (Bergen, 1996; Finkelhor and Yllo, 1985). Other women experience what has been labelled "sadistic" or "obsessive" rape; these assaults involve torture and/or "perverse" sexual acts and are often physically violent. Pornography is frequently involved with sadistic forms of rape (Bergen, 1996; Finkelhor and Yllo, 1985).

On the other side of this debate, some have argued that marital rape should not be subsumed under the heading of domestic violence because doing so in the past has led to rape in marriage being overlooked as a distinctive problem (for more on this debate *see* Bergen, 1996; Russell, 1990). It is necessary to recognize marital rape as a distinctive problem because for many women who are battered and raped, the sexual violence is particularly devastating and that trauma must be addressed specifically by service providers (Finkelhor and Yllo, 1985). Additionally, it is problematic to assume that marital rape survivors are all battered wives, because this ignores the reality that some women are raped by their husbands but do not experience other forms of violence. It must be reiterated that most of the research on marital rape has been conducted with battered women. This methodological problem may overstate the extent to which women are both battered and raped by their partners. Indeed, Russell (1990) found that four per cent of women in her sample who had ever been married had been raped by their partners, but not battered. In what Finkelhor and Yllo (1985) have called "force—only rape", husbands use only the amount of force necessary to coerce their wives; battering may not be characteristic of these relationships. Forty per cent of Finkelhor and Yllo's sample of women were victims of "force—only rape." Thus, to categorize marital rape only as an extension of domestic violence excludes these women and their experiences. As we will address later, it is important for advocates who are involved in trying to end violence against women to see marital rape both as a form of rape and of domestic violence in order to assist survivors.

This assistance may be particularly necessary given that women who are raped by their husbands are likely to be raped many times—often 20 times or more before they are able to end the violence (Bergen, 1996; Finkelhor and Yllo, 1985; Russell, 1990). Marital rape survivors not only experience a higher number of assaults, but research indicates that they are more likely than women raped by acquaintances to experience unwanted oral and anal intercourse (Peacock, 1995). Husbands often rape their wives when they are asleep, or use coercion, verbal threats, physical violence, or weapons to force their wives to have sex. Importantly, some researchers have found that compared to batterers, men who batter and rape are particularly dangerous men and are more likely to severely injure their wives and potentially escalate the violence to murder (Browne, 1987; Campbell, 1989).

Risk Factors

Most researchers of marital rape agree that rape in marriage is an act of violence—an abuse of power by which a husband attempts to establish dominance and control over his wife. While the research thus far reveals no composite picture of a husband-rapist, these men are often portrayed as jealous, domineering individuals who feel a sense of entitlement to have sex with their "property". Given this, women appear to be particularly at risk for being raped by their partners under some circumstances. As was previously indicated, women who are battered are at greater likelihood of being raped by their partners (Frieze, 1983). Additionally, pregnancy appears to be a factor that places women at higher risk for both physical and sexual abuse (Bergen, 1996; Browne, 1993; Campbell, 1989). Being ill or recently discharged from the hospital are also risk factors for women (Campbell and Alford, 1989; Mahoney and Williams, 1998). As research with battered women has previously revealed, women are at particularly high risk of experiencing physical and sexual violence when they attempt to leave their abusers for this represents a challenge to their abusers' control. Finkelhor and Yllo (1985) found that two-thirds of the women in their sample were sexually assaulted at the end of the relationship. Other researchers have found that women who are separated or divorced from their partners appear to be at high risk for sexual abuse (Dobash and Dobash, 1992; Kurz, 1997; Russell, 1990). Some researchers have noted other risk factors including drug and alcohol use by the abuser, and previous experiences of sexual abuse among the victims. However, these factors are perceived as more controversial and the research is far from conclusive (Frieze, 1983; Russell, 1990; Whatley, 1996).

Effects of Rape

Despite the historical myth that rape by one's partner is a relatively insignificant event causing little trauma, research indicates that marital rape often has severe and long-lasting consequences for women. The physical effects of marital rape may include injuries to the vaginal and anal areas, lacerations, soreness, bruising, torn muscles, fatigue and vomiting (Adams, 1993; Bergen, 1996). Women who have been battered and raped by their husbands may suffer other physical consequences including broken bones, black eyes, bloody noses, and knife wounds that occur during the sexual violence. Campbell and Alford (1989) report that one-half of the marital rape survivors in their sample were kicked, hit or burned during sex. Specific gynaecological consequences of marital rape include vaginal stretching, miscarriages, stillbirths, bladder infections, infertility and the potential contraction of sexually transmitted diseases including HIV (Campbell and Alford, 1989).

Some researchers have compared the psychological effects of being raped by one's partner to other forms of violence. Given that women who are raped by their partners are likely to experience multiple assaults, completed sexual attacks, and rape by someone that they once presumably loved and trusted, it is not surprising that marital rape survivors seem to suffer severe and long-term psychological consequences (Kilpatrick, Best, Saunders, and Vernon, 1988; Frieze, 1983). Similar to other survivors of sexual violence, some of the short-term effects of marital rape include anxiety, shock, intense fear, depression, suicidal ideation, and post-traumatic stress disorder (Bergen, 1996; Kilpatrick *et al.*, 1988; Russell, 1990). Compared to women raped by strangers and those whom they don't know well, marital rape survivors report even higher rates of anger and depression (Koss, Dinero, Siebel, and Cox, 1988). Long-term effects often include disordered eating, sleep problems, depression, problems establishing trusting relationships, and increased negative feelings about themselves (Bergen, 1996; Frieze, 1983). Research has also indicated that the psychological effects are likely to be long-lasting—some marital rape survivors report flashbacks, sexual dysfunction, and emotional pain for years after the violence (Bergen, 1996; Whatley, 1993).

Counselling of Survivors of Rape

There are four important issues for psychotherapist/mental health counsellors to explore when counselling a survivor of rape:

- Socio-cultural influences on a woman's response to rape,
- Her history of victimization,
- The specific nature of her assault, and
- Her experiences with victim-blame.

Psychotherapists/counsellors who work with survivors of rape should consider a woman's reaction to rape within a socio-cultural context. Psychotherapist/counsellors should remain sensitive to cultural differences in a survivor's access to services, her feelings of safety when reporting crimes, or how disclosures following rape may be received in her community. The therapist/counsellors should consider how cultural factors shape a survivor's view of gender roles, which in turn influence the meaning she imparts to the rape experience. For example, in south Asian culture women, due to culture, may be more likely to blame themselves for causing the rape. Latina women may be more likely to blame themselves for causing the rape, if they subscribe to the cultural belief that women contribute to rape by their behaviour and dress and are responsible for controlling male sexuality as well as their own (Low & Organista). It is critical that therapists/counsellors assess for cultural influences in their conceptualization of a survivor's rape experience and to choose strategies that are appropriate for use with clients from diverse cultural groups (Hansen, Gama, and Harkins, 2002).

Therapists/counsellors providing treatment for survivors of sexual assault and rape should be aware of a client's history of victimization. There is a considerable body of research demonstrating that early sexual abuse and maltreatment are significant risk factors for rape as an adult (Kessler and Bieschke, 1999; Koss and Kilpatrick, 2001; Sanders and Moore, 1999; Tjaden and Thoennes, 1998). One explanation for these findings is that rape in childhood or adolescence can lead to the experience of low self-worth and powerlessness, resulting in poorer general functioning, lack of protection against high-risk situations, and greater risk of multiple times victimization (Breitenbecher and Gidycz, 1998). In one study with a national sample of female college students, women who had been raped in adolescence or early in college were more likely to report engaging in high-risk, health-related behaviours (e.g. physical fights, smoking, binge drinking, two or more current sexual partners) than were college women in general; these behaviours may also put them at risk for multiple victimization (Brener, McMahon, Warren, and Douglas, 1999).

The treatment issue is related to the specific nature of the assault. As rapes are generally classified as stranger, acquaintance, date, partner, or marital rapes, psychotherapists/mental health counsellors need to understand a client's response to rape in the context of her prior relationship to the perpetrator. For example, women perceive their risk of being raped by a stranger as much higher than by an acquaintance, date, or partner (Nurius, Norris, Dimeff, and Graham, 1996); yet there is a much greater likelihood of a woman being raped by someone she knows (Tjaden and Thoennes, 1998). Despite the fact that women fear stranger rapes more than acquaintance or date rapes, the effects of both crimes in terms of negative psychological effects are similar (Cowan, 2000; Shapiro and Schwartz, 1998). Women survivors of acquaintance, date, or partner rapes, however, tend to engage in more self-blame and are less likely to label their experiences as rape when compared with those who experienced stranger rapes (Koss and Kilpatrick, 2001). When working with survivors of rape perpetrated by someone they know, mental health counsellors can validate clients' fears and reactions, and specifically assist them in challenging their self-blaming tendencies regarding their role in the rape.

The Therapist/Mental health counsellors must further consider issues specific to women who were sexually assaulted while under the influence of alcohol or other drugs. Rape is highly associated with alcohol use by both perpetrator and victim. This finding is particularly strong for college students. In a recent national survey of college students conducted by Ullman, Karabatsos, and Koss (1999), half of all women had experienced some type of sexual victimization. During these incidences, 53 per cent of perpetrators and 42 per cent of victims reported using alcohol at the time of the assault. In a study by Schwartz and Leggett (1999), women who reported being raped when they were too intoxicated to give consent tended to blame themselves, questioned their role in the assault, and did not label the attack as rape even when the incident clearly met the criteria of a felony crime. Many women who are raped while intoxicated may not be aware that most legal jurisdictions define rape as sexual acts committed without a woman's consent, including when she is incapable of giving consent due to intoxication. The counsellors can educate women who are raped while intoxicated regarding the legal definitions of rape so, that they can appropriately label their experiences and make informed decisions regarding the initiation of legal proceedings. Women may be hesitant to label the event as rape or to report the crime to the police due to their memory impairments. On the occasions when such rapes are reported, prosecutors may be reluctant to pursue these cases since the legal system requires evidence of a struggle to prove that sexual activity was non-consensual (Easton, Summers, Tribble, Wallace, and Lock,

1997). It is, therefore, important for mental health counsellors to consider the multiple violations that a survivor of drug-facilitated sexual assault has experienced: she was drugged against her will, forced into sexual activity without her consent, has no memory of the rape, may receive sceptical reactions from law enforcement, and may receive limited support from prosecutors in pursuing legal recourse.

Last, mental health counsellors can increase their awareness of the societal tendency towards victim-blame. Many survivors experience negative reactions from others and are often blamed for causing the rape. Termed a secondary victimization (Feldman, Ullman, and Dunkel-Schetter, 1998), the experience of insensitivity and minimization by others can have a considerable effect on a woman's recovery. Victim-blaming and negative social reactions are common for all rape survivors, but are particularly pronounced for women who are raped by someone with whom they have a prior intimate relationship. In comparing social reactions to survivors of the four types of rape, Cowan (2000) found that victim-blame was most likely to occur in cases of partner and date rape. Even though these survivors are similarly affected despite their relationship to the perpetrator (Cowan; Resnick *et al.*, 2000; Schwartz and Leggett, 1999), they receive more blame and less support than survivors of stranger rapes. Women who are survivors of rape committed by someone they know and trust, therefore, may be particularly at risk for negative social, medical, or legal reactions.

Treatment Approach for Rape Survivors

The treatment approach described that follow draws from best practice guidelines for the treatment of PTSD (Foa *et al.*, 1999). The multimodal format for rape survivors encompasses four treatment strategies designed to address specific PTSD symptoms:

1. To provide education about commonly experienced PTSD symptoms through psycho education;
2. To facilitate the client's retelling of the event through exposure-based techniques;
3. To challenge the client's maladaptive beliefs about her role in the event through cognitive restructuring; and
4. To enhance her coping skills through anxiety management techniques.

1. Psycho Education

All supported treatments for rape-related trauma include an educational component (Foa *et al.*, 1999; Marotta, 2000). While this approach alone does not reduce symptoms in the long-term (Rauch, Hembree, and Foa, 2001), it has been demonstrated to be most effective when combined with TF CBT, Narrative Exposure therapy, exposure-based techniques, cognitive therapy, and anxiety management. Early in treatment, clients can be provided with education about PTSD symptoms. Clients experience relief as they recognize they are not "crazy", but are experiencing manifestations of PTSD, a reaction to trauma experienced by most women who are raped (Rauch *et al.*). Psychotherapist/counsellors can also provide clients with written materials outlining rape survivors' commonly experienced thoughts and feelings (e.g. fear, guilt, anger, shame, embarrassment, betrayal, powerlessness, depression) to review as homework.

As clients view their symptoms as a response to trauma rather than as pathology (Bratton, 1999; Lubin and Johnson, 1997), they can strengthen esteem and a sense of self-worth. To this end, mental health counsellors can teach the client to separate her PTSD symptoms and reactions from her view of herself as an individual. Through psycho-education, clients can identify strengths that the trauma did not disrupt, including intellect, perseverance, and coping skills (Lubin and Johnson). Clients may also be empowered through education regarding the impact of socio-cultural processes that perpetuate rape. Further, they can discuss and dispel commonly accepted rape myths including the belief that the survivor somehow invited the rape and is responsible for the crime. These psycho-educational segments can be structured in the form of a mini-lecture used to begin and end the session to balance the intensity of each session (Williams and Sommer, 1994).

2. Exposure Therapy

The goal of this phase of treatment is to assist the survivor in working through painful memories by confronting specific situations, emotions, and thoughts that have become associated with the rape and which currently evoke intense anxiety and fear. As survivors recount thoughts, feelings, and memories surrounding the rape, a highly formalized, structured approach is needed to help them face this emotionally charged material (Johnson and Lubin, 2000). Narrative Exposure Therapy (NET)

Common Thread, Prolonged Exposure (PE) incorporates imagined and *in vivo* exposure and is particularly well suited to address the PTSD symptoms of intrusive thoughts, flashbacks, and trauma-related fears (Foa *et al.*, 1999).

When survivors are asked to confront their fears, it is understandable that they will be resistant to this strategy. The counsellors can express empathy by acknowledging a survivor's fears and conveying positive expectations for her recovery (Draucker, 1999). Mental health counsellors also need to spend adequate time in educating clients about the rationale for this phase of treatment. As suggested by Foa, Rothbaum, and Steketee (1993), counsellors can explain the use of PE to clients in the following way:

- Memories, people, places, and activities now associated with the rape make you highly anxious, so you avoid them.
- Each time you avoid them you do not finish the process of digesting the painful experience, and so, it returns in the form of nightmare, flashbacks, and intrusive thoughts.
- You can begin to digest the experience by gradually exposing yourself to the rape in your imagination and by holding the memory without pushing it away.
- You will also practice facing those activities, places, and situations that currently evoke fear.
- Eventually, you will be able to think about the rape and resume your normal activities without experiencing intense fear.

After explaining the rationale for the use of these techniques, counsellors can utilize imaginal exposure to assist clients in repeatedly recounting the memories associated with the rape until the thoughts no longer induce intense fear and anxiety (Foa *et al.*, 1999). As clients close their eyes, they are asked to describe the rape as if it were happening in the present, including all details, feelings, thoughts, and behaviours. They are asked to visualize and describe the rape as vividly as possible. As part of this process, mental health counsellors will often instruct clients to select a number ranging from 0 to 100 that best represents their current level of anxiety or discomfort. Termed Subjective Units of Distress (SUD), these self-ratings are elicited prior to, during, and after the rape description as a method for assessing progress in reducing anxiety over time (Meadows and Foa, 1998). The rape scenario is repeated several times per session, long enough for the discomfort and anxiety to be experienced and then decreased. Meadows and Foa (1998) recommended that these descriptions be audiotaped, as clients may then listen to the tapes as daily homework assignments. Writing about the event in a journal is also recommended (Harris, 1998; Resick and Schnicke, 1993). Through the use of journaling, clients can recount the details and emotions associated with the event, and then read these entries aloud in session. As this exercise is completed over the course of several weeks, clients are asked to increase the level of detail and emotion with each repetition (Harris). Mental health counsellors should assist clients in processing their emotions following the use of imaginary exposure to decrease intensity prior to the end of the session. They can also acknowledge the difficulty of this phase of treatment and can reinforce a client's willingness to face and work through her fears. According to Foa *et al.* (1995), clients are empowered when they recognize their successes in confronting anxiety-producing memories and in tolerating the resulting emotions.

The third component of PE is the use of *in vivo* exposure. As described by Meadows and Foa (1998), the survivor is asked to focus upon those activities and situations associated with the rape that are now safe, but that she currently fears or avoids, thus causing significant disruptions in her daily functioning. Mental health counsellors can assist survivors in creating a list of avoided situations and then in hierarchically ordering these items so that they range from least to most distressing. A SUD rating is assigned to each situation. Starting with the situation that causes the least distress, the client remains in that situation for a minimum of 30 minutes. This time period is deemed long enough for her to experience anxiety, challenge and evaluate her ideas about the actual danger present in the situation, and let the anxiety decrease. She is asked to rate her anxiety through SUD ratings and to note reductions in these ratings as she experiences these feared situations and activities. For example, a college student who refuses to attend classes due to her fear of all men who resemble her perpetrator can practice studying in the library with a friend as a step towards resuming class attendance. Over the course of several sessions, she can progress through the hierarchy until she is able to resume her normal activities and routines.

The use of PE is effective for women survivors of rape who have intact memory of the attack, but these techniques need to be modified for use with women who experience memory impairment. A survivor can be reassured that she does not have to access and re-experience the rape in order for recovery to occur, but she does need to recognize the significance and impact of the rape in her life (Williams and Sommer, 1994). Clients who cannot recall the actual rape will not be able to recount or journal about the concrete details surrounding the event. While writing in a journal is a helpful way for clients whose memories are intact to process their experiences, writing is not a recommended strategy for survivors in accessing memories of trauma (Feldman, Johnson, and Ollayos, 1994). However, survivors may benefit from re-experiencing the emotions and thoughts that occurred immediately prior to and following the memory loss. *In vivo* exposure may also be helpful for clients who avoid feared cues associated with the rape, regardless of their memory impairment of details of the actual event.

If a survivor has no verbal memories of the rape, emotions associated with the event may be accessed through non-verbal means. As suggested by Harris (1998), "the body remembers what the mind forgets" (p. 96). Techniques for use with survivors of drug-facilitated sexual assault or alcohol-induced memory impairment can, therefore, include alternative, experiential approaches drawn from art, music, or dance/movement therapies (*see* Johnson, 2000, for a review). The use of art has been recommended for survivors of rape as a means to access emotions that have been visually encoded (Backos and Pagon, 1999; Hargrave-Nyakaza, 1994). Art described as a visual dialogue (Spring, 1994), can give the survivor with no verbal memory something tangible to hold onto during the counselling process and can also represent a survivor's progress in counselling. Further, Stuhlmiller (1994) suggested that survivors with memory impairment may also benefit from movement and activity to rebuild body awareness and access imagery and emotions related to the rape.

3. Cognitive Therapy

Cognitive approaches have demonstrated efficacy in treating survivors of rape (Foa *et al.*, 1993; Meadows and Foa, 1998; Resick and Schnicke, 1993) and are particularly recommended for addressing symptoms of numbing, detachment, loss of interest in activities, irritability, guilt, and shame (Foa *et al.*, 1999). In cognitive therapy, clients are taught to identify the thoughts or beliefs they experience during negative emotional states. The counsellor and client then collaboratively evaluate the validity and challenge the helpfulness of these ideas and subsequently replace irrational beliefs with rational or beneficial thoughts (Meadows and Foa). This process can also be incorporated with thought stopping, in which maladaptive beliefs are stopped and replaced with positive thoughts

(Muran and DiGiuseppe, 2000). Resick and Schnicke also used cognitive restructuring principles in their Cognitive Processing Therapy (CPT) designed for rape victims. As part of the CPT approach, survivors are assisted in identifying and then challenging maladaptive beliefs and "stuck points" related to five areas: self-blame, power, esteem, trust, and intimacy. In the paragraphs that follow, literature related to these five issues is presented.

Self-blame and guilt—The counsellors can play a critical role in assisting survivors in challenging self-blame, even when victim-blame is perpetuated by society and significant others in their lives. In one study of survivors of rape, all women experienced victim-blame from their support systems, but the women who experienced the highest distress following rape were those who incorporated these negative reactions into their views of themselves (Regehr, Marziali, and Jansen, 1999). Of women who blamed themselves for the crime, some survivors assigned blame to their behaviour, while others attributed blame to their character (Muran and DiGiuseppe, 2000). Those who attributed blame to their behaviour (e.g., "I could have gone home earlier that night") experienced fewer symptoms than those who blamed their character ("I deserved this" or "I am a bad person"). The issue of guilt is often related to self-blame. Trauma-related guilt issues can include perceived responsibility for causing the rape, beliefs that decisions made and actions taken during the rape were not justified, or the belief that one knew what was going to happen and did not do enough to prevent the crime (Kubany, 1998). As self-blaming and guilt-related beliefs are reviewed during counselling sessions, these thoughts can be replaced with more logical self-statements that reflect the client's strengths and power (Kubany, 1998). For example, she can replace the thought "I made a stupid decision to go to my date's apartment, and since I could have prevented it, I deserved what happened to me" with "I may have made a decision I wouldn't make now, but the rapist is responsible for this crime. I will do everything I can now to regain the power he took away from me." As part of reducing self-blame and guilt, survivors can continue to examine the socio-cultural forces that perpetuate victim-blame, and they can use this knowledge in restructuring their beliefs about their role in the rape. This type of cognitive restructuring can also help to assuage the negative effects of victim-blame frequently encountered by survivors of rape.

Power and control—Treatment should be designed to assist survivors in restoring personal power that was temporarily disrupted during the assault. Due to the perpetrator's violent use of power and control, however, women may initially view all issues related to power as negative and may attempt to avoid regaining personal power (Carey, 1998). Through cognitive restructuring, clients' negative views of power and control can be replaced with empowering beliefs that equate power with recovery. While the client was indeed powerless at the time of the rape, she can learn to make the distinction between this temporary lack of control and her ability to make decisions in the present regarding the direction of her recovery. Survivors who develop a sense of agency have more positive treatment outcomes; Regehr, Marziali, and associates (1999) found that rape survivors who were able to view themselves as active agents in determining the results of events in their lives experienced fewer symptoms of PTSD and depression than did women with an external locus of control. As an important part of regaining a sense of power, mental health counsellors can encourage clients to take an active role in treatment by providing choices and flexibility regarding counselling goals and in the timing and pacing of sessions. Clients who claim the direction of their treatment are empowered to be the "authors and arbiters of their own recovery" (Draucker, 1999: 18).

Self-esteem, intimacy, and trust—It is important to explore the impact of rape on a survivor's self-image. Resick and Schnicke (1993) recommend asking clients to examine their meanings of the rape, and what effect it has had on their view of themselves. Clients' answers to these questions can reveal a pattern of stuck points (e.g. "I am unlovable because this happened to me") that can be challenged and reframed. Survivors' difficulties with self-esteem are interconnected with issues of trust and intimacy. If a survivor questions her judgement, engages in self-blame, and experiences victim-blame following rape, she may experience problems in trusting both herself and others. As rape is a trauma intentionally inflicted upon a woman by another individual; critical issues to explore in counselling will include disruptions in her capacity for intimacy and her ability to trust others (Draucker, 1999).

As clients challenge maladaptive beliefs in recovery, they can eventually learn to view the rape and its aftermath as a traumatic but growth-enhancing experience (Williams and Sommer, 1994) that provides them with a more flexible worldview (Koss and Kilpatrick, 2001). According to Frazier and Burnett (1994), 57 per cent of adult rape survivors in their sample cited positive changes that resulted from their rape experience (e.g. improved interpersonal relationships, enhanced self-awareness, and spiritual growth). Studies in resilience theory demonstrate that resilient individuals are those who grow and develop as a result of trauma. Rather than being stunted by life difficulties, they recover from traumatic events with an increased sense of empathy, enhanced coping skills, and greater capacity for intimacy (Young-Eisendrath, 1996). Regehr, Cadell *et al.* (1999) found similar qualities in a study of survivors of sexual assault who displayed the most resilience in recovery. These women possessed a sense of safety and trust, a positive view of self, a sense of power, positive relationships, the ability to employ cognitive reframing, and a refusal to engage in self-blame. Survivors who strengthen these qualities and skills in recovery will also develop the ability to cope more effectively with future life demands. Further, they may become empowered to engage in advocacy and activism in working to reduce the prevalence of sexual violence (Robinson and Howard-Hamilton, 2000).

4. Anxiety Management

While there are a variety of anxiety management techniques, Stress Inoculation Training (SIT) is one of the most researched and comprehensive anxiety management programmes for survivors of sexual assault and rape (Meadows and Foa, 1998). The goal of SIT is to promote a set of coping skills that help to reduce general anxiety, hypervigilance, hyperarousal, sleep disturbances, and difficulty in concentration (Foa *et al.*, 1999). These coping skills include muscle relaxation training, controlled breathing exercises, role playing, covert modelling, and positive thinking and self-talk, assertiveness training, guided self-imagery and dialogue, and thought stopping. Krakow *et al.* (2001) recently examined the use of an anxiety management technique in reducing PTSD-related sleep disturbance and nightmares. In a randomized, controlled study of women survivors of sexual assault who experienced nightmares and insomnia, participants were asked to consider their nightmares as learned habits that are influenced by what they think about during the day. Through the use of imagery rehearsal, women were asked to select one of their disturbing dreams, to change the dream, and to describe the new dream in writing. Over the course of three sessions, survivors were asked to describe the new dream using self-imagery, and to rehearse the new dream throughout the week for at least 5 to 20 minutes. According to Krakow and colleagues, the survivors in the treatment group experienced a significant decrease in overall PTSD symptoms when compared with survivors in the control group. Further, as the survivors who learned to use self-imagery gained a greater sense of control over their nightmares, they also implemented these techniques as a successful method for coping with other problems in their lives. Clients are empowered as they develop these and other anxiety management techniques to facilitate recovery from rape-related trauma.

Conclusions

In conclusion, Psychotherapists/counsellors can provide sensitive treatment for survivors of rape by balancing their focus on PTSD symptom reduction with support, validation, and client empowerment (Draucker, 1999). While the recommended strategies and methods described in this model are straightforward, the actual process of recovery from rape-related trauma is long and difficult (Koss and Kilpatrick, 2001). Survivors are vulnerable to victim-blame, self-blame, unwillingness to disclose the rape to others, and an overall lack of support in addition to PTSD symptoms and other significant negative psychological and physiological outcomes. By integrating the support that survivors need with a structured treatment approach for rape-related trauma symptoms, counsellors can best assist survivors of rape in their journey towards recovery.

References

American Psychiatric Association. (2000). *Diagnostic and Statistical Manual of Mental Disorders* (4th ed., text rev.). Washington, DC: Author.

Ahrens, C.E., and Campbell, R. (2000). Assisting rape victims as they recover from rape: The impact on friends. *Journal of Interpersonal Violence*, 15, 959-986.

Backos, A.K. and Pagon, B.E. (1999). Finding a voice: Art therapy with female adolescent sexual abuse survivors. *Art Therapy: Journal of the American Art Therapy Association,* 16, 126-132.

Bourque, L.B. (1989). *Defining rape*. Durham, NC: Duke University Press.

Bratton, M. (1999). *From Surviving to Thriving*. New York: Hawthorn Maltreatment and Trauma Press.

Breitenbecher, H.B. and Gidycz, C.A. (1998). An empirical evaluation of a programme designed to reduce the risk of multiple sexual victimization. *Journal of Interpersonal Violence,* 13, 472-489.

Brener, N.D., McMahon, P.M., Warren, C.W., and Douglas, K.A. (1999). Forced sexual intercourse and associated health-risk behaviours among female college students in the United States. *Journal of Consulting and Clinical Psychology*, 67, 252-259.

Brownmiller, S. (1975). *Against Our Will: Men, Women, and Rape*. New York: Bantam.

Campbell, R., Raja, S., and Grining, P.L. (1999). Training mental health professionals on violence against women. *Journal of Interpersonal Violence*, 14, 1002-1013.

Carey, L.A. (1998). Illuminating the process of a rape survivors' support group. *Social Work with Groups*, 21, 103-116.

Clum, G.A., Nishith, P., and Resick, P.A. (2001). Trauma-related sleep disturbance and self-reported physical health symptoms in treatment-seeking female rape victims. *Journal of Nervous and Mental Disease*, 189, 618-622.

Cowan, G. (2000, May). Beliefs about the causes of four types of rape. *Sex Roles: A Journal of Research*, 807-824.

Donovan, J.W. (2000). Gamma-hydroxybutyrate, Gamma-Butyrolactone, and Butanediol: Abuse and effects. *Journal of Toxicology: Clinical Toxicology*, 38(2), 184.

Draucker, C.B. (1999). The psychotherapeutic needs of women who have been sexually assaulted. *Perspectives in Psychiatric Care*, 35, 18-29.

Dunn, P.C., Vail-Smith, K., and Knight, S.M. (1998). What date/acquaintance rape victims tell others: A study of college student recipients of disclosure? *Journal of American College Health*, 47, 213-220.

Easton, A., Summers, J., Tribble, J., Wallace, P.B., and Lock, R.S. (1997). College women's perceptions regarding resistance to sexual assault. *Journal of American College Health*, 46, 127-132.

Feldman, P.J., Ullman, J.B., and Dunkel-Schetter, C. (1998). Women's reactions to rape victims: Motivational processes associated with blame and social support. *Journal of Applied Social Psychology*, 28, 469-503.

Feldman, S.C., Johnson, D.R., and Ollayos, M. (1994). The use of writing in the treatment of PTSD. In M.B. Williams and J.F. Sommer (Eds.), *Handbook of Post-traumatic Therapy* (pp. 366-385). Westport, CT: Greenwood.

Foa, E.B., Davidson, J.R.T., and Frances, A. (1999). Expert consensus guideline series: Treatment of post-traumatic stress disorder. *The Journal of Clinical Psychiatry*, 60 (Suppl.16), 1-31.

Foa, E.B., Hearst-Ikeda, D., and Perry, K.J. (1995). Evaluation of a brief cognitive-behavioural programme for the prevention of chronic PTSD in recent assault victims. *Journal of Consulting and Clinical Psychology*, 63, 948-955.

Foa, E.B., Rothbaum, B.O., and Steketee, G.S. (1993). Treatment of rape victims. *Journal of Interpersonal Violence*, 8, 256-276.

Frazier, P.A., and Burnett, J.W. (1994). Immediate coping strategies among rape victims. *Journal of Counselling and Development*, 72, 633-639.

Hansen, L.S., Gama, E.M.P., and Harkins, A.K. (2002). Revisiting gender issues in multicultural counselling. In P.B. Pedersen, J.G. Draguns, W.J. Lonner, and J.E. Trimble (Eds.), *Counselling Across Cultures* (5th ed., pp. 163-184). Thousand Oaks, CA: Sage.

Hargrave-Nyakaza, K. (1994). An application of art therapy to the trauma of rape. *Art Therapy: A Journal of the American Art Therapy Association*, 11, 53-57.

Harris, M. (1998). *Trauma Recovery and Empowerment: A Clinician's Guide for Working with Women in Groups.* New York: Free Press.

Johnson, D.R. (2000). Creative therapies. In E.B. Foa *et al.* (Eds.), *Effective Treatments for PTSD: Practice Guidelines from the International Society for Traumatic Stress Studies* (pp. 302-314). New York: Guilford.

Johnson, D.R., and Lubin, H. (2000). Group psychotherapy for symptoms of PTSD. In R.H. Klein and V. Schermer (Eds.), *Group Psychotherapy for Psychological Trauma* (pp. 141-169). New York: Guilford.

Kessler, B.L., and Bieschke, K.J. (1999). A retrospective analysis of shame, dissociation, and adult victimization in survivors of childhood sexual abuse. *Journal of Counselling Psychology,* 46, 335-341.

Kimerling, R., and Calhoun, K.S. (1994). Somatic symptoms, social support, and treatment seeking among sexual assault victims. *Journal of Consulting and Clinical Psychology*, 62, 333-340.

Koss, M.P., and Kilpatrick, D.G. (2001). Rape and sexual assault. In E. Gerrity, T. Keane, and F. Tuma (eds.), *Mental Health Consequences of Torture* (pp. 177-193). New York: Plenum.

16

Violence Against Women

Nature, Consequences and Rehabilitation Strategies

Shalini Mittal and *Tushar Singh*

Introduction

March 8th every year is celebrated as International Women's Day, but even then the incidences of violence against women have been continuously increasing to pandemic proportions. The society still has a patriarchal structure where women are considered secondary to males who use violence against women to control them and assert their power. Violence against women is a collective term used to refer to violent acts that are primarily or exclusively perpetrated against women. Often it is considered to be a hate crime. In India, several legislative provisions have been made to protect women and to punish those involved in such incidences (i.e. Dowry Prohibition Act, 1961, Protection of Women from Domestic Violence Act, 1994, Immoral Traffic (Prevention) Act, 1956, Muslim Women (Protection of Rights on Divorce) Act, 1986, Criminal Law (Amendment) Act, 2013 etc.). Despite the provisions and enforcement of such strict legislation, many cases of gender violence go unreported. Women face different types of violence throughout their lifetime ranging from domestic violence, rape, molestation, dowry death and kidnapping. A global review of WHO (2013) has indicated that 35 per cent of women worldwide have been a victim of at least some form of abuse including physical, sexual, intimate partner and non-partner violence. However, the data from United Nation's national violence studies show that almost 70 per cent of women have suffered physical and sexual violence in their lifetime, by their intimate partners (UN Women, 2012). In fact, violence against women is not confined to a single culture or country. Literature, art, and historical documents have evidence that women across many cultures throughout the history were forced into sexual encounters (Brownmiller, 1975; Zeitlin, 1986).

Types of Violence against Women

Violence against women can be of many types: physical, sexual, psychological and economic. Minor forms of victimization in the form of sexist statements, sexually tainted whistles are quite common. Other more serious forms of violence especially rapes are also deeply embedded in our society. In 1992, Linda L. Marshall constructed Severity of Violence against Women Scales that helped in conceptualizing different dimensions and levels of the severity of violence against women. These are threats of violence, acts of violence and sexual aggression. Each of these dimensions differs in the level of severity from mild to moderate and serious acts of violence. Threats of violence refer to symbolic violence and may involve mild, moderate and serious acts of violence (e.g. driven dangerously with you in the car, shook a fist at you, threaten to destroy property, threatened to kill you, respectively). Similarly, acts of physical violence may be minor, mild, moderate and serious (e.g. pushing or shoving you, pulling hair, slapping with the back of his hand, and choking, respectively). Sexual Aggression involves forcing the women into sexual encounters (e.g. physically forced you to have sex). Below mentioned are some of the major forms of violence against women:

1. ***Violence by an intimate partner***: Violence by an intimate partner refers to physical violence inflicted by an intimate partner where the woman might be beaten, coerced into sex or otherwise abused.
2. ***Sexual violence***: Women often have to face sexual exploitation in the form of rape, attempted rape, marital rape, the practice of child marriage, human trafficking.
3. ***Female genital mutilation/genital cutting***: Refers to several types of traditional cutting operations performed on women and girls. Such practices are predominant in certain countries of Africa and Middle East.
4. ***Dowry murders***: Dowry murders refer to a practice where the husband or the in-laws kill the woman for the want of dowry. Although dowry as a practice is prevalent in many countries, dowry murders are mostly prevalent in South Asian countries.
5. ***Violence during pregnancy***: Often pregnant women have to face

physical violence that can have serious health problems for the mother and the child. Practices of female infanticide, prenatal sex selection and systematic neglect of girl child are widespread in Middle East, South and East Asia, North Africa.

6. ***Honour killing***: In many cultures, the relatives kill women who engage in activities that are thought to be a threat to the honour of the family. Such practices include engaging in premarital sex, adultery, marrying up men of their choice (love marriage). Even women who are only suspected of engaging in such activities are killed along with victims of rape.

Impact of Violence

The incidences involving violence against women are perpetually increasing. So, it becomes increasingly necessary to understand the needs and sufferings of these victims. There is sufficient evidence to show that victims of violence against women suffer from various physiological, psychological and social problems.

1. ***Physiological impact***: The victims of violence may suffer from the physical trauma that refers to physical injury caused due to an external force. They may suffer from several physical injuries ranging from minor bruises to fractures of the bones to more severe internal injuries. Acid attacks and other physical acts of violence may even cause disfigurement. Sexual violence poses a risk of many health risks including increased incidences of abrasion, bleeding and the possibility of HIV/AIDS and other sexually transmitted diseases. It may also lead to miscarriage, pre-term labour, and low birth weight. Many times victims even die because of the severity of the injuries.
2. ***Financial impact***: Costs of victimization are often high. In addition to physical injuries, victims of violence against women are forced to pay off huge medical bills. Their personal belongings may be damaged, destroyed or even stolen. Sometimes, victims move to a different location away from the site where the violence occurred. In such cases, they are forced to incur relocation expenses. They also face a loss of wages due to incapacitation, taking time off from work to repair the damage, participation in criminal proceedings and seeking medical health treatment.

3. ***Social impact***: Often there is a social stigma attached to certain crimes, such as rapes. As a result, such victims are not accepted well in the society. They may become a subject of gossip and may be avoided by others. Often victims are even blamed for their plight and as a result they often face isolation. Sometimes, they may even have to bear with unwanted sympathy and in other cases with complete lack of sympathy. They may suffer from disturbances in their relationships with others, especially with husbands, boyfriends or family members. These disturbances may even lead to ending of these relations. In addition, often rape victims have problems finding a marriage partner.
4. ***Psychological and emotional impact***: Violence leaves scars that heal slowly. The severity of the harm caused varies from one person to another and depends on the severity of the violence. The consequences manifest themselves in various health problems and psychological problems. Victims experience feelings of shock, terror and numbness because of victimization. Often, because the society blames them for what happened, they experience shame, helplessness and even guilt. They may have difficulty trusting others in addition to experiencing intense sorrow, anger and rage and anxiety. According to Rees *et al.* (2011), women who have had a history of violence had worse mental health in terms of both, current mental health problems and occurrence of mental health problems throughout the lifetime. In addition, there was an increased likelihood of these women to have physical and mental disability and reduced quality of life. The experience of serious sexual assault and rape has been found to be associated with mental health disturbances in a significant proportion of victims (Kilpatrick *et al.*, 1985). In fact, for the rape victims, the trouble does not end with the ending of the actual rape. After the incident, the victim must escape from the assailant and alert others about her distress (Burgess and Holmstrom, 1980). A study by Khanna (2008) noticed that women who suffered sexual violence were traumatized by how the forensic exam was conducted. Many reported that it felt like another form of sexual violence. Women of aggravated assault were more likely than rape victims to report that they feared for their lives during the assault (Riggs, Kilpatrick and Resnick, 1992). There is sufficient evidence to suggest that depression and post-traumatic stress disorder is

common among victims of violence against women. Stein *et al.* (1988) suggested that a high percentage of women who experience sexual assault suffer from a major depressive episode. In a study conducted in Spain, 330 patients who were affected by psychological traumas such as sexual assault, domestic violence, and terrorism, were examined. Among them, 54.5 per cent were diagnosed with PTSD, which was more frequent in victims of sexual assault and terrorism (Echeburua *et al.*, 2003). Some victims of crimes that are repetitive in nature, such as domestic violence, develop learned helplessness that can produce feelings of helplessness, hopelessness, can limit efficient performance in a variety of areas, inhibit motivation, and can produce emotional reactions that are similar to symptoms of clinical depression (Seligman, 1980). Victims may also experience sequelae of victimization such as Rape Trauma Syndrome and Battered Women Syndrome.

Rape Trauma Syndrome

Rape Trauma Syndrome is a group of behavioural, psychological and physical symptoms that are experienced by victims of rape and are clustered into the acute phase and long-term reorganization process. The phrase 'Rape Trauma Syndrome' was coined by Dr. Ann Wolbert Burgess and Dr. Lynda Holmstrom in 1974 following a comprehensive study of alleged rape victims at Boston City Hospital between 1972 and 1973. The syndrome occurs in two phases. The acute phase begins during the rape itself and continues for next 2-3 weeks. During this phase, the victims experience a number of somatic manifestations such as physical trauma, skeletal muscle tension, gastrointestinal irritability and genitourinary disturbances along with several emotional reactions, such as feelings of fear, humiliation, embarrassment, anger, revenge and self-blame. The victims may exhibit an 'expressed emotional style' which is characterized by feelings of fear, anger and anxiety that are revealed through crying, sobbing, smiling, restlessness and tenseness. In other cases, the victims may exhibit a 'controlled emotional style' which is characterized by hidden feelings that are reflected in their calm and composed effect. The acute phase is followed by the second phase known as the long-term reorganization process. This stage may last for a period of six months to a year or longer. The first major symptom of this phase is the increased motor activity that is reflected by a change in residence. Many victims move to a different location away from the place where the rape had occurred; they change their telephone numbers. Victims also turn to family members and friends for support during this phase. The victim does all this in an effort to retain a normal existence and to ensure their safety. The second major symptom is the occurrence of nightmares that are usually of two types: firstly, those in which the victim wishes to do something, but then wakes-up before they could take an action; secondly, those in which the victim takes an action and fights with her attacker; and the third major symptom is the 'traumatophobia' which refers to a phobic reaction to a traumatic situation. Fear of people behind them, fear of crowds, fear of indoors, and fear of outdoors are some examples of traumatophobia.

Battered Women Syndrome

The term 'Battered Women Syndrome' was coined by psychologist Lenore Walker for a set of distinct psychological and behavioural symptoms that occur as a result of prolonged exposure to situations of intimate partner violence. She suggested two particular theories about battered women: firstly, the cycle theory of battering and secondly, an adaptation of Martin Seligman's theory of learned helplessness (Walker, 1984). Cycle theory of violence suggests that spousal abuse occurred in cycles characterized by varying degrees of severity. In the first tension building stage, the victim will have to face verbal and emotional abuse along with minor incidents of physical violence (e.g. slapping). In order to avoid such situations in future, the victim will try to placate the abuser but, on the contrary, such behaviour reinforces violent tendencies. This passivity leads to the second stage of acute battering incident during which the victim's sense of fear and perceptions of danger are maximum along with the risk of death or serious injury although the severity of violence may vary. Then the third phase of loving contrition follows, during which the abuser tries to convince the victims that they would change, and such incidents would not happen in future. Walker suggested that even if a victim experiences the cycle once, that will be enough for her to develop battered women syndrome and adopt behavioural patterns that reflect learned helplessness.

Walker also utilized an adaptation of Seligman's learned helplessness theory to explain why battered women fail to leave their abusers. Walker suggested that like the electric shock, prolonged exposure to battering situations leads to a kind of psychological paralysis that is similar to the concept of learned helplessness proposed by Seligman. Over the time, the woman's motivation to respond and to bring about a change diminishes.

Rehabilitation of Victims of Violence

Violence against women causes severe physical and mental health issues for such victims. However, support services are typically meagre. It is very essential to understand the needs and problems of these victims so as to help them retrieve control over their lives. The laws protect the rights of the offender well. However, to recognize and safeguard a victim's right to rehabilitation is equally important. Rehabilitation is to restore to useful life, through therapy and education or to restore to good condition, operation or capacity. For the rehabilitation process to be successful, it is crucial to identify the resources that a victim has for coping. Resources are sources, utilization of which would lead to increased well-being.

1. ***Personal resources***: Optimistic, capable, healthy and affluent individuals are perceived to be resourceful. These resources are crucial in the face of challenging or threatening situations. In addition to actual competence, perceived competence is equally essential for an individual to cope. If the individual underestimates one's personal resources, effective adaptive strategies are less likely to develop. It is known as perceived self-efficacy (Bandura, 1992). Low self-efficacy is associated with depression, anxiety and helplessness. Individuals with high self-efficacy can identify their personal resources better and hence, are better able to cope and return to a normal level of functioning.
2. ***Social resources***: Social support has been found to be beneficial in coping (Rodin and Salovey, 1989). Social support may refer to the actual resources provided by others to the victims or the social support perceived by the receiver. Both, actual and perceived social support, have been found to play a crucial role in coping along with engagement in activities with others. West, Frank, Anderson and Stewart (1984), found that the unsupportive behaviour of others was associated with poorer psychological adjustment of the victims.
3. ***Psychological resources***: Psychological beliefs such as optimism, personal control, a sense of meaning have been found to be protective of physical and mental health in the face of

threatening situations. Such psychological beliefs have special significance in helping the people to cope with intensely stressful and life threatening situations (Taylor and Brown, 1984). Several pieces of research indicate that dispositional optimism is positively related to positive changes and benefits after stressful situations (Curbow, *et al.*, 1993; Davis *et al.*, 1998).

Approaches to Rehabilitation of Victims

Modes of Victims' Right to Rehabilitation

There are various modes of victims' right to rehabilitation that include access to justice and fair treatment, i.e. compensation, reparation, and victim assistance.

- *Compensation*: In cases where the court feels that there is a need for rehabilitation of victims, compensation may be recommended. In India, compensation of victims of crime may be given by courts under section 357 of Code of Criminal Procedure (Cr. P.C.). However, the victim does not have a guaranteed right except that they may get some assistance in the form of payment for compensation. Compensation provided under section 357A of Cr. P.C. is general in nature and covers all crimes, but there is also a scheme meant specifically for rape victims. National Commission of Women has proposed a Criminal Injuries Compensation Board for the payment of compensation to victims of rape.
- *Reparation*: Reparation as means of compensation is very broad and inclusive in scope. It involves acknowledging that serious wrongs have been done and that the injured person is qualified for remedy and redress by right. It not only includes monetary and non-monetary compensation, but also restitution, rehabilitation, satisfaction and guarantees of non-repetition.
- *Victim assistance*: Apart from providing compensation, victim assistance is crucial for rehabilitation of victims. It includes services like crisis intervention, counselling, emergency shelter, criminal justice advocacy and emergency transportation.

Coping with the Trauma

Psychologists have proposed various models to explain the process of victimization and subsequent coping attempts that may be different for different victims.

1. ***Levison's Coping Model***: Casarez Levison (1992) proposed a model of coping for victims, which follows the person from the pre-crime state, to the crime and immediate after-effects, early coping and finally, reorganization. The model includes the following stages:

   Stage 1: *Pre-victimization/Organization*—This stage focuses on the adaptation level of the victim prior to victimization. This includes the person's economic, social, personal and psychological resources. It focuses on how the person dealt with stressors of the daily life prior to victimization.

   Stage 2: *Victimization/Disorganization*—This stage focuses on the criminal event itself and first few hours to 2 days after the criminal event. During this stage, the person is the victim and may experience traumatic stress, disorganization, physical or psychological injury along with feelings of anger, shock, disbelief, helplessness and hopelessness.

   Stage 3: *Transition/Protection*—During this stage, the victims are in need of maximum support from their social networks and professionals. This support will help them to cope better. However, some victims may use maladaptive coping strategies such as alcohol and drug abuse. If the stressors continue, the victims will not be able to cope appropriately and move on to the final stage. On the contrary, they will reach a state of total exhaustion.

   Stage 4: *Reorganization/Resolution*—This stage focuses on consolidating and restoring the victim to a stable functioning person. It may take 6-12 months for some victims to reach this stage while others might take years. This stage involves returning to normal relations and daily life routine. People may have to face feelings of denial and acceptance around their experience. Stage of reorganization does not mean returning to the pre-victimization state. It simply means that victims will have to incorporate the understanding of their victimization experience into their understanding of themselves and the world.

2. ***Psycho-social Coping Model***: Psycho-social Coping Model that was developed by Dussich (1985), serves as a general theory for understanding all forms of victimization and for facilitating recovery, which uses behavioural and legal concepts. This theory suggests that the physical, social and psychic interactive space within each individual tries to survive is the coping environment and is known as the coping milieu. Coping milieu is different for different problems and persons. The model begins with the coping milieu and the individual's personal resources that include repertoire, social assets (social class, sibling position, role etc.), psychic assets (e.g. intelligence, personality, education, skills), physical assets and time. The individual has these personal resources and confronts the problem in the milieu. Several continua make-up each problem which the individual evaluates at a moment in time. This heuristic that allows the individual to freeze time for problem appraisal is known as 'problem freeze'. The different problem moment continua are the time continuum (length of time for which the problem has existed), due continuum (time remaining for problem resolution), evolution continuum (the speed with which the problem became known), person continuum (number of persons in the problem), severity continuum (complexity of the problem), familiarity continuum (the extent to which the problem is known to the person), context continuum (the extent to which the problem is in or out of context), and the threat continuum (the extent of threat to a person's well-being). The psychosocial coping process has 4 phases each being a continuum within which the individual can make choices with failure most likely to be at one end and success most likely to be at the other end. The first is the prevention phase that begins with the awareness that a problem is possible. During this phase, denying the likelihood of a problem will more likely cause failure whereas reasonable anticipation of a problem will more likely cause success. The second is the preparation phase that starts with the awareness that a problem is imminent. This awareness will cause the person to engage in an appraisal, rehearsal, worrying and practicing. This behaviour is more likely to cause success. On the other hand, the absence of an appraisal, rehearsal, worrying and practicing is more likely to cause failure.

The third action phase begins when the problem is present. In the face of the problem, learned resourcefulness, diminished vulnerability, and self-delivered reassurance will help the person to cope. On the other hand, learned helplessness, disappointment in protective authorities and increased expectations of vulnerability will lead to failure in coping. The fourth phase reappraisal phase starts when the problem is over. During this phase, replay and assessment will result in secondary coping whereas the absence of replay and assessment will result in no secondary coping.

Scott, Oberst and Dropkin's coping framework (1980): Scott, Oberst and Dropkin (1980) proposed a coping framework that suggests five tasks of psychological recovery which are as follows:

1. *Mourn the Loss*: According to this model, the first task for psychological recovery should be to mourn the loss, be it of a sense of invincibility or physical attractiveness. It is crucial for the recovery that the seriousness of the loss must be realized fully.
2. *Confront the Loss*: The second task is to deal with the loss by confronting it. They should actively face the problem and not run away from it.
3. *Confront the Possible Denial*: Following victimization, often victims avoid going outside, interacting with others or avoid facing the problem. Such avoidance may lead to feelings of anger, isolation, depression and bitterness. Hence, it is important for the victim to recognize such forms of denial and deal with them.
4. *Reframe the Experience*: The fourth task involves redefining the experience of victimization. During this task, it is crucial for the victims to acknowledge the loss incurred, but they must find renewed hope and mastery in newly found skills.
5. *Integrate the Experience*: The final task of psychological recovery involves incorporating and integrating the experience of victimization and disfigurement into their over-all self-concept.

Transtheoretical Model of Change

The Transtheoretical Model of Change (TMC) (Prochaska, DiClemente and Norcross, 1992) focuses on the fact that different victims react differently and have different needs following the experience of violence and hence, emphasis should be on proving focused intervention to each victim. This model helps to the level of services that may be needed by the victim. Services should range from information sharing to intensive individual therapy. This should include pamphlets, psychological intervention, paraprofessional support, information. In addition to the primary victim, the victim's support network, and society too should be targeted. This will help the victims to assess their situation faster and relieve them the distress of searching for new resources.

Education of victim: It is crucial to educate the victim about the process of coping with the trauma. Victims should also be educated about the criminal justice procedure, professionals involved in their case and their respective roles. Apart from this, they should be educated about the goals and processes of therapy clearly so as to make an informed choice. For this purpose, information booklets, pamphlets, and information seminars may be used.

Education of support system: Natural supports should also be educated about how to provide emotional, informational and appraisal support. They should also be educated to help them better understand the traumatisation process and the possible reactions of the victims. They should also be trained on how to react their friend or partner's victimization.

Peer support groups: Not all victims require professional help. In such cases, peer support groups turn out to be quite cost-effective. These groups should also be linked to professionals in some way to help the victims get easy access to them whenever required.

Professional support groups: Professionally supervised support groups are useful for more severely traumatized victims who may not be ready to enter more active treatment programmes. In such cases, professional support groups help them build-up the strength required to enter into more active treatment programmes.

Therapy: Individual and group therapy provided by professionals proves helpful for the victims experiencing severe trauma. Such professionals can help identify the symptoms of trauma and provide therapies that best suits the needs of the victims. Some victims may need short-term intervention while others might require therapy for a longer time.

Paraprofessionals: Paraprofessionals working in victims' services serve an important function in examining the victims and the interventions that may prove beneficial. Taking into consideration the actual and perçeived social support may help victims, paraprofessionals help victims fill this gap, identify and understand their own problematic reactions that may stand in the way of successful recovery.

Conclusion

Violence against women has been showing an upward trend globally. Despite several people's efforts to bring about gender equality, availability of legislative provisions that protect the rights of women, they still hold a secondary position to males in this patriarchal society. Art, literature, newspapers and other documents bear witness to the fact that the incidences of violence against women have been increasing. It is discernible that victims do experience emotional, behavioural and cognitive changes as a result of victimization. The severity of the trauma not only depends on the severity of the crime itself but also, on the pre-victimization state of the individual, their coping strategies, and the interventions provided to them. However, compared to the amount of trauma experienced by these victims, support services are meagre. A prevalent attitude among law enforcement agencies seems to be that solving the cases is the major priority. Moreover, the rights of the offender are well protected, but little is spoken of the victim's rights. To ensure that the victim returns to being a normal functioning individual, it is necessary to safeguard their right to rehabilitation. The legal system can help the victims receive justice, compensation, and reparation as a part of the rehabilitation. The focus of the rehabilitation programme should be on helping the individual identify her personal, social and psychological resources required for coping and on identifying the individual needs of the victims. To ensure complete recovery, therapy best suiting the needs of the victims should be provided. In addition to this, victims, as well as their support network and society as a whole, should be educated about the traumatisation process, criminal justice system, goals and process of therapy. This will not only help the victims to identify and understand their own problematic behaviours but also help cultivate increased sensitivity towards victims in the society. Such an inclusive rehabilitation process will not undo the victimization experience nor will it restore the victim to the pre-victimization stage. But, it will help the victims to integrate the understanding of the victimization experience into their understanding of themselves and the world and gradually return to a daily life routine.

References

Bandura, A. (1992). Exercise of personal agency through the self-efficacy mechanism. In R. Schwarzer (Ed.), *Self-efficacy: Thought Control of Action* (pp. 3-38). Washington, DC: Hemisphere.

Burgess, A.W. and Holmstrom, L.L. (1980). Rape typology and the coping behaviour of rape victims. In S.L. McCombie (Ed.), *A Rape Crisis Intervention Handbook: A Guide for Victim Care* (pp. 27-40). Plenum Press, New York.

Burgess, A. and Holmstrom, L. (1974). Rape trauma syndrome. *American Journal of Psychiatry,* 131, 980-986.

Brownmiller, S. (1975). *Against Our Will: Men, Women and Rape*. New York: Bantam Books.

Casarez-Levison, R. (1992). An empirical investigation of coping strategies used by victims of crime: Victimization redefined. In E. Viano (ed.), *Critical Issues in Victimology: International Perspectives* (pp. 46-57). New York: Springer Publishing Co.

Chockalingam, K. (1993). Restitution to victims of crime in India: Recent developments. *Indian Journal of Criminology,* 21(2), 72-81.

Curbow, B., Somerfield, M., Baker, F., Wingard, J. and Legro, M. (1993). Personal changes, dispositional optimism, psychological adjustment to bone marrow transplantation. *Journal of Behavioural Medicine*, 16, 423-443.

Davis, C.G., Nolen-Hoeksema, S. and Larson J. (1998). Making sense of loss and benefiting from the experience: Two construals of meaning. *Journal of Personality and Social Psychology*, 75, 561-574.

Dussich, J.P.J. (1985). *New Perspectives in Control Theory: Social Coping of Youth Under Supervision.* Southern Illinois University, Carbondale.

Echeburua, E., Corral, P. and Amor, P.J. (2003). Evaluation of psychological harm in the victim of violent crime. *Psychology in Spain,* 7 (1), 10-18.

Khanna, R. (2008). Communal Violence in Gujarat, India: Impact of sexual violence and responsibilities of healthcare system. *Reproductive Health Matters,* 16 (31), 142-152.

Kilpatrick, D.G., Best, C.L., Veronen, L.J. *et al.* (1985). Mental health correlates of criminal victimization. A random community survey. *Journal of Consulting and Clinical Psychology*, 53, 866-873.

Prochaska, J.O., DiClemente, C.C. and Norcross, J.C. (1992). In search of how people change: Applications to addictive behaviours. *American Psychologist,* 47(9), 1102-1114.

Rees, S., Silove, D., Chey, T., Ivancic, L., Steel, Z., Creamer, M. and Forbes, D. (2011). Lifetime prevalence of gender based violence in women and the relationship with mental disorders and psychological function. *JAMA: Journal of American Medical Association*, 306 (5), 513-524.

Riggs, D.S., Kilpatrick, D.G. and Resnick, H.S. (1992). Long-term psychological distress associated with marital rape and aggravated assault: A comparison to other crime victims. *Journal of Family Violence,* 7 (4), 283-296.

Scott, D.W., Oberst, M.T. and Dropkin, M.J. (1980). A stress-coping model. *Advanced Nursing Science*, 3, pp. 9-23.

Seligman, M.E.P. (1980). A learned helplessness point of view. In L. Rehm (ed.), *Behaviour Therapy for Depression*, (pp. 123-142). Academic Press: New York.

Stein, J., Golding, J., Siegel, J., Burnam, M. and Sorenson, S. (1988). Long-term Psychological Sequelae of Child Sexual Abuse. *The Los Angeles Epidemiologic.*

Taylor, S.E. and Brown, J.D. (1988). Illusion and wellbeing: A social psychological perspective on mental health. *Psychological Bulletin,* 110, 192-210.

UN Women (2012). *Violence against women prevalence data: Surveys by country.* Accessed at http://www.endvawnow.org/uploads/browser/files/vawprevalence_matrix_june2013.pdf on 11-05-2015.

Walker, L.E. (1984), *The Battered Woman Syndrome,* Springer Publishing Company, New York.

West, D.G., Frank, E., Anderson, B. and Stewart, B.D. (1984). *Social Support and Post Rape Symptomatology.* University of Pittsburgh School of Medicine (unpublished manuscript).

World Health Organization (2013). *Global and regional estimates of violence against women: Prevalence and health effects of intimate partner violence and non-partner sexual violence.* Accessed at http://apps.who.int/iris/bitstream/10665/85239/1/9789241564625_eng.pdf on 11-05-2015.

Zeitlin, F. (1986). Configurations of rape myth. In S. Tomaselli and R. Porter (Eds.), *Rape: A Historical and Social Enquiry* (pp. 122-151). New York, Basil Blackwell.

17

Effectiveness of Reality Therapy in Multiple Perspectives

Nisha Kumari and *Anubhuti Dubey*

Introduction

Reality Therapy, an approach to psychotherapy and counselling was disseminated by William Glasser in 1960s. It holds a different view from traditional psychiatry, psychoanalysis and health model schools of psychotherapy. It concentrated on three Rs of psychiatry, i.e. realism, responsibility, and right-and-wrong. Reality Therapy asserts that the people are undergoing socially universal human circumstances rather than a mental illness. When the person fails to accomplish basic needs his behaviour deviate from the norm. The Reality Therapy does not take interest in a person's past—as gratifying fundamental needs is part of a person's present life. The Reality Therapy approach focuses on the here-and-now actions of the people and the ability to craft a better future. Moreover, unlike other forms of psychotherapy this therapy does not see to unconscious mental processes also.

Glasser (1965) argued that in a hurry to tag the population as mentally ill; the social component of psychological disorders has been extremely unnoticed. The reality therapy makes an attempt to branch out the client from the behaviour. Since a person go through the distress consequential from a social problem does not make him sick; it merely makes him out of synergy with his psychological needs. Actually, reality therapy lends a hand to people to scrutinize their wants and needs, assess behaviours, and build plans for satisfying their needs. Reality Therapy is a practical method that can be used by therapists, counsellors, teachers, parents, and others. Reality Therapy is most prominently applied in psychotherapy. It also consists of broken learning behaviour educated from years of not getting desires met and unlearning dysfunctional methods people have used to endure in the past.

Basic Conceptualization of Reality Therapy

The objectives of undertaking psychotherapy are usually to gain insight, to see connections, and to reach a higher level of self-awareness. However, the initial goal of reality therapy is behavioural change resulting in greater need satisfaction. People go through other forms of psychotherapy because they feel that something was amiss in their lives. But the reality therapist considers such individuals are not fulfilling their needs successfully, and as a result they experience discomfort, anxiety, depression, guilt, fear, or shame. Nevertheless, owing to the skilful use of reality therapy, it is likely to facilitate a person appraise whether behavioural change is looked for and feasible and whether adjusting to the burdens of the "real world" would be appropriate and satisfying. When the clients choose that change is advantageous to them, they are assisted to get on to better options intended to continue or add to their need gratification.

Reality Therapy is rooted in control theory, a system of brain functioning (Powers, 1973). Control theory maintains that the human brain functions like a thermostat that seeks to regulate its own behaviour in order to change the world around it. Glasser (1981, 1985) modified this theory to the clinical setting and devised it in a manner that makes it functional to therapists, counsellors, and others. The work of William Powers (1973) was greatly theoretical.

Human needs are innate, general, and universal, and not restricted to one specific race or culture. All human behaviour is intended to gratifying the four psychological needs, i.e. need for belonging, power, fun (or enjoyment), and freedom, with the physical need for survival. As an outcome of the satisfaction of these needs the person feels a sense of control that other theories propose to as self-actualization, self-fulfilment, or becoming a fully functioning person.

Psychological needs are positioned into the cerebral cortex, or new brain. For the reason people learn to cooperate and function as a unit, unearth belonging in families, schools, jobs, social clubs, and religious organizations. Hence, it is one of the objectives of psychotherapy to facilitate clients to fulfil this prime human drive. In addition, human beings hunt for power in the form of achievement, competence and accomplishment. The need for power does not entail to the taking advantage of another person. Satisfying the need for power means accomplishment or achievement. Even though power stimulates human beings to compete, it is not right that when somebody fulfils a need for power, someone else must suffer defeat.

A further aim of psychotherapy is to help out the clients to fulfil their needs for power without retreating someone else's right to do the same. The need for fun or enjoyment is also a prominent need of human beings. The effective gratification of this need leads the person away from boredom, apathy, and depression. Therefore, one of the goals of reality therapy is to facilitate people fulfil the need for fun or enjoyment within boundary and without violating the right of others to meet this same need.

The need for freedom, independence, or autonomy is another psychological need propagated in reality therapy. The need for independence means that if human beings are to perform in an entirely human way, they must have the opportunity to make choices and to behave in their own manner, without unnecessary, irrational restrictions. So, another goal of reality therapy is to facilitate clients discover need-satisfying choices for attaining autonomy.

Primary Human Drives

The choice theory suggests that human being is motivated to satisfy one or more of the five basic and genetically encoded needs. These needs are—survival, love and belonging, power (or achievement), freedom (or independence), and fun (or enjoyment). Humans are not directly acted upon by each independent need. Instead, sometimes survival needs are linked with needs for love or power, and each individual experiences a unique blend of human need states. In contrast to the other four needs, the first human need, survival, is a physical need. Glasser (1998) had written about the five basic human needs at length in the Choice Theory.

1. ***Survival***: In our daily routine lives, the need to survive and the concept of survival is quite far-flung unless we encounter any life-threatening condition. Even during times of war and terror, usually, only a marginal population of the world directly experience grave conditions. Survival as an intellectual concept is quite distinct from the survival as a personal experience. Glasser mentions that individual survival needs are expressed through their total behaviour including thoughts, behaviours, feelings, and physiology.
2. ***Love and Belonging***: According to Glasser, the need for love

and belongingness is the primary human need. In the basis of Glasser's assumptions on the priority of the human need to love and belong, the influence of love and belongingness can be seen everywhere. *Romeo and Juliet,* play of William Shakespeare concern with the power of love. The choice between love and survival, Romeo and Juliet clearly express their preference and they choose to give up survival rather than giving up love. In the context of choice theory, suicide is generally a choice that emerges out of a conflict between survival and another basic need. Human need for love and belongingness involves sexual love, friendship love, and romantic love, that is why it appears to be most profound and physically powerful.

3. ***Power***: Wubbolding (2000) has mentioned that the needs for power are often viewed in a negative way. He likes to apply achievement, inner control, or accomplishment as more optimistic descriptors of this basic human need. People take pleasure to having at least a little power. Having some power and authority is intrinsically rewarding rather than being completely powerless. People in the world recognize wealth and status as immense power. From the outlook of choice theory, in the absence of excessive striving for power or experiencing oneself as powerless consequence in unhappiness and a need for counselling. Dissimilarity with some reality therapy practitioners (R.E. Wubbolding, personal communication, May 6, 2003), Glasser (1998) considers an excess need for power to be a deeply destructive force within culture.
4. ***Freedom***: Sometimes, the need for freedom is referred to as independence (R.E. Wubbolding, personal communication, May 6, 2003). As Glasser (1998) states, "freedom concerns us mainly when we perceive that it is threatened". According to choice theory, it is the fact that many teenagers reply to the clarion call for freedom which suggests that teenagers are often being denied freedom by their parents. It has been seen that many parents all-over the world use the psychology of external control with their children. Thus, it should not be surprising to discover teenager's striving hard to meet their basic human needs for freedom. Choice theory suggests that creativity in humans is directly connected to freedom.
5. ***Fun***: Glasser (1998) is of the view that "the need for fun became built into our genes". He honestly associates the need for fun

to play, and, even further, he associates playing to learning, emphasizes that "the day we stop playing is the day we stop learning." Glasser has also mentioned that fun "is the easiest need to satisfy" and "is best defined by laughter". In our everyday life we always notice that when we met our need for fun with the day we almost met our other needs which are somehow associated with the need for fun. Many people articulate that their primary needs, i.e. need for love and belongingness are genuinely tangled with fun.

Classroom Behaviour in the Context of Primary Needs

Reality Therapy provides students a dose of reality. The idea behind five basic needs for the students are considered such as—

1. ***Need for power***—accomplishment and success.
2. ***Need for love and belonging***—experience of appreciated by others.
3. ***Need for freedom***—self-government and self-sufficiency.
4. ***Need for fun***—amusement, happiness and satisfaction.
5. ***Need for survival***—sustenance, protection, and some other basic needs.

Students always perform on these needs. Many of them have learned inadequate ways to fulfil their needs which disrupt a classroom. A good teacher should investigate student's desires and then assists them to meet those desires. If students think that they have some power to control their own learning, they will not experience that they should do something out to get their wants fulfil. According to reality therapy, a teacher needs to get out of the controlling style and into a role of teamwork and inspiration. In many situations when students are controlled by others they consider it in a negative way and charge others for their troubles and begin loosing inspiration.

Glasser mentioned that student's actions are made up of these four components: performing, thoughts, sense and functioning. It is noticed that a large amount of students prefer to opt the first two actions rather than the later two because they are generally controlled by their parents. In that situation when students does not feel these five basic needs they will have face difficulty to choose the accurate behaviour and definitely would not feeling well and will have a dysfunctional performance. In brief, broken performance results in that condition when a student is sad and is not receiving their major needs met.

Origin and History of Reality Therapy

The origin of Reality Therapy is linked with Glasser's disappointed view with psychoanalytic psychiatry. William Glasser develops reality therapy which is generally based on his experience with clients. However, Glasser more or less completed all of his training from conventional psychoanalysis. William Glasser and his mentor and teacher, psychiatrist G.L. Harrington produced Reality Therapy at the Veterans Administration Hospital in Los Angeles in the early 1960s. In 1965, Glasser published the book entitled *'Reality Therapy'* in the United States. The term consists of a procedure that is people-friendly and people-centred and has nothing to do with giving people an amount of reality (as a risk or penalty), but rather helps people to be aware of how flight of the imagination can divert them from their choices they manage in life. Glasser asserts that in order to live a more pleasing and satisfying life the past should be resolved and moved because in general the past is not something to be dwelled upon. By the 1970s, the concepts were extended into what Glasser then called "Choice Theory", a term used in the title of several of his books. By the mid-1990s, the still growing concepts were described as "choice theory", a term conceived and planned by the Irish reality therapy practitioner Christine O'Brien Shanahan at the 1995 IRTI Conference in Waterford, Ireland and then adopted by Glasser. The growing practice of reality therapy remains a foundation of the larger body of his effort. According to Choice theory, we all have the capacity to choose many of our future behaviours and hold ourselves deliberately responsible for how we are acting, thinking, feeling, and also for our physiological states. So in this way each of us is a self-governing and self-regulating being. Choice Theory tries to clarify, or give an explanation that how we all have attempts to organize our world and those within that world.

Current Status of Reality Therapy

In the present time, reality therapy as an efficient therapeutic modality acknowledged with many applications. For example, an unpublished document of the Department of Defence used at a 1981 Conference on Drug Abuse in the Armed Forces stated that over 90 per cent of the more than 200 armed forces clinics that treat drug and alcohol abuse

use reality therapy as their preferred therapeutic approach. In 1968, the Institute for Control Theory, Reality Therapy, and Quality Management had been founded in Los Angeles that progress the training of reality therapy applied to psychotherapy, counselling, schools, agencies, and management. A certification course had been increasingly started, and for the practice of reality therapy the initial certificates had been distributed in 1975.

The title Reality Therapy Certified (RTC) is distributed to those persons who implemented an 18-month training programme. That programme has been involved workshops; video and audio taping, supervised practice, small group practice, feedback, and other experiences. The Institute for Reality Therapy organizes the certification procedure. In 1988, Glasser enquired of Robert E. Wubbolding to become the first administrator of training for the Institute. In that ability, Wubbolding had been monitored the certification procedure and the faculty training programmes. A lot of the work of practitioners of reality therapy has been extended beyond the world of psychotherapy. In 1968, Glasser had written *Schools without Failure*, in which he emphasized that the children who have not the capability to control their world effectively (i.e. succeed in school), become hurt so much and consequently more often they stop trying to learn.

At the current time, the Institute for Reality Therapy and its instructors instruct the concepts in Glasser's *The Quality School* (1990b) to schools in the United States and somewhere else. In this pioneering work, Glasser applied the ideas of W. Edwards Deming (1982) to education. The main problems with the educational system are not the disturbance of the students, poorly salaried teachers, unused computers, lack of community participation, or dozens of other problems. But the major problems are symptoms of the unseen fact that Americans have established on ordinary work, behaviour and efforts on the part of students. The lack of quality education leads the nation at the risk. Glasser revealed that if the education of control theory or reality therapy has given properly it could improve the quality of performance in school. For the use of Deming and Glasser's principle in a quality school, everyone has been trained.

From the very beginning to till now reality therapy continuously remaining the counselling and therapy tool. It is trained in almost many countries besides the U.S. and Canada, and the Institute had been ties to Japan, Korea, Ireland, Norway, the United Kingdom, Australia, New Zealand, Hong Kong, Singapore, and the former Yugoslavia. After the publication of Glasser's *Stations of the Mind* (1981) and *Control Theory*

(1985), many people have heard about control theory and its delivery organization, reality therapy. Furthermore, Glasser had reconceptualized the fundamentals of reality therapy under two general categories: environment and procedures (1990a). Robert Wubbolding (1992) had extended these thoughts by discussing them as a series of therapy and the WDEP system (Wants, Doing, Evaluation, and Planning). Robert Cockrum (1989) mentioned that "William Glasser has never been content to allow his theories to be taught or used without constant scrutiny, addition and sometimes even major changes." *The Journal of Reality Therapy* was launched in 1981, edited by Lawrence Litwack. After that time, more than 200 essays, articles, and research studies had been published on the applications of reality therapy. In 1994, almost 4500 people had finished the reality therapy certification process worldwide, with the numbers growing every year. Reality therapy is seen a slow but steady increase in acceptance as a practicable and appreciated psychotherapy theory and learning system.

Techniques of Reality Therapy

Reality Therapy is acknowledged as a form of psychotherapeutic and psychological approach. Basically, it helps us to identify that what we want to achieve in life and what steps could we take to get them. According to reality therapy all our aims and desires are based on five basic needs: power, love and belonging, freedom, fun, and survival, and after fulfilling them they give us utter satisfaction. Furthermore, the reality therapy techniques revolve around these needs.

1. ***Supporting***—It is very necessary for the reality therapists that they assist clients to focus on what they want from their life. In this way by helping them they achieve it in a positive and beneficial way and the reality therapist directly communicate support. Glasser working with clients on specific tasks that in his own way he communicates support to them.
2. ***Encouraging***—Reality therapists should be optimistic and encouraging with clients. Theoretically, it has been found that focusing on the person or, in unusual cases, on the person's past, the reality therapist revealed successes and positive identity. Moreover, there is an emphasis on relationship between therapist and client.
3. ***Listening***—Several non-reality therapists have seen reality

therapy as a directive and confronting therapy. In fact, reality therapists put emphasis on listening. Their listening should be more in the form of a friend's listening to another friend and less in the form of non-directive Carl Rogers listening. Furthermore, reality therapists deliberately prefer to listen to client's successes, plans, and efforts to connect with others, and they decrease listening to client's talk about symptoms or depressing past experiences.

4. ***Accepting***—One of the core value of this therapy is the accepting nature of therapist. Reality therapists must accept the truth that all clients want to fulfil their five basic human needs. In the therapy session it helps in providing a brilliant establishment of empathy and helping relationship within the clients. However, reality therapists should never accept client statements that externalize liability. It is probably considered that many students and professionals mistakenly seen reality therapy as being strictly confrontational. But, actuality reality therapists do not use strict confrontation, it is generally considered to use teaching techniques when clients externalize liability. So, it can be emphasized that, reality therapists simply accept client's needs and then educate them choice theory.
5. ***Trusting***—Trust is the foundation of reality therapy. Reality therapists try to communicate trust in several ways. It strengthens the relationship of therapist and client. As such, in the studies of Glasser he primarily started building a trust relationship.
6. ***Respecting***—The most important point of this type of technique is that the reality therapists always respect people's desires. For example in one of the Glasser's study he presents the following excerpt from a case in which Glasser is working with a man who was married and have desire to become a woman describes his excellence on both connecting with clients and respecting them: I could turn him over to someone else, but we've made a good connection. He may think I am afraid to deal with his problem, and we will lose the connection. It is that connection that is all important. Even his wife will look for that connection—that I really want to help him; that I respect him even though he wants to be a woman (2000).
7. ***Negotiating differences***—Reality Therapy focuses more about that how can he negotiate differences. It is truth that almost many people have the same five basic human needs. It is the basic

assumption of choice theory that all individuals will have desire to fulfil these needs in a distinctive manner which is different from each other. The reality therapists provide help to clients that they negotiate the differences between what they want from life and what they are getting from life. In couple's therapy, Glasser considered a concept called "the solving circle" to assist clients beneficially negotiates their differences.

Steps in Reality Therapy

There are six basic steps which can be used to execute the therapy—

1. ***To build an Environment***—Building such kind of environment in which the client feels relaxed, safe and sound, unwrapped and free to present his opinions is the initial step for the therapist. It must be a situation in which the client experiences a need satisfying environment. Moreover, client should feel to be treated, appreciated and also listened to. In the built environment the therapist should be satisfying the clients by fulfilling their both aspects of fun and learning. For the success of therapy, it is necessary that the therapist should establish a rapport with the client.
2. ***Interaction with the Client***—This step is called an interaction process in which the therapist comes closer to know the needs of a client such as the way he keeps the complete picture in front of the helper. In fact this step consists the process which involves listening to the client. And after that the therapist moves ahead to plan to meet client's needs.
3. ***Evaluation of the Current Behaviour***—This is the third step in which the therapist wholly evaluated the present behaviour of the client. The therapist wants to know that exactly where and why the client is lacking to achieve his aim. At that place the helper should ask the client that whether his present behaviour is assisting him to come closer to his aim or not. If the client says yes then the present behaviour needs to go on further till it needs slight changes. But if the client says no then the responsibility of the helper is to bring in a major change in the client's opinion and hence in his act also. It is necessary for the client that he knows what he wants. The therapist should assist him to direct his opinion in a constructive direction. The helper

should asked some question to pin point a trouble and work on it such as—what he wants ?, what are his actions to achieve them?, Is the present behaviour assist him or not? The answers of these questions will help in channelize the creation of a possible plan of his action or achievement.

4. ***Possible Behavioural Planning***—The helper should try to plan as such the possible behaviour of the needy that help him to re-connect himself to his own social world. Having awful relationship is often the cause for a client to be unable to find his quality world.

   This is that step where the therapist's plan is built up with the consent of the client. Client's approval is most important such as the success of the therapy depends on the truth that—if the plan satisfies client's needs then he will show interest to bring about a change in his behaviour. At this place the therapist should help the client to focus on the things that are under his control (belief and behaviours). The essence of the reality therapy depends on the fact that one has to focus on changing one's own actions, belief and thinking to come closer to the aim.
5. ***Commitment to the Plan***—This step involves client's commitment to the plan. If the client wants to commit verbally, he can do this but it is better that he gives it in writing to bring in little importance in the plan of action. This would keep reminding the client his liability that he has to bring a change in his actions to build a constructive world. The client is accountable for the plan that works effectively such as the steps taken for action are worked out in his presence and with his consent only.
6. ***A Complete Evaluation***—The last step of the therapy suggests that if the plan does not bring a change in the client's world then it is better to modify the probable plan of the behaviour according to client's needs. It should be continued till the client is completely satisfied and he comes closer to get his quality world back. The entire portrait rotates around the client as he has to finally feel relaxed in his world. It is helper and the client who can better judge to take decision about the success of the plan, nobody can other than them.

Therapist should focus on these following key points—

1. Past should be ignored because 'present' is important.

2. The therapist should consider that not to complain on the client's symptoms. Because, it may be possible that it puts a negative impact on client.
3. Therapist should focus on the total behaviour of the client.
4. Therapist should develop a sense of liability in client for the plan of action to work.
5. It is also important to be considered that the therapist increases the capability of the client to take up the change.
6. The therapist should try to focus on those things which remain under the control of the client.
7. With the help of therapist client should have the choice to refuse or revise the plan of behaviour.
8. Throughout the therapy session the therapist should have a lot of endurance to deal with the client.
9. The client should increase faith in the efficiency of the plan.
10. The helping relationship between the therapist and the client must be pleasant and encouraging.

Application of Reality Therapy

Reality Therapy can be utilized in several areas such as reality therapy has been applied as a form of psychotherapy instrument, a personal growth programme, a tool for organizing or training employees, a classroom strategy, and an educational reform strategy. It has been effectively used to severe mental state such as bipolar disorder, catatonia, and depression. It has been applied in marriage therapy and also with suicide ideation and fear, family issues such as caring for elderly parents, identity issues, and school achievement (N. Glasser, 1980). Moreover, some other fields in which reality therapy has been applied effectively involve child abuse, adolescent rebellion, incest survival, bereavement, parental relations, and eating disorders (N. Glasser, 1989), self-help (Good, 1987), mental health (Garner, 1983), and recovery programmes (Reuss, 1985).

From its early foundation reality therapy is based on outcome research. Studies of Glasser (1965) revealed that the treatment of long-term hospitalized psychotic patients in the Veterans Administration Neuropsychiatric Hospital in Los Angeles has included 210 patients and their problems were categorized into many types of schizophrenia such as; paranoid schizophrenia, catatonic schizophrenia, hebephrenic schizophrenia and undifferentiated schizophrenia. Every patient was hallucinated, and delusional, and spent most of their time inactively sitting and waiting. In average there stayed 210 patients in the hospital for the fifteen years. Approximately two years after the reality therapy programme was initiated, out of 210 the 100 men had been released.

Some other studies have shown development in self-esteem, a decline in court referrals (Shea, 1973), and excellence in classroom behaviour (Hart-Hester, Heuchert, and Whittier, 1989). Yarish (1985) describes considerable differences in client's perceived locus of control as an outcome of their treatment with reality therapy. Honeyman (1990) studied on addicted people and found constructive outcome. Parish, a leading researcher studied the effects of reality therapy on undergraduate students and teachers, and frequently shown its positive effects (Parish, 1988, 1991). Likewise, some other studies have found beneficial impact with graduate students (Peterson, Woodward, and Kissko, 1991), and in residential youth programmes (Bratter, Bratter, Maxym, Radda, and Steiner, 1993).

A large amount of research evidences prove the usefulness of reality therapy. It is helpful to examine several forms of assessment. Initially, convincing evidence for the efficiency of reality therapy lies in the increasing amount of professional people who seek credentialing in this area. Become certified as a reality therapist almost 500 people completed the 18-month programme during 1994. This certification process requires assurance of personal time and resources. The personal choice to get training is most often made after using some of the ideas learned through self-study or short guidance sessions. Such persons come from teaching, social work, counselling, psychotherapy, corrections, management, and many other helping disciplines.

The relevance and appropriateness of reality therapy are validates through that evidences which are come from case studies. Tollefson (1980) describes an example of a case study of a boy named Henry. Henry drinking too much and his family are also chemically dependent. He had spent his 17 years in mental hospitals. For his anti-social behaviour, hostile, and threatening behaviour he was arrested and first hospitalized after high school. The boy has been constantly deteriorated, and continuously become violent and impulsive. His abusive behaviour and aggressive nature plagued him and those around him. Tollefson (1980) mentioned that "He also became untidy", urinated into his own mouth, and became infected playing with his feces. After a long time he remained in this state and continuously became inferior, "aggressive, apprehensive, regressed, autistic, confused, disorderly, and poor in appearance". Whenever other patients try to harm him in minor ways he withdrew into a corner of the ward, "coming out only to steal coffee or cigarettes". Anyone approaching his corner was greeted with bellowing, curses, and threats. The therapists spend a lot of time attempting to set up a relationship by speaking only in brief to Henry. After constantly asking simple questions by the therapist, Henry had increasingly begun to answer briefly. After some sessions, Henry began leaving his corner for concise conversations with the therapist. The therapist used reality therapy procedures more openly when its success began to be more obvious. He asked questions about whether the way Henry had acted on the ward was assisting him. At initial session, he would put his head between his legs and say 'No' and finally he was able to perform more and more self-evaluations of both positive and negative behaviours, he would come into the therapist's office and after that he should sit in a chair and make plans. In spite of occasional regressions progress continuously occurs. It has been noticed that Henry increasingly began to cooperate with other patients and made off-ward trips that improved his self-perceptions (self-esteem, power, achievement). Finally, he was started to go to the commissary, the library, and the gym without incident. This situation increased his need-satisfying and other patients and staffs were also satisfied to him. The therapist was finally success to change Henry as he improved constantly and using his plan and enduring to raise his self-respect and take more liability for his own behaviour. In this way such case illustrates the use of reality therapy with an excessively disturbed being. So, it may be said that the system is reasonably appropriate to client's extensively encountered by practitioners.

Honeyman (1990) examined the effects of reality therapy group treatment on addicts. The client's self-perceptions were inventoried upon access to treatment and at the second week, fourth week, and sixth week.

Following are some significant changes in the client's perceptions about themselves:

1. Improved self-esteem as an outcome of coming to sense client's own power.
2. Increased wakefulness that they were taking more liability for their behaviour.
3. Greater confidence that they were not capable to control their drinking.
4. Knowledge to relate to others in selfless ways rather than repressive ways.
5. Deep alertness of addict-identity.
6. Recognition of the significance of a superior authority.

Honeyman (1990) summarized that as a measure of concurrent validity, the Minnesota Multiphasic Personality Inventory (MMPI) profiles of the 24 client (showed) a general decline in (negative) symptom behaviour demonstrating that clients are in more control of their lives at the time of discharge. The above data represent an effort to get beyond the essential, but extremely intellectualized results of several scientific studies that argue to be based on hard data.

Reality Therapy as a Classroom Strategy

Reality Therapy as a classroom strategy assists students to be responsible and investigate their own problems and then solve them. Glasser is of the view that students are able to control their behaviour because they are rational beings. Such as, sincere students are usually observed on their first day of school. When teachers help students to learn excellent performance choices, the students become responsible person and have the ability to fulfil their wants in the real world. Students are required to recognize their behaviour and they should take significant decision regarding that behaviour.

One of the most important things about reality therapy is that this therapy places the liability on the student rather than the teacher. Despite of their family backgrounds and home situations all students are projected to obey the rules. The teacher's task is to help students to become accountable and industrious members of classroom. According to reality therapy, teachers should frequently stress student liability for their own behavioural choices not to punishing students. Classroom meetings become an important part to addressing problems. For the improvement of students they should sit in a close surroundings and talk about classroom situations and troubles. The teacher's responsibility is to give surroundings information as wanted and to keep back opinions. Each and everyone student should take part in the construction of classroom rules, consequences, and actions. It is necessary that each student is expected to agree with the rules and outcomes. These rules are flexible in nature and on the other hand, could be changed with another gathering as the circumstances change.

Use of Reality Therapy in Different Settings

Reality Therapy has been applied in almost all kinds of situations. It can be used in private practice to prisons. In private practice it is generally utilized for short-term course, but in institutions where people are confined for years, it is applied as long as clients are required to be in the course or until their treatment is enough to allow them to be returned to society. However, this therapy can be used with individuals, groups, and families.

Individual Therapy

A large amount of clients who willingly go through Reality Therapy receive treatment on a one-to-one basis. Just like any other therapy, the therapist described about the entire process that he used in treatment. After that clients are asked to tell their story. Then clients start to discuss their trouble feelings and how they are worried about something that has happened to them, how the society create problems, how they have desire to change their outer worlds. Several clients have already a sense of interior control and desire to change their own behaviour. They confess that they are unhappy, irritated, embarrassed, or blameworthy and they try to find better choices. Moreover, unintentional clients are occasionally unwilling, aggressive, reserved, or submissive. The therapist has tried to make emotional contact using skills essential to most therapies such as: active listening, reflection, clarification, and many other processes useful in establishing a pleasing therapeutic setting. The therapist allowing the clients to tell their story that assist therapist to determine client's perceived locus of control. For example, how much liability the client has taken for past behaviour and how much liability he or she can practically take for instant upcoming choices. Therapist should have a lot of patience that he listen client's opinion of his or her story also have determination about the perceived locus of control. The therapist assists the client to set aims for the therapy by asking them what they wish to have happen as a consequence of the relationship. More particularly, it is sensible to ask what the person wishes to gain from the individual session. This question can hardly be overvalued. The understood message of the therapist is that various changes can be made instantly and that there is expectation. Sometimes, a glimmer of daylight is greeted with surprise for disappointed, unhappy person who are living in psychological darkness. Therapist's Focus on the present behaviour of the client, rather than the past behaviour assists clients to become aware of their actions that are the part of their behaviour over which they have most control. On the basis of the style of therapist, they are asked occasionally to make judgements on their requirements. Here some questions are raised. Such as are they realistic? Are they advantageous wishes, or would have their wishes met be dangerous to them? Are client's overall behaviour and their particular actions helping them? Therapist then asked to clients to make plans that complete the distinctiveness of successful planning. Simple arranged sheets are often used. In private practices, the best possible execution occurs through a joint judgement by therapist and client based on whether the client has been capable to take up more effectual need-fulfilling behaviours in his or her life.

Group Therapy

Reality Therapy is particularly a successful therapy that is effectively utilized for groups. Generally, reality therapy begins with the psychological connection between the therapist and people. Wubbolding (1991b) has revealed that how reality therapy is incorporated into the stages of groups (Corey, 1994). The requirements of the clients should be addressed at every stage of group development, though it is impossible for all requirements that they constantly to be met to the same amount. At the initial stage the need for belonging is met in everyone that they feel included in the group. The therapist asks what people would like from the group. Entire behaviour is also explored: life trend, particular actions, useless and useful self-talk, way of thinking, and even physiological behaviours. Further the power need of group development is approached in the second stage when apprehension, inconsistency, and conflict become exterior. The operational phase of group development and belonging is addressed in the third stage when the group members come to consider that others in the group can be of some help to them. Authority or success is the evident that participants have a desire to change. The organizer assists them to make a decision that they should work as hard as it become possible to change their behaviour. Advance planning assists to deal with fun and belonging needs in the last stage. Further discussion of development touches on the need for autonomy. Final termination of the group can come about in several ways that are based on the choice of the group members.

Marriage and Family Therapy

Reality Therapy which comes from control theory describes about the way human brain functions, is a greatest instrument for marriage and family therapy. It can also add a practical organization and rescue system and it can be incorporated into systems theory. Wubbolding (1988) has explained that how reality therapy is useful for family therapy. The objectives of reality therapy that are based on family therapy consist of the following:

1. ***Obtain at least a small amount of need fulfilment***—Likewise other applications the helper helps family members through satisfying their psychological needs without interference with the rights of other family members.
2. ***Modify levels of perception***—Helper provides help to family members that they become less judgemental about each other.
3. ***Utilize quality time***—Simultaneously spend time in a non-critical manner, doing pleasurable activities, making a warehouse of positive perceptions that serve as a foundation for the healthy relations essential for upcoming problem solving and for negotiating decisions.
4. ***Change behaviour***—Therapist's most noticeable aim is to assist family members, modify in the way of their action towards each other equally in the therapy session and in the existing life of the family. Human beings are like that organism who prefer behaviours to fulfil their requirements, because they are control systems. It is essential that the utilization of reality therapy in family counselling ensures that every member and the family as a group look at that things which are required, their effort to work as a family, and the efficiency of their individual overall behaviours and the family's overall behaviour. The action planning would be successful only in that case when these beginning components are present.

Contributions of Reality Therapy

It is considered that reality therapy has its nearly short-term focus and the truth that it deals with conscious behavioural problems. In reality therapy client's self-assessment, a plan of achievement and an assurance to following through are the foundation of the therapeutic process because insight and wakefulness are not enough. Reality Therapy focuses on powerfully encouraged clients to engage them in self-assessment that they come to a decision: what they are doing is working or not, and to assign themselves to do what is essential to make changes. The existential foundations of choice theory are a most important strength of this approach. As an outcome of reality therapy, people are seen as doing their best they can rather than seen as being desperately and vulnerably miserable. They are making the preferences they expect that will consequently satisfying their requirements.

The reality therapists provide help to clients and conduct a searching inventory that what the clients are doing. If clients find out that their current behaviour is not working then they are much more likely to consider acquiring a new behavioural inventory. It is considered that reality therapy has been effectively applied in addiction treatment and recovery programmes for over 30 years. It involves working with addicted populations that exemplifies how this notion is practically utilized. In various conditions it would be unsuitable to begin long-term therapy with addicted people because they investigated into unconscious dynamics and also have rigorous investigation of their past. In this way, reality therapy is most prominently focussed on making changes in the present and it is an effective, short-term approach.

References

Bratter, B., Bratter, T., Maxym, C., Radda, H., and Steiner, K. (1993). The John Dewey Academy: A residential quality school for self-destructive adolescents who have superior intellectual and intuitive potential. *Journal of Reality Therapy,* 9, 42-53.

Cockrum, J.R. (1989). Reality therapy: Interviews with Dr. William Glasser. *Psychology*, 26, 1, 13-16.

Corey, G. (1994). *Theory and Practice of Group Counselling*. Pacific Grove, CA: Brooks/Cole.

Deming, W.E. (1982). *Out of the Crisis*. Cambridge, MA: MIT.

Garner, A. (1983). Living with mental patients. *Journal of Reality Therapy*, 2, 27-31.

Glasser, W. (1965). *Reality Therapy: A New Approach to Psychiatry.* New York: Harper and Row.

Glasser, W. (1968). *Schools Without Failure*. New York, NY: Harper Collins.

Glasser, N. (ed.). (1980). *What are You Doing*? New York, NY: Harper Collins.

Glasser, W. (1981). *Stations of the Mind*. New York, NY: Harper Collins.

Glasser, W. (1985). *Control Theory*. New York, NY: Harper Collins.

Glasser, N. (ed.). (1989) *Control Theory in the Practice of Reality Therapy.* New York, NY: Harper Collins.

Glasser, W. (1990a). A Diagram of the Brain as a Control System (chart). Los Angeles, CA: Institute for Reality Therapy.

Glasser, W. (1990b). *The Quality School*. New York, NY: Harper Collins.

Glasser, W. (1998). *Choice Theory: A New Psychology of Personal Freedom.* New York: Harper Collins.

Glasser, W. (2000). *Reality Therapy in Action.* New York: Harper Collins.

Glasser, W. (2002). *Unhappy Teenagers: A Way for Parents and Teachers to Reach Them.* New York: Harper Collins.

Good, E.P. (1987). *In Pursuit of Happiness.* Chapel Hill, NC: New View Publications.

Hart-Hester, S., Heuchert, C., and Whittier, K. (1989). The effects of teaching reality therapy techniques to elementary students to help change behaviours. *Journal of Reality Therapy*, 8, 13-18.

Honeyman, A. (1990). Perceptual changes in addicts as a consequence of reality therapy based on group treatment. *Journal of Reality Therapy*, 9, 53-59.

Parish, T. (1988). Helping teachers take more effective control. *Journal of Reality Therapy*, 8, 41-43.

Parish, T. (1991). Helping students take control *via* an interactive voice communications system. *Journal of Reality Therapy*, 11, 38-40.

Peterson, A., Woodward, G., and Kissko, R. (1991). A comparison of basic week students and introduction to counselling graduate students on four basic need factors. *Journal of Reality Therapy*, 9, 31-37.

Powers, W. (1973). *Behaviour: The Control of Perception.* New York, NY: Aldine Press.

Reuss, N. (1985). Alternatives to cocaining. *Journal of Reality Therapy*, 4, 8-11.

Shea, G. (1973). The effects of reality-therapy-oriented group counselling with delinquent, behaviour-disordered students. *Dissertation Abstracts International*, 34, 4889-4890.

Tollefson, W. (1980). Coming out of the corner. In *What are You Doing?* New York: Harper Collins.

Wubbolding, R. (1988). *Using Reality Therapy.* New York: Harper Collins.

Wubbolding, R. (1991b). *Using Reality Therapy in Group Counselling* (videotape). Cincinnati, OH: Centre for Reality Therapy.

Wubbolding, R. (1992). *Reality Therapy Training Manual.* Cincinnati, OH: Centre for Reality Therapy.

Wubbolding, R.E. (2000). *Reality Therapy for the 21st Century.* Muncie, In: Accelerated Development.

Yarish, P. (1985). Reality therapy and locus of control of juvenile offenders. *Journal of Reality Therapy*, 6, 3-10.

18

A Call for Culture Specific Mental Health Therapies

Anubhuti Dubey

The contemporary world has reached at certain point of development and maximization of pleasure through materialistic gains that also started creating stresses and anxieties in people as such pleasures are not long lasting as the material gone the pleasure derived from it also disappears which led a vacuum in the life of people. Hence, there is a pressing need to enhance the availability and quality of mental health services in traditional societies like India also where the society is gradually becoming materialistic to some extent. The problems of loneliness, different types of anxieties and insecurities, cut throat competitions etc. begin to impact the individual at a very tender age just like other parts of the globe. Therefore, traditional mental health treatments are and should be modified to better match clients' cultural contexts. For instance, in one of the reports of a research team of World Health Organization (WHO) (1979), it is examined that unique aspect of Asian Indian culture may differentially impinge on mental health issues such as acculturation, rates of psychopathology, and manifestation of psychiatric symptoms. In one such of the descriptions a site of Agra, in India was cited where the researchers had expressed grief that there is "ignorance about the nature of mental illness" and "misconceptions and superstitious beliefs about mental illness" which lead people to seek help from 'faith healers'. Angel and Thoits (1987) maintain that although the clinical features of an illness may be invariant, culture have an effect on the phenomenological experience and identification of illness. For instance, South East Asians hail from such cultural background in which people do not correlate mental disorder with negative feelings and emotional difficulties (Tung, 1985). Patients have been offered an array of therapeutic alternatives in developing countries. In these 'developing' sites, multiple medical systems are commonly available and people often 'shop around' among a range of therapeutic alternative whereas in the 'developed' sites western biomedical care dominates (though not equally so in every case) and there is less use of diverse therapies (WHO, 1979). Halliburton (2004) reported in his article the quantitative and qualitative material from research on patients' experiences and methods of healing in three forms of therapy for psychopathology in the State of Kerala, India: ayurvedic (indigenous) psychiatry, allopathic (western) psychiatry and religious healing (at a Hindu temple, a Muslim mosque and a Christian church, all of which have reputations for healing mentally ill persons). A careful scrutiny of individual patients' retrospective narratives of his/her illness histories had shown that patients had thoroughly different experiences with the same therapies. For example, a number of patients affirmed that they get respite from their illness only *via* ayurvedic therapy, while others asserted that they find no help from this type of treatment. Likewise differing experiences were reported for the other two healing systems. This finding, combined with the finding that all three therapies produced positive levels of short-term improvement, suggests that having a number of therapies to choose from makes it more likely that a person will find a treatment that 'fits'—that is, one that works for him or her because it meets the personality, desires or concerns of the patient (such as personal religiosity or concerns about the effects of treatment). WHO studies themselves acknowledge wide use of non-Western therapies at developing country research sites (Jablensky *et al.*, 1992; Sartorius *et al.*, 1986; WHO, 1979). Therapies other than Western biomedicine are certainly available in the developed sites, but these studies indicate that alternative medical systems are widely available and relatively easier to access in the developing locations.

India is a multicultural traditional society where people visit religious and traditional healers for general and mental health related problems. A considerable number of epidemiological surveys done in India on mental disorders have confirmed the prevalence of mental morbidity in rural and urban areas of the country and there degree is akin to global rates. There are many unique and esoteric forms of healing in India, some of which may not be helpful to any patients and some of which include healers of spurious credentials or ability. Raguram *et al.* (2002) found that patients they examined improved significantly during their stay at the temple, which they felt was due to the temple providing a supportive, reassuring environment that constitutes a place of asylum.

There are "culturally recognized" or "culturally accepted" symptoms. For example—In Eastern societies particularly in Indian subcontinent, 'It is more usual to explain chest pains or heart problems, often as a "heavy heart" or a "burning heart", which are accepted symptoms of deep sadness, while in the West, a consultant would begin by fastening the complainant to a heart monitor as they would not automatically relate it right away to depression or anxiety." And this is one of the reasons a number of individuals brawl with psychological treatments includes culture or race. Cultural factors can play out in many ways. In multicultural and multiethnic nations the therapists have to learn to be culture sensitive. For example, some African-American patients find it difficult to speak with white therapists, some Asians feel uncomfortable talking about their emotions, and there are other culture-specific barriers to communication.

Conclusion

Although this volume cannot assert to have demonstrated that having generally existing varied therapy systems aids the likelihood of improvement for mental disorders, it invites thought to a concern that cross-cultural psychiatrists, clinical psychologists and medical anthropologists should consider about culture specific psychotherapies as an attempt to explain the better recovery rates for serious mental illnesses.

It is not easy to establish a division between 'legitimate' and 'spurious' therapies, but thorough and cautious, qualitative research on the experience of patients may facilitate this issue. Therapy with Indians in the changing contemporary world should be geared towards achieving a balance between the individualistic demands of Western culture and the interdependence of the Indian family (Durvasula and Mylvaganam, 1994).

References

Angel, R.J., and Thoits, P. (1987). The impact of culture on the cognitive structure of illness. *Culture, Medicine and Psychiatry*, 11(4), 465-494.

Durvasula, R.S., and Mylvaganam, G.A. (1994). Mental health of Asian Indians: Relevant issues and community implications. *Journal of Community Psychology*.

Raguram, R., Venkateswaran, A., Ramakrishna, J., and Weiss, M.G. (2002). Traditional community resources for mental health: A report of temple healing from India. *British Medical Journal*, 325, 38-40.

Tung, T.M. (1985). Psychiatric care for Southeast Asians: How different is different? In T. Owan (ed.), *Southeast Asian Mental Health: Treatment, Prevention, Services, Training, and Research* (pp. 5-40). Washington, DC: U.S. Department of Health and Human Services.

World Health Organization. (1979). *Schizophrenia: An International follow-up Study*. New York: Wiley.

Index